ON FAIRNESS AND EFFICIENCY

The privatisation of the public income during the past millennium

George Miller

The POLICY PRESS

First published in Great Britain in October 2000 by

The Policy Press
34 Tyndall's Park Road
Bristol BS8 1PY
UK

Tel +44 (0)117 954 6800
Fax +44 (0)117 973 7308
e-mail tpp@bristol.ac.uk
http://www.policypress.org.uk

British Library Cataloguing in Publication Data

A catalogue record for this book is available from the British Library

ISBN 1 86134 221 7

George Miller is Professor of Epidemiology at the University of London
Queen Mary and Westfield College, and a member of the Medical Research
Council's Senior Clinical Scientific Staff.

Cover design by Qube Design Associates, Bristol.

Illustration on front cover supplied by kind permission of Tate Gallery,
London.

Printed and bound in Great Britain by Hobbs the Printers Ltd, Southampton.

Contents

List of tables

Preface

Soon after coming to power in May 1997, Prime Minister Tony Blair outlined his vision for Britain: "... nothing less than the model 21st century nation; a beacon for the world ... the best place to live, the best place to bring up children, the best place to lead a fulfilled life, the best place to grow old" (*The Times*, 1 October 1997, p 8). To realise this glorious prospect, declared New Labour, the nation must modernise with a sense of greater purpose. Obsolescent practices which hobble must yield to better ways of moving forward. It follows, therefore, that if Britain wishes to become 'the beacon for the world', it must rethink its concepts of what is *fair* and what is *efficient*.

Tony Blair quickly established the Social Exclusion Unit to spearhead the task of renewal and revitalisation of the nation's deprived neighbourhoods, which numbered in the thousands. Its report of 1998 "made clear that these neighbourhoods suffered from serious multi-faceted problems that would require action on all fronts" (Social Exclusion Unit, 2000, p 5). But there is a strong case to believe that these problems are themselves but facets of a much more fundamental issue which goes to the heart of Britain's political economy. The nation is by no means alone in this respect, but it serves well as an illustration of the problem.

To borrow a rhetorical device from New Labour's manifesto of 1997 – 'Rent, Rent, Rent!'. The original call, for 'Education, education, education', resounded intelligibly throughout the nation, but in sharp contrast, a call for Rent reform would these days elicit little response apart from perplexity. Yet what the nation does with its surplus income after all Wages have been paid to Labour and all Interest paid to Capital, in other words what it does with its Rent, is the fundamental issue that is not being addressed. The nature of Rent, why it matters so much for the success of Britain's Welfare State, and why its mistreatment within Welfare Capitalism perpetuates so much unfairness, inefficiency and material deprivation, have not been grasped.

Originally regarded properly as the public's income for social purposes, Rent has been slowly privatised over the past millennium, to the lasting detriment of justice. In the process, Rent has acquired historical, legal, political, public health and social dimensions which are as important to appreciate as its economic dimension. For reasons that had little to do with economic efficiency, Rent became attached to landholding along with other privileges such as the rights to vote and to sit in parliament. The franchise and membership of parliament have now been wrested from 'land', but not yet Rent. Hence any meaningful discussion of Rent must be set within the context of land in its various economic, legal and social senses. This book presents Rent and land from all relevant aspects as I see them, in order to set out the case for reform. As a clinical scientist I have dared to interpret economics, history and law as they relate to Rent in order to achieve my purpose, which is to identify inequities in Wealth that undermine the health of the nation.

Part I opens by highlighting the strong impact that material deprivation has on health, fulfilment of life and life expectancy, not only in Britain but essentially wherever the association has been sought. To be deprived of the benefit of Rent will be no different in these respects from other forms of deprivation tied to denial of work, a decent wage, or a fair return on investment. Chapter Three sets out the law of Rent and the inefficiencies which flow from its privatisation, including unemployment. Chapter Four considers the effect of unemployment on health. Chapter Five reviews the record of 20th century reforming governments which sought redistribution of wealth through taxation, in lieu of Rent foregone, in order to tackle four of William Beveridge's giant evils: Ignorance, Disease, Idleness and Want. The fifth giant, Squalor, is the subject of Chapter Six, which describes the adverse consequences of privatised Rent for housing of the less well off. Chapter Seven outlines proposals for Rent reform needed to secure universal social inclusion in a universal Welfare State that serves as a model for the 21st century.

Part II looks back, tracing the evolution of the present state of affairs over the past millennium in order that we can grasp the roots of the problem. Chapters Eight and Nine describe how Rent came to be privatised in law, incorporated with that most fundamental of privileges, the right to govern, within the bundle of rights and privileges called land. Chapter Ten reviews the jumble of taxes on wages and interest devised by early governments as they gradually privatised Rent, and by later administrations which steadfastly refused to turn over Rent for public revenue. Chapters Eleven and Twelve remind us of the consequences of social exclusion in all its forms, including denial of the benefits of Rent, for society's poorest in times gone by. Also described here are the long struggles to wrest the franchise and the right to sit in parliament from the landed constituency, essential prerequisites for the eventual return of Rent to the State as public revenue. Chapters Thirteen and Fourteen describe the last serious attempt to right a great wrong, the unsuccessful political struggle to redress the inequity of privatised Rent, played out between 1880 and 1920. In this way, Part II reveals the underlying continuities which run through the past, explaining much of our present predicament, and without the appropriate legal, social and economic reforms will be the harbinger of future troubles.

Acknowledgements

My indebtedness to the scholarship of others is obvious, a debt which I have tried to acknowledge in the references cited. I particularly wish to express my thanks to Dr Ann Williams and Dr John Hudson for their valuable criticism of early drafts of sections covering Anglo-Saxon England and Feudalism after the Norman conquest. Fred Harrison, Professor Mason Gaffney, Dr Roger Sandiland and Sir Kenneth Jupp reviewed the manuscript, providing much needed encouragement. Of course, all opinions and errors of fact are my own.

The Robert Schalkenbach Foundation of New York generously supported the costs of publication. It is no exaggeration to say that the book would not have seen the light of day but for the unswerving support and skills of Marian Fitt who prepared the typescript. The hope is that the end product will appeal to all who have a genuine concern for the Welfare of their society.

George Miller
May 2000

In memory of my parents,
Mary and George

Part 1:
Looking through the welfare state

Introduction

The plaster is not as large as the sore. (Attributed to Sir Matthew Hale)

Any system whereby the State undertakes to protect the health and well-being of each and every citizen, especially those in financial or social need (Fowler, 1990), is bound to be treasured. Such, for all its faults and abuses, is Britain's Welfare State. Although having many subsidiary purposes, above all the Welfare State aims to serve in the collective defence of the mental, physical and social health of all, primarily by re-distributing the wherewithal in cash and in kind to those in need from those for whom the loss presents no perceptible risk of material deprivation. The State strives for an all-embracing system to prevent neglect and exclusion, based on the mutual understanding that the utility of the last pound is less to the rich family than to the poor family, and that the transfer from the former to the latter is a positive benefit. The embodiment of empathy in citizenship, an expression of fellow feeling between families of the nation who have never met, the system ennobles as it strives to succeed.

Fine sentiment, but all is not goodness and light in the land. Sir Henry Phelps Brown, distinguished economist and member of the Royal Commission on the Distribution of Income and Wealth between 1974 and 1978, warned: "The case for the Welfare State is overwhelming to those who remember some of the city streets, or the cottages in the villages, as they were before the First World War.... But there are limits to the extension of welfare, and reactions against it. It presupposes that people will accept the reasonableness of contributing; but fellow-feeling does not extend universally, and in any case the contributions are merged in a sum of taxation whose burden is resented. This resentment has mounted as the visible expenditure has grown..." (Phelps Brown, 1991, pp 526-7).

Born in 1906 in the market town of Calne in Wiltshire, Phelps Brown may well have had memories of those pre-First World War conditions to which he referred. He wrote these words in the 1980s, 40 years on from the birth of Britain's universal Welfare State, an era for which Derek Fraser added a cautionary postscript, "The Decline of the Welfare State 1973-1983?", as he updated his book on British social policy (Fraser, 1984, pp 250-3). The same period was the focus of Paul Pierson's *The dismantling of the welfare state?* (Pierson, 1994). Eighteen months before his death in December 1995, Phelps Brown would have seen reports of a speech made by the Conservative Michael Portillo, then Chief Secretary to the Treasury, in which he said: "A civilised nation depends on the values of neighbourliness and concern for others. But as people learn to look to the State for a solution to every social problem, people tend to think less of what their responsibilities are ... their compassion is exercised by proxy: through paying taxes" (*The Independent*, 28 June, 1994).

Many questioned the extent to which the social improvements alluded to by Sir Henry could be credited to the Welfare State, rather than advances in science and technology, the generation of wealth and other successes since 1918. For some the Welfare State had not done enough; for others it had over-reached itself. For some it was under-funded; for others its spending was inefficient and out of control. For those such as Mr Portillo it was the epitome of Big Government – over-expansive, over-taxing and over-bureaucratic. For others the Welfare State had yet to be nurtured to full maturity, when it would truly stand in the service of economic stability and justice: the flagship of morality on the turbulent waters of politics.

Much of the never-ending debate centres round when shortage becomes need. On one criterion, however, all should be able to agree: when shortages curtail life there is need indeed. Thus the disclosure of a five to seven year difference in life expectancy between families at opposite ends of the scale of social class presents society with an enormous challenge, especially when the difference appears to have increased in recent years (Drever and Whitehead, 1998). The headlines have been eye-catching: 'Ministry admits ... Poor suffer more illness than rich' (*The Guardian*, 24 October, 1995); 'The poor get poorlier' (*The Guardian*, 26 February, 1997); 'Hunger and cold: facts of life for 11 million Britons' (*The Independent*, 22 July, 1997); 'Heart illness risk for poor' (*The Guardian*, 24 July, 1997); 'Death rate gap widens to worst for 50 years' (*The Guardian*, 11 August, 1997). In 1977 the Labour administration's Secretary of State for Social Services appointed a Research Working Group to examine social inequalities in health, headed by Professor Sir Douglas Black, Chief Scientist at the Department of Health. His Report concluded that the poorer health experience of the 'lower occupational groups' applied to all stages of life, and that the remedy lay beyond the ambit of medicine (Townsend et al, 1992). The brief dismissal of this group's work by the incoming Conservative administration has entered the annals of history. The aftermath, as declared in the headlines, was 'Inner-city poverty and death rates rise' (*The Independent*, 21 November, 1994).

A living wage

With the return of a Labour administration in 1997, Tessa Jowell, Britain's first Public Health Minister in the Department of Health, re-addressed these issues, intending to report by mid-1998 in time for the 50th anniversary of the launch of the National Health Service. In the meantime, Prime Minister Tony Blair's Labour administration published its green paper, *New ambitions for our country: A new contract for welfare*, which declared that "the welfare system has failed to keep pace with profound economic, social and political changes" (Department of Social Security, 1998, p 9). Government talked of overhauling "the machinery of welfare (that) has the air of yesteryear" (Department of Social Security, 1998, p 9). The objective of this exercise was to equip the Welfare State not merely to prevent outright destitution (the first way), or to alleviate poverty (the second way), but to prevent need (the third way). "Work is at the centre of our reform programme", declared the Green Paper: "Work for those who can; security for those who cannot" (Department of Social Security, 1998, p iii). So perhaps the Welfare State requires re-definition as it enters its third age: a system whereby the State undertakes to protect the health, well-being and right to work of its citizens, in order to prevent financial and social deprivation.

There is nothing to criticise in such aims, but neither is there anything new in them. Words like these echo across the ages. "The great business of the nation (is) ... to keep the poor from begging and starving and ensuring such, as are able, to labour ... ". So wrote Sir Josiah Child in 1669. William Beveridge, the designer of Britain's Welfare State after 1945, wrote to his mother Annette in 1904: "Granted that many parents have now the responsibility of feeding their children without the power of doing so (owing to low wages), the remedy is not to remove the responsibility but to give the power" (Harris, 1977, p 55). In order to empower (and the credo of Labour's reform is 'empowerment not dependency') (*The Economist*, 28 March, 1998, p 35), Beveridge urged industrial re-organisation to ease the problems of unemployment. His proposals included the labour exchange (forerunner of the modern job centre), public works at times of industrial recession, improved training and technical education. By 1914 two million men were seeking work annually through 423 labour exchanges (Harris, 1972, p 295).

In 1941, following the great recession of the 1930s, Archbishop William Temple wrote: "The present threat of unemployment to the maintenance of home and family must be ended" (Temple, 1976, p 102). Had he foreseen the outcome of later research provoking the headline 'Unemployment kills ...' (*The Guardian*, 25 January, 1996), Archbishop Temple may well have added 'life' to 'home and family'. Nevertheless, large discrepancies persist between the dearth of jobs paying a living wage and the surplus of workers seeking employment. While there is obvious sense in ensuring the possession of skills suited to employment in a modern age, the age-old recurring problem is not so much a lack of workers willing to take jobs, but a lack of accessible jobs paying a family wage to willing workers. In 1998 the government reported that "one in five working age households have no one in work" (Department of Social Security, 1998, p 3).

If only the hardship of joblessness could be rectified permanently by measures on which the government pins its faith, such as personal advice on how to find work, the subsidy of low pay, the removal of disincentives to work created by the taxation and benefits systems of previous administrations, training for work, and the provision of childcare for mothers when working outside the home, all would then be well. But the problems of worklessness and low pay go much deeper than such measures suggest and the government cares to admit. In fact, worklessness, low pay and impoverishment go to the roots of the political economy, being largely products of a peculiar blend of economic forces, old and not so old, consisting of a vestige of Feudalism, exploitation of this very important vestige under Capitalism, and well-meaning but misguided and counter-productive taxation policies to fund the State. How this mix came to be, and its consequences for the distribution of health and wealth, are of fundamental importance for all.

Impoverishment is a symptom, the causes of which are not confined to poor families and poor neighbourhoods. The enigma of Capitalism, as William Beveridge realised, is that although the system is eminently capable of producing wealth to abolish want, its mode of production creates and perpetuates want by distributing national resources most inequitably between families, neighbourhoods and regions. This is the key word – *inequitably*, rather than 'unequally'. There is an inbuilt injustice within Capitalism as practised. Like so many, Beveridge was never able to discover how to create a distribution of wealth and income under Capitalism which was consistent with justice and did not jeopardise the process of production. His greatest accomplishment, the universal Welfare State, has manifestly not been the answer. Whatever else may have been achieved, taxation of wages and interest for Welfare has undoubtedly been counter-productive, and over the past 50 years the prospects for health and the life expectancy of those who have least, have not been moved any closer to the standards set by those who have most. In this fundamental respect Welfare has not proven to be the antidote for the poison within the fruits of Capitalism. But why not? Why was Gordon Brown, New Labour's Chancellor of the Exchequer, confronted in 2000 with the same task as his predecessors, the harmonious marriage of fairness and efficiency?

Standard texts on economics list several causes of temporary worklessness and low income. One such cause, structural unemployment arising from the closure of traditional industries, was the focus of New Labour's *National strategy for neighbourhood renewal* in 2000 (Social Exclusion Unit, 2000). Though these causes are of undoubted importance, even in aggregate they do not come anywhere near to explaining why, almost a century after Beveridge first showed interest in the problem, Britain's government finds itself confessing: "For those able to undertake it, paid work is the surest route out of poverty.... But one in five working age households have no one in work" (Department of Social Security, 1998, p 3). A fundamental reason, which also explains much of the inequitable distribution of resources under Capitalism, cannot be understood until Rent (see below) is understood. To appreciate the immense social and economic significance of Rent is in large measure to come to grips with the essentials of British society and its offshoots. We need to understand how Rent's social value was undermined during its long process of privatisation and monopolisation under Feudalism. We need to acknowledge its exploitation under laissez-faire Capitalism, and ultimately to recognise its treacherous behaviour under private ownership in Welfare Capitalism. But the pathway to understanding and communication is bedevilled by semantics: the very word 'Rent' works against clarity of exposition.

Rent

In common parlance 'rent' is the tenant's periodical payment to the landlord for the use of land and any buildings on the site. This is the *commercial* rent of the world of private business. But there is also *economic* Rent (hereafter simply 'Rent') as defined originally for classical economics, which is the surplus in the national income remaining after all Wages have been paid to Labour and all Interest paid to Capital, and which goes to those holding land in one way or another. Had there been an economist in that earlier epoch when the surplus income in the economy was reserved largely for local and national purposes, this might then have been called something like the 'common wage' or, to revive and adapt a good old English word that trips more easily off the tongue, 'commonage'. But economists first described this surplus income in a much later age when it was well and truly privatised as that part of the national income going to those holding land. So we are stuck with Rent.

The confused semantics that arises when 'rent' has one meaning in common coinage and another in political economy is bad enough, but when, as happened, it becomes bandied about in economics to mean whatever professors want it to mean, the situation takes a much more serious turn for the worse. As the economy moved on from the agrarian age, the special social significance of Rent was trivialised by economists serving late 19th century industrial enterprise and allowed to fade into oblivion, a reflection of the ascendancy of Business or Market Capitalism over Welfare Capitalism. New professors usurped the term to describe certain features of the new economy as perceived by them. The result was 'rent of ability', 'quasi-rent', 'rent of status' and a new meaning given to economic rent itself (see Chapter Thirteen). The term became corrupted by loose usage while Rent as a form of income was subsumed into Interest as 'profit', a blind eye being turned to its social nature. For those who wish to stress Rent as a social fund the obscuration of the term in this sense and its ambiguity when used without qualification are inconveniences, to say the least.

The record of Rent, ancient and modern, and its role in the Welfare State have all the richness of English history, a richness I have sought to convey. Therein lie the origins of over-privilege under Feudalism, its conversion into a highly marketable commodity under Capitalism, its covert existence under Welfare Capitalism, and the perpetuation of under-privilege with its abridged lifespan in a society which still knows social class. These insights expose the contradictions which frustrate Welfare policy and suggest a more constructive way forward.

The everyday level of debate about Britain's Welfare State, the nation's salve for deprivation and sub-health, must desist from agonising about when shortage becomes need. Nor can discussion be restricted to recommendations about specific responses, of which there have been legion. More thought needs to be given to what keeps the debate alive, that deeply disturbing feeling that the Welfare State is but a filmy tableau, needing only a puff to expose a fundamental injustice rooted in the political economy. We speak of 'inequalities' in income and health because we choke on that taboo word 'inequities'. What we are confronted by with every puff, though dare not but dimly acknowledge, is evidence for injustice in the land of fair play.

History forewarns that any serious attempt to introduce the long-neglected but fundamental issue of Rent into Britain's debate about social exclusion, fairness and efficiency and its Welfare State risks re-kindling a bitter controversy which raged fiercely 100 years ago. Deeply contentious in 1900, the proposition that Rent is properly a form of public income is likely to be just as hotly debated in 2000, especially by those who hold fast to Rent as private income within Capitalism.

The global perspective

The setting of this book is Britain, but the concerns addressed are global. In 1948 the General Assembly of the United Nations adopted the Universal Declaration of Human Rights (United Nations, 1948). Though not amounting to international law, the Declaration derives force to the extent that nations ensure conformity between its ideals and their own legislative and other actions. Article 25 has this to say:

1. Everyone has the right to a standard of living adequate for the health and well-being of the family … and the right to security in the event of unemployment, sickness, disability, widowhood, old age or other lack of livelihood in circumstances beyond his control.
2. Motherhood and childhood are entitled to special care and assistance. All children … shall enjoy the same social protection.

Set against this measure, there remain millions of families living out a sub-standard existence. The secondary and tertiary explanations for this state of affairs are legion, but a primary factor is hidden within Article 17:

1. Everyone has the right to own property alone as well as in association with others.
2. No one shall be arbitrarily deprived of his property.

True enough – but what in moral or natural law distinguishes private property from communal property? What is this supra-national or universal law to which everyone must answer if Article 17 is to conform with Article 25? For if this law is violated, and what is morally communal property is sequestered as private property for the benefit of some privileged citizens to the detriment of others, the intentions in Article 25 will be seriously compromised. The fact is that this natural law is indeed flouted, Article 25 is put into jeopardy, and the United Nations' objectives are thwarted.

Two treaties inspired by the Declaration of Human Rights were published in December 1966. The International Covenant on Civil and Political Rights and the International Covenant on Economic, Social and Cultural Rights were adopted by the General Assembly and offered to member nations. Britain ratified the Covenant on Economic, Social and Cultural Rights on 20 August 1976. The USA cannot bring itself to do so, finding something disturbing in its stand on such universal rights as those to work, to fair wages, to a decent living, to education and freedom from hunger. Underlying much of the reticence is the right to private property as presently constituted for Business Capitalism. Welfare Capitalism is the loser.

Unemployment, an inequitable distribution of income and wealth, and a resultant shortening of the lifespan of the under-privileged will persist until honest debate plumbs the murky depths. In London in late 1998, Sir Donald Acheson, former Chief Medical Officer, declared: "... it has become clear that the range of factors influencing inequalities in health extends far beyond the remit of the Department of Health and that a response by the Government as a whole will be needed to deal with them" (Acheson, 1998, p v). Elsewhere he stated: "The weight of the scientific evidence supports a socioeconomic explanation of health inequalities. This traces the roots of ill health to ... income, education and employment as well as the material environment and lifestyle.... We have identified a range of areas for future policy development ... (which) include: poverty, income, tax and benefits ..." (Acheson, 1998, p xi). Given strict terms of reference, his group left policy development to their political masters. Yet the intransigence of social class differences in death rates to Welfare policies, described in the following chapters, demands a critical appraisal of the political economy.

ONE

The poor and their health:
the early record

I care not how affluent some may be,
provided that none be miserable in consequence of it.
(Thomas Paine, *Agrarian Justice*)

"In the north part", reported Ralph Maddison in 1623, "many do perish for food ... because of want of monies and want of employment and labour for the poor" (Slack, 1992). Grim experience had long taught the unemployed and those who lived with them that lack of work, material deprivation and poor health stalked the land hand in hand. Governments were only too well aware of the petty crime, begging and sickness that accompanied harsh economic conditions. Bristol typified English cities and towns during the 16th and 17th centuries. Even in good years the ratio of burials to baptisms tended to be higher in the poor parishes on the outskirts than in the wealthier parishes of the city centre. When a series of failed harvests created great hardship in 1597 the inner parishes appeared not to have been seriously affected, whereas burial rates trebled in the poorer parishes of St Mary Redcliffe and Temple. During the plague of 1603, of the 35 out of 42 burials in the parish of Christ Church that could be identified by later researchers, 24 were of those carried out of an impoverished community of about 70 in the 'Pithay', an over-crowded filthy alley near the poor-house. By contrast, only 11 burials were of the dead from the 240 communicants in up-market Broad Street, Wine Street and Tower Lane. When plague returned to Bristol in 1645, burial rates in All Saints and St Nicholas parishes, where the streets were paved and drained, just about doubled. In St Mary Redcliffe and Temple, where the lanes were littered with decaying sewage, burial rates increased eight-fold (Slack, 1977).

Whether rich man, poor man, beggar man or thief, all are born to die. The monks who composed the mural paintings of the 14th and 15th centuries, the 'dances of death', were well aware of the flimsier hold of the poor than the rich on life on this earth, but this must have appeared inconsequential compared with the eternity faced by all souls in the life hereafter (Mackenbach, 1995). They were more concerned to have mortals do penance before facing their Maker, especially the great, the belief being that higher standards would be expected at the Last Judgement of those who were blessed with the comforts of this life. For secular society, however, the constant threats of sickness and death were of more immediate import. In the Geneva of the 17th century, the average life expectancy of the highest social classes, 36 years, was twice that of the lowest classes (Perrenoud, 1975). Among British ducal families, 69% of children born between 1480 and 1679 survived to age 15 or beyond (Hollingworth, 1965). In the poor London parish of St Botolph's, the respective survival rate of those born between 1583 and 1599 was 30% (Forbes, 1979). In 1805 Dr Hall could state confidently: "... for the purpose of investigating the manner in which they (ie the people in a civilised state) enjoy or are deprived of the requisites to support the health of their bodies and minds, they need only be divided into two classes, viz the rich and the poor" (Hall, 1805, p 2). Among his evidence was the following experience.

> When the Equitable Insurance Office at Blackfriars Bridge was first established, the premiums taken were according to the ratio proposed by Dr Price, who formed it from the accounts of the annual deaths taken from the bills of mortality kept in different cities of Europe. These deaths were about 1 in 22, annually, of all the people, taken indiscriminately. Proceeding thus, the profits of the Society were so great, that in a few years they realised their enormous capital, upon which, their premiums were lowered.... The Society, notwithstanding, continued to increase in riches. The cause of the phenomenon, therefore, was a matter of inquiry, on which it was found that they had adapted their premiums to the deaths of the rich and poor taken together; and it soon occurred that none but the rich were insured. Their extraordinary profit, therefore, must arise from the circumstances of there being fewer deaths annually among the rich than among the poor, in proportion to the numbers of both ... it seems probable, that the deaths of the poor are to those of the rich as two to one, in proportion to the numbers of each. (Hall, 1805, pp 11-12)

The Victorian actuaries

In 1861, actuaries with the London Assurance Corporation and the Scottish Widows Fund Assurance Society published *Peerage Families' Experience Tables*, based on the lives of the British peers, their children, and the children of their first sons between 1800 and 1855. In 1864, the Reverend John Hodgson and the Guardian Life Assurance Society published *Observations on duration of life among the clergy of England and Wales*. These calculations were based on 107,000 years of life shared between more than 5,000 clergymen born after 1759, of whom 3,100 had died by 1860. The *Peerage* tables showed that children of the aristocracy at that time could expect to live 12 years longer than the average male (40 years) or female (42 years). The clergy were similarly long-lived. These figures were improved upon in 1874 by Charles Ansell of the National Life Assurance Society, who sent a questionnaire to men of the church, medicine and law, gathering information on more than 50,000 persons. The results showed once again the advantages in health and longevity enjoyed by the wealthy. For every 1,000 children born alive to the peerage, 880 were still living at 10 years of age. For every 1,000 births to the upper classes and the general population the survivals were 850 and 700, respectively. Contrasts were particularly marked during early childhood. The annual mortality for children under five years was 28 per 1,000 for the upper classes, but 66 per 1,000 for the general population (Humphreys, 1887, pp 259-63).

Assistant Registrar General Noel Humphreys assembled his paper on 'Class Mortality Statistics' for the Royal Statistical Society in 1887 (Humphreys, 1887). Telling his audience that the decline in the English death rate per year since 1875 (to 20 per 1,000 from the earlier 23 per 1,000) was proof of the power of public health, he proposed that the time had come to monitor the extent to which this improvement was shared by the working classes. Forty years previously, Friedrich Engels had extracted data from the famous *Report on the sanitary condition of the working classes* to illustrate the appalling state of affairs in Britain's towns around 1840 (Engels, 1993, pp 117-18). In Liverpool, the average life expectancy of the gentry and professional classes was 35 years; that of businessmen and skilled workers was 22 years; and that of the labourers and service classes as little as 15 years. These same statistics were given prominence in *The Lancet* of 1843 (*The Lancet*, 1843). Engels quoted the findings of Dr P.N. Holland in a district of inner Manchester, Chorlton-on-Medlock, published in 1844. Dr Holland categorised houses and streets into three classes. Residents of second and third class streets had mortality rates 18% and 68% higher, respectively, than those of first class streets (Commission of Enquiry into the State of Large Towns and Populous Districts, 1844).

The evidence from the Registrar General

Viscount Melbourne's Whig administration introduced civil registration of births, marriages and deaths in 1836. The following year the General Register Office for England and Wales was established at Somerset House under Lord John Russell's relative, Thomas Lister. George Graham took over on Lister's death in 1842. William Farr, statistical superintendent to both men, regularly published death rates by occupation, and his successor Dr Ogle developed this approach using data for 1880 to 1882. Among men aged 25 to 65 years, allowing for differences in age between occupational groups, Ogle found that the death rate of clergy was 40% less than the national average, while for teachers and lawyers it was 28% and 16% less than the average, respectively. On the other hand for cab drivers, innkeepers, street sellers and London's general labourers it was respectively 48%, 52%, 88% and 105% above the national average. Specific occupational and locality effects were also clear. Agricultural labourers had a death rate about 30% less than average, while that of doctors was 12% above the nation's average. To disentangle the effect of poverty from those of occupational risks and locality, Humphreys wished to look at the situation in childhood and infancy. He therefore turned to some remarkable figures assembled by Dr Grimshaw, Ireland's Registrar General.

Victorian Dublin: its rich and poor

The late-Victorian slums of Dublin were the worst in Europe. The wages of the poor were extremely low even by contemporary standards. In the early 1880s, with the city still recovering from the Phoenix Park murders of Lord Frederick Cavendish and his Under-secretary, Thomas Burke, Dr Grimshaw placed the 347,000 citizens of Dublin into four classes: the Professional and Upper Classes, the Middle Classes (householders of 'second class localities in the city', civil servants, bankers and so on), the Artisan and Small Shopkeeper Class, and the General Service Class which included those in workhouses. The workhouse deaths were one of several problems faced by Grimshaw. They accounted for as many as 16% of all deaths in the city because the wards and infirmaries of the workhouses were caring for far more than the pauper class. Poor clerks, domestic servants, shop assistants and small shopkeepers also died there as inpatients. Ignoring this element of misclassification, but after adjustment for differences in the age structure of the four classes, Dublin's Professional and Upper Classes were shown to have a death rate 37% lower than the average for England and Wales, while the General Service Class had a rate of 66% above this average. Annual mortality rates in the under-fives (per 1,000) were 22 in the Professional and Upper Classes, 71 in the Artisan Classes, and 110 in the Service Class. Thus the effect of poverty in early childhood was to raise the death rate by a factor of five in Dublin at that time. Of equal interest, an inverse gradient between class and mortality was revealed: intermediate classes had intermediate death rates, a characteristic which has persisted into the 1990s and found wherever it is sought. Mr Humphreys stressed that it was time to collect such information for England and Wales, but this had to wait for 16 years.

The army, Empire and the poor

Governments responded slowly to increasing concerns for the well-being of the Victorian poor, until at the turn of the century the administration was suddenly galvanised into action by an event which left a proud nation bewildered – the second Boer War. Only two years previously in 1897 Britain had turned Queen Victoria's Diamond Jubilee into an immense celebration of Empire. The mood even caught Dublin. When the Queen visited the city in 1900 vast crowds turned out to cheer her. Little were the people aware that this seemingly invincible Empire had just about reached its zenith. In his contributions to the *New Monthly Magazine*, collected in 1825 into his *The spirit of the age*, William Hazlitt had perceptively portrayed many influential men of his day, among them Jeremy Bentham, Samuel Taylor Coleridge, Horne Tooke and Sir Francis Burdett (Hazlitt, 1906). Many were patriots for their time, but none an Imperialist. Devotion to country abounded in Britain, but not yet any heady commitment to Empire-building. Yet only 70 years on and the nation would not have forgiven any writer on the great men of that age who overlooked soldiers such as Lord Kitchener of Khartoum, Lord Roberts of Kandahar, Lord Worseley of Cairo, General Charles Gordon also of Khartoum, or Field Marshal Viscount Garnet Wolseley of Tel-el-Kabir. Britain's Empire covered a quarter of the earth's habitable surface, its colonies, dominions and protectorates connected by sea lanes plied by a British fleet possessing more mercantile and fighting ships than the rest of the world together. The British army, however, appeared much more than it was. The record in the Crimea had been awful and the colonial wars had been strong on bravado and heroism but outdated on methods of warfare. Even as late as 1898 the massacre of 10,000 Sudanese for the loss of 28 men of the 31st Lancers was no measure of the army's real fighting capacity. The second Boer War came as a nasty shock.

The British army drew its volunteers overwhelmingly from families in which the breadwinner was a manual worker, often bringing home under 30 shillings (30s) a week when in employment – about 47 '1993 pounds' (Newman and Foster, 1995, p 305). Having suffered some early reverses in the Boer War, the army turned events in its favour only by placing its infantry on horseback and overwhelming the enemy with large contingents from Canada, Australia and New Zealand. Alarmed, the Director General of the Army Medical Service wanted to know why 40% to 60% of volunteers were deemed to be physically unfit, mostly because of 'want of physical development, defective vision, disease of the heart, or bad dentition'. It was the memorandum from the Inspector General of Recruiting, however, which put the cat among the pigeons. This spoke of a gradual deterioration in the quality of volunteers over the years. The suggestion that the situation was worsening prompted the Secretary of State for the Home Department to write to the Presidents of the Royal Colleges of Physicians and Surgeons for their opinions. Hence the name given to the ensuing official enquiry – the Inter-Departmental Committee on Physical *Deterioration* (Inter-Departmental Committee on Physical Deterioration, 1904).

The Royal Colleges were wary. The question of physical deterioration was a subject of virulent debate at that time, and they were rightly loathe to criticise their colleagues in public health. Public health medical officers had laboured for decades to improve the health and reduce the high death rates of the urban poor. Underpinning their work was the 'sanitary movement', which held that improvements in housing, the quality of the air and water, and other environmental factors would benefit the health of these people very considerably. Their whole purpose was being undermined, however, by the growing School of Scientific Naturalism, a product of the imagination of Francis Galton.

The rise of eugenic theories of poverty

Born near Sparkbrook, Birmingham in February 1822, Galton was cousin to Charles Darwin, the famous scientist born in Shrewsbury 13 years earlier. Darwin studied medicine in Edinburgh but failed to complete the course owing to an aversion to surgery. Galton took the same studies at London and Cambridge universities but he too did not complete the courses, having inherited sufficient wealth to indulge in travel and exploration as a gentleman of independent means. His journeys in the Kalahari region of Africa earned him election to the Royal Geographical Society and the Royal Society by the age of 35. In 1859 Darwin published his *On the origin of species by means of natural selection.* Inspired by this work, Galton set about applying its basic concept to the human condition. In his book *Hereditary genius*, published in 1869, he proposed that human mental and physical attributes were inherited, and seized upon the idea that the physical and mental stock of the human population could be improved by selection of parenthood.

Around 1880 the Anthropometric Committee of the British Association for the Advancement of Science was conducting a five-year survey of 53,000 persons of all ages and both sexes throughout the UK, including children of all social backgrounds. The investigators gained access to the 'industrial' and 'reformatory' schools established for poor children under a series of statutes beginning in 1854. Local magistrates sent 'juvenile offenders' to reformatories, while the 'innocent but neglected' went to industrial schools. At the other end of the social spectrum covered by the survey were the scholars of the public schools. The average height of boys aged 11 to 12 years was found to be 140 cm in the public schools, as compared with 127 cm in the poor schools. Working with the Anthropometric Committee, Galton promoted the view that the relative social positions of the children and their parents in this survey were a direct consequence of biologically (genetically) determined attributes and abilities, running in parallel with their height. He argued that different types of employment 'selected out' different levels of inherited mental ability and physique, and that social inequalities and contrasts in wealth were scientifically explained by social contrasts in inherited characteristics.

After toying with 'viriculture' as the name for his new science, Galton opted for 'eugenics', from the Greek for 'well-born'. This indeed was a 'science' for the new Imperialism, with its notions of racial superiority. Emboldened by those who enthused about his notions, Galton used the Huxley Memorial Lecture of 1901 to propose in a quite arbitrary manner that the British population could be divided into fifths, each representing a segment of the natural distribution of 'genetic worth' in the community. The Liverpool shipowner, merchant and sociologist Charles Booth had spent many years grading the population of London in terms of eight occupational classes, and Galton dared to superimpose his supposed classes of inherited worth on Booth's occupational grades, thereby forcing his notion of the equivalence of 'genetic' and 'civic' worth. Galton had no notion of genetics as we understand it today, and lacked any understanding of the time scale on which evolution operates. His views did not go unchallenged, but nevertheless they were a gift to those seeking reasons not to offer relief to those in poverty, and an affront to the public health movement.

Many brilliant but socially prejudiced men were attracted to Galton, including the mathematician Karl Pearson. In his Huxley Lecture given just before the Inter-Departmental Committee on Physical Deterioration, Pearson claimed:

> We are ceasing to breed intelligence as we did 50 years ago.... The mentally better stock is not reproducing itself at the same rate as it did of old: the less able, less energetic, are more fertile than the better stocks. ... The only remedy is to alter the relative fertility of the good and bad stocks in the community. Let us have a census of the effective size of the families among the intellectual classes now and a comparison with the effective size of families in the like classes of the first half of the century.... Compare in another such census the fertility of the more intelligent working man with that of the uneducated hand labourer. You will ... find that grave changes have taken place in relative fertility during the last 40 years. We stand, I venture to think, at the commencement of an epoch which will be marked by a great dearth of ability ... intelligence can be trained but no training or education can create it. You must breed it.... (Inter-Departmental Committee on Physical Deterioration, 1904, p 38)

The working classes were being told by their betters that their position in life, their susceptibility to disease and early death, were consequences of their genetic inferiority.

For Galton and the eugenicists, class differences in death rates during childhood were due to the innate inferiority of the working classes. This degeneracy included their alleged lack of moral fibre and self-control. In seeking to improve the health and stamina of the poor, Galton claimed, the public health movement was strengthening their capacity to breed their inferior biological properties into the population at a rate exceeding that at which the upper classes were reproducing their own superior inherited traits. Galton made contributions to science, including meteorology, but public health had little for which to thank him. His was mainly a diversionary contribution allied to an age-old question: is it poverty that causes ill health, or ill health that causes poverty? These possibilities are obviously not mutually exclusive, but so stubbornly have disbelievers in the ill effects of poverty resisted what the poor have known from time immemorial, that only recently could it be claimed that such doubts have finally been laid to rest by dogged research dating from the Committee on Physical Deterioration.

Army officers, drawn largely from the peerage and landed gentry, generally held a low opinion of the ranks. P.H. Stanhope recorded how on 4th November 1821, the Duke of Wellington had said to him that the British army "is composed of the scum of the earth – the mere scum of the earth" (Floud et al, 1990, p 31). The Director General of the Army Medical Service, Sir William Taylor, told the Inter-Departmental Committee of 1903 that men who drifted into recruitment were largely 'rubbish', 'not fit or disinclined to work', and 'the condition of those rejected is only representative of the state of the wastrels of the large towns who live by casual labour'. A breath of fresh air must have entered the committee room with the anatomist, Professor Daniel John Cunningham of Edinburgh University. Stressing that much he had heard from other witnesses was 'pure presumption', he stated in no uncertain terms: "the inferior bodily characteristics which are the result of poverty ... and which are therefore acquired during the lifetime of the individual, are not transmissible from one generation to the next. To restore, therefore, the classes in which this inferiority exists to the mean standard of the national physique, all that is required is to improve the conditions of living, and in one or two generations all the ground that has been lost will be recovered."

The call for research to guide policy regarding the poor

In its inquiry into the 'causes of degeneracy in certain classes, and the means by which it may be arrested', the Inter-Departmental Committee considered nurture as well as nature. Thought was given to over-crowding, atmospheric pollution, conditions in the factories, the effects of alcoholism, the alleged tendency of the poor to have more children than the rich, the importance of nutrition, the consequences for mothers of working in pregnancy and during their children's infancy, breast feeding, and 'parental ignorance and neglect'. The lack of objective evidence became only too apparent.

Advice on what to do about the socio-economic circumstances of the poor was beyond its remit, but nevertheless the Committee recommended labour colonies for the unemployed and the provision of public nurseries. Parents unable to live an independent existence to a standard stipulated by the State could be compulsorily detained in such colonies while their children were placed in the nurseries or boarded in industrial schools. The education system was seen as offering the remedy by overcoming ignorance, providing good school meals and ensuring medical inspection of the pupils, though of course teachers could not do anything about the underlying social conditions beyond the school gate. There was also, incidentally, a call for the prohibition of the sale of tobacco in sweet shops, in order to protect children from the temptation to smoke.

To monitor the effectiveness of these and other Welfare measures, there should be anthropometric surveys of the type recommended by Professor Cunningham, together with a council to examine the findings and advise government accordingly. The Committee realised that destitute people were treated for sickness at the public expense through the Poor Law system of infirmaries, infirmary wards in the general workhouses, asylums for the mentally ill and domiciliary care supervised by the Poor Law medical officers. Yet the Poor Law commissioners, and later the Local Government Board responsible for overseeing the system, had never collected any national statistics on the amount of sickness treated in this way or on the outcome. A register of sickness should therefore be compiled on the returns from the Poor Law institutions. Finally, the Committee noted that although the Registrar General's statistics on national birth and death rates were valuable for many purposes, they threw no light on whether the health of the poor had altered over the years because the figures were not broken down by social class: "We lament even today the failure of government to heed such advice, because we now are sadly lacking on information regarding sickness rates by social class" (Inter-Departmental Committee on Physical Deterioration, 1904, pp 84-93). The Registrar General was unable to tackle the lack of data on sickness, but his office could look at birth rates and death rates by social class. The man who took up the challenge was Dr Thomas Henry Craig Stevenson, native of Strabane, County Tyrone in Ireland, educated at University College London, and Superintendent of Statistics at the General Register Office from 1909.

Were the poor more fertile than the rich?

Dr Stevenson and Dr Arthur Newsholme, Brighton's Medical Officer of Health, used the Census of 1901 to classify London's boroughs according to the average number of domestic servants per family, as a guide to affluence (Newsholme and Stevenson, 1906). For every 100 families there were 81 servants in Hampstead, 22 in Holborn, and eight in Poplar, for example. After adjustments for differences between the boroughs in age distribution and frequency of marriage, the annual birth rate per 1,000 population was found to be 20 in Hampstead and other well-serviced boroughs, 26 in Holborn, and 32 in Poplar. The poorer certainly appeared to be more fertile. Newsholme and Stevenson believed these social contrasts to reflect greater use of birth control in affluent boroughs rather than true differences in fertility, though they had little supportive evidence. Nevertheless, such statistics certainly motivated the economist John Maynard Keynes to advocate promotion of birth control for the masses. During the 1920s he associated himself publicly with the Society for Constructive Birth Control and the New Generation League, fearing that over-population with people from the working classes would have undesirable economic consequences (Toye, 1997).

Stevenson's scheme of the Edwardian social classes

Stevenson took another step forward when in 1913 he presented an analysis of fertility by social class derived from the national census of 1911 (General Register Office, 1913, p 44). He used the stated occupation of the breadwinner to derive social class, a technique with its limitations, but none fatal for his purpose. Stevenson organised occupations 'into a number of groups, designed to represent as far as possible different social grades'. The classification had three basic categories: Class I being 'upper and middle', Class III covering skilled workmen (the aristocracy of labour), and Class V those in unskilled work. Time and again Stevenson was faced with occupational descriptions that could place the holder of the job either in Class I or III, or in Class III or V, depending on the grade (not recorded at this census). A draper, for example, could be the head of a large firm or an apprentice. His solution was to place such cases into two indeterminate Classes, II and IV, giving the five-class system still in use today:

Class I   Professional
Class II   Intermediate (nurse, teacher, manager etc)
Class III   Skilled worker
Class IV   Partly skilled (farm worker etc)
Class V   Unskilled manual worker

The poor and the social anthropologists

Stevenson's classification of occupations has been criticised for its supposed lack of underlying initial theory (more on this later). Had Stevenson been alive to reply he would doubtless have retorted that the theory he was testing was not his but that of Francis Galton – that those of lowest genetic worth, as indicated by the occupation for which they were suited, were also the most fertile. Social class differences in birth rates were a big issue in those days, and occupation was a strong indicator of Edwardian social class. Stevenson was making a legitimate contribution to the fields of sociology and social anthropology, expanding ever since the 1860s. Here we need to set his work in its contemporary social context.

As Foreign Secretary, Viscount Palmerston was forced to deal with Greece in 1850. Don Pacifico, a native of Gibraltar (British since 1713) had suffered at the hands of a mob led by the sons of the Greek Minister of War. Palmerston sent in the fleet, and international repercussions called for parliamentary debate. A passage in his speech encapsulated the contentment of an aristocracy approaching calmer political waters after its buffeting during the radical 1830s and 1840s: "We have shown the example of a nation in which every class of society accepts with cheerfulness the lot which Providence has assigned to it, while at the same time every individual of each class is constantly striving to raise himself in the social scale – not by injustice and wrong, but ... by the steady and energetic exertion of the moral and intellectual faculties with which his Creator has endowed him. To govern such a people as this is indeed an object worthy of the ambition of the noblest man who lives ..." (Argyll, 1892, pp 128-9). Yet the plight of the poor was pitiful, though largely curtained from the gaze of the general public, as described by Henry Mayhew in his book of the following year, *London labour and the London poor.*

There was a longstanding tradition of voluntary aid for the poor during hard times in Britain, as exemplified by the Society for Bettering the Condition and Increasing the Comforts of the Poor, founded by William Wilberforce and friends in 1796. The Society for Organising Charitable

Relief and Repressing Mendicity appeared in 1869, soon to be called the Charity Organisation Society. A significant number of social workers and theorists drawn to this movement, among them Charles Stewart Loch, Bernard Bosanquet and the Reverend Samuel Barnett (later Canon), had come under the influence of a moral philosophy cultivated at Balliol College in Oxford. To find the origins of this movement we have to go back to Benjamin Jowett of that College, who was largely responsible for introducing England to the thoughts of the German philosopher Georg Wilhelm Hegel. Many schools of philosophy traced their roots to Hegel, including Marxism ('Left Hegelians') and the 'adapted Hegelianism' of the British School of Absolute Idealism developed by Jowett's pupils Thomas Hill Green and Edward Caird.

Green (Stevens and Lee, 1973, pp 498-9), who died prematurely of a congenital heart disorder in 1882, is of particular interest for the origins of Britain's Welfare State. He was born in 1836, son of the rector to the Yorkshire parish of Birkin, east of Leeds. His mother's uncle, Archdeacon Hill of Derby, had given the living of the parish to her husband. In 1860 Green was lecturer and fellow of Balliol under Jowett. His interest in social problems led him to develop active interests in the education of the poor and in the temperence movement. In 1867 he spoke for the Reform Bill and in 1870 he supported Forster's Education Bill. This shy and hence seemingly aloof academic had a charismatic earnestness which captivated many of his students, including the reforming economist Arnold Toynbee. Insofar as it is ever possible to trace the ideas behind a movement like the Welfare State to one source, then Green and his colleagues must be strong candidates. With Jowett, Green was largely responsible for creating a tradition at Balliol which influenced many men who came after them, not least William Beveridge when he arrived there on a mathematics exhibition in 1897. Edward Caird, Master of Balliol between 1893 and 1907, was the man Beveridge was to know while at Oxford. Beveridge later recalled Caird's advice: "Go and discover why, with so much wealth in Britain, there continues to be so much poverty and how poverty can be cured" (Harris, 1977, p 41).

Charles Booth: pioneer of social investigation

Charles Booth was cousin by marriage to another great personality in the British social and Socialist movements, Beatrice Potter. A daughter of Richard Potter, chairman of the Great Western Railway, and Lawrencina Heyworth, daughter of a successful Liverpool merchant, Beatrice arrived in London a wealthy young woman. She joined the Charity Organisation Society as a social visitor in 1883. Three years later Charles Booth resigned as managing director of his business and invited Beatrice to join him as a research worker to examine the dimensions of poverty in London. They were among many caught up in the attack of national conscience during the depression of the 1880s. Was it right that so much poverty existed in the midst of affluence?

On 17 May 1887, Booth presented a paper to the Royal Statistical Society on his early work in the London Borough of Tower Hamlets (Booth, 1887). The 450,000 inhabitants were placed in 32 occupational categories for male heads of households and seven for female heads of households. The security and level of income of men in any occupation varied widely, so Booth devised eight classes of 'means and position' as follows:

A. Lowest Class: "(so-called) labourers, loafers, semi-criminals, a proportion of the street sellers, street performers and others." Booth excluded those in workhouses from this count. They represented between 1% and 2% of local society.

B. Casual Earnings: "shiftless, hand-to-mouth, pleasure loving and always poor" as a class. Booth put 11% of Tower Hamlets in this category.

C. Intermittent Earnings: "This is a pitiable class, consisting largely of struggling, suffering, helpless people". These were the victims of economic recession, some 7% of the community, and most suitable as recipients of charity "on some evidence of thrift as a precondition".

D. Small Regular Earnings: "No class deserves greater sympathy than this one; its members live hard lives very patiently ... The hope of improved condition ... lies only in their children ... State aided technical education would be of great value ...". In Tower Hamlets 15% were such little hopers.

E. Regular Standard Earnings: "The best class of street sellers ... the best off amongst the home manufacturers, and some small employers". Just over 45% of the population Booth judged to be of this type, and claimed that they owned "a good deal of property in the aggregate".

F. Higher Class Labour: "... a well-to-do and contented body of men"; the foremen and skilled artisans.

G. Lower Middle Class: "... hard working, sober, energetic class", consisting of clerks and the "lower professional classes".

H. Upper Middle Class: "the servant keeping class".

So, for example, of 1,354 male heads of households who were street sellers and their dependents, 8% were 'loafers'. 8% were 'shiftless and pleasure loving', 34% were of the pitiable type, 11% were enduring a hard life patiently, and 40% were 'of the best of their type'. Of large employers, half were Lower Middle Class and half were Upper Middle Class. Taking as 'poor' a 'bare' income of 18s to 21s a week to support a moderate family, Booth put 35% of the population at either this level or below; they were mostly of the 'loafer' or 'shiftless and pleasure loving' types.

Booth's early opinion of the Lowest Class was revealing. The Lowest Class were of 'low character', leading a 'savage life', with drink as their only 'luxury'. They were the "battered figures who slouch through the streets, and play the beggar or the bully, or help to foul the record of the unemployed". They "render no useful service and create no wealth: they oftener destroy it". They "degrade whatever they touch, and as individuals are almost incapable of improvement". As for their state, "There appears to be no doubt that it is hereditary to a very considerable extent". Their children were 'street Arabs', found "separated from the parents in pauper or industrial schools, and in such homes as Dr Barnardo's". Booth thought that all was not completely lost, however, and that "those able to wash away the mud may find some gems in it" (Booth, 1887). To this condemnation Galton added that their condition merely reflected their low inherited civic worth.

What struck Booth powerfully was the sense of helplessness. On the one hand were pitiable wage earners unable to regulate or obtain the value of their work, and on the other the rich who were 'helpless to relieve want without stimulating its sources' (ie creating idleness, lack of thrift, and wastefulness on 'drink'). There was also the helplessness of the manufacturer or dealer who could 'work only within the limits of competition'. Here was the Victorians' dilemma as they saw it – how to help the deserving poor without encouraging the undeserving poor. From this helplessness, Booth believed, sprang "Socialistic theories; passionate suggestions of ignorance". (Booth was never a Socialist, moving from the Liberal radicals in his youth to the Conservative Party in 1905.)

Booth concluded that the discipline of economics was divorced from realities. The Cambridge economist, Professor Alfred Marshall, was in the audience and denied that his profession confined itself to abstract theory. He felt that it was hampered by a lack of surveys such as Booth's. Marshall claimed that the wealthy were willing to pay their taxes in order to improve the conditions of London, but feared that to do so would only attract more labour into the city. The result would be more overcrowding, competition for jobs, a forcing down of wages owing to the increased supply of labour, and an increase in rents. He suggested that one reform might be to permit migration into London only on condition of a demonstrated ability to pay for a decent, healthy room. The reduced supply of labour would then drive up wages to a level sufficient to meet the rent of decent accommodation. How to enforce such restrictions on movement, Marshall did not discuss. A Mr Fordham pointed out that wages in agriculture were much below those in London, so he did not see how the flow into London could be reversed. Another gentleman thought the poor should be directed to opportunities for advancement in the colonies (Booth thought the colonial authorities would not welcome London's 'loafers and semi-criminals').

Professor Leoni Levi questioned whether Booth's definition of poverty, at 18s to 20s per week for the head of household to care for a moderately sized family, was not over-generous, because others in the family were likely to be earning something. Furthermore, if their expenses included 'unnecessary luxuries', there were no grounds for sympathy. Another speaker stressed how *official* pauperism had declined enormously in London in recent years: whereas in 1871 there were 50 in every 1,000 Londoners on the pauper roll, in 1887 there were not more than 25 per 1,000. The conditions of relief had altered, he admitted, but he claimed that this change had encouraged greater self-reliance. By this he meant that the workhouse operated an increasingly harsh regime in London's East End, so that fewer of the poor would submit themselves. He overlooked the reality. Poverty had not declined; only pauperism.

The poverty line

Booth covered many of the comments raised in his 17-volume *The life and labour of the people of London*, which appeared in stages between 1889 and 1903. He blazed a trail in social enquiry, inventing the method as he went along, including his concept of 'poverty line'. He came to view most poverty as involuntary and not the fault of its victims. Inspired by Booth's initiative, Seebohm Rowntree undertook a similar survey of York in 1899. He classified families with two to four dependent children into those with a weekly income of less than 18s, 18s to 21s, 21s to 30s, and more than 30s (18s in 1900 had the approximate purchasing power of £32 in 1993). Families with fewer than two children were placed one income bracket higher; conversely families were put into one income bracket lower when there were more than four children. This is what

Rowntree had to say about the living conditions of moderate-sized families with an income of 17 shillings and 8 pence (17s 8d) after payment of rent:

> A family living upon the scale allowed for in this estimate must never spend a penny on railway fare or omnibus. They must never go into the country unless they walk. They must never purchase a halfpenny newspaper or spend a penny to buy a ticket for a popular concert. They must write no letters to absent children, for they cannot afford to pay the postage. They must never contribute anything to their church or chapel, or give any help to a neighbour which costs them money. They cannot save, nor can they join a sick club or trade union, because they cannot pay the necessary subscriptions. The children must have no pocket money for dolls, marbles or sweets. The father must smoke no tobacco, and must drink no beer. The mother must never buy any pretty clothes for herself or for her children, the character of the family wardrobe, as for the family diet, being governed by the regulation, 'Nothing must be bought but that which is absolutely necessary for the maintenance of physical health, and what is bought must be of the plainest and most economical description.' Should a child fall ill, it must be attended by the parish doctor (ie Poor Law medical officer); should it die, it must be buried by the parish (ie a pauper's grave). Finally, the wage earner must never be absent from his work for a single day. If any of these conditions are broken, the extra expenditure involved is met, *and can only be met*, by limiting the diet; or, in other words, by sacrificing physical efficiency (ie going hungry). (Rowntree, 1941, p 103)

The diet selected for this family by Rowntree was "more economical and less attractive" than that given to paupers in workhouses. Rowntree and Booth both recognised that their definition of poverty was in reality incompatible with life without charity, theft or public assistance. 'Primary poverty' was a standard of bare subsistence rather than living: the wonder was that they thought it useful to employ. Even so, Rowntree found 10% of families in York to be in primary poverty, and 18% to be in 'secondary poverty', by which he meant that their total earnings would have been enough for 'bare subsistence' had they not used some of the income on wasteful expenditure such as the occasional pretty dress or pint of beer. Rowntree concluded from his own work and that of Booth that around 1900 between 25% and 30% of the town populations of the United

Kingdom were living at or below a level of bare existence (Rowntree, 1906, pp 300-1).

From birth rates to death rates by social class

This was the social broth in which Galton's eugenic hypothesis was cultured. Knowing the limited quality of the data at his disposal, Stevenson re-phrased the hypothesis: "Does the rate at which married men 'reproduce themselves' differ significantly according to their occupation?" Taking illegitimate births, the same question was asked of unmarried women. The Registrar General's office then added the all-important supplementary question, do *death* rates in infancy differ according to the parent's type of work?

Stevenson's occupational classification was designed to shape the Census data as best he could to conform to Booth's scheme as adopted by Galton. He faced many anomalies, one being the occasional inconsistency between status accorded to the post and financial situation of the post holder, as happened for example with commercial clerks. Largely out of a reflected glory from the status of the post in earlier years, male clerks were placed initially in Class I with doctors and lawyers. Clerks of the city were highly valued for the beautiful copperplate handwriting with which they compiled the ledgers. The elite of the profession were the corresponding clerks, often fluent in several languages and responsible for communication with clients overseas. Part of their status came from the need to mimic the appearance of their masters: black coated, white collared, and topped off with black hat. In 1874, however, Remington and Sons produced the first typewriters for sale, and by the 1890s most offices had a lady clerk at her machine. Yet old habits died hard, and many businesses retained a marked preference for handwritten correspondence prepared by their male clerks. In 1891 there were 71,000 clerks living in London, earning about 30s a week and with little or no capital. One contemporary observer described their status: "Though their pay is lower than that of the lowest class of artisans they are nevertheless expected to live well, to dress trimly, and generally to bear themselves as gentlemen" (Kynaston, 1995, p 32). Such errors of classification would lead to an under-estimate of the social class gradient in mortality. Clerks were relegated in future years to arrive finally among Class III: 'skilled workers'.

Stevenson demonstrated that around 1911, the year of the momentous Parliament Act (see Chapter Fourteen), there was an 'astonishing' contrast in death rates at nine to 12 months of age, almost three times higher in Class V than Class I. He regarded this excess as a measure of the unnecessary loss of life associated with poor conditions of living. Poor women had more babies than wealthy women, but they also lost more in infancy. Having demonstrated the utility of his approach, Stevenson then examined what it said about death rates in men by occupational class, a topic of much interest for public health then as it is now (Stevenson, 1923). All the evidence pointed to an excess mortality in Classes IV and V, but there was a need to quantify and monitor contrasts between classes, as pointed out by Professor Cunningham. Stevenson's findings open the next chapter.

Political medicine – the early years

In 1911, amelioration of the gaps in health and vitality between rich and poor appeared an eminently practical proposition for public health professionals. The major causes of death in the labouring classes were all amenable to preventive measures: tuberculosis, chronic bronchitis, pneumonia and rheumatic heart disease, for example. Politicians and economists were not nearly so sanguine: indeed, economists largely pulled out of the exercise and left the task to other professions. There were many in these years who were content to argue that economics must be technical and descriptive, without any philosophical or ethical dimensions (Geiger, 1933, p 487). Questions of economic welfare should be referred to another department. This desire on the part of some economists to withdraw into an ivory tower (with notable exceptions – Coats, 1990), where they could divorce their pursuit of economic ends from moral considerations, was, to say the least, unhelpful. In no small way the failure of Welfare Capitalism to close the gaps in health across the occupational groups (see below) can be laid at the door of that ivory tower of economics in the earlier years of the 20th century.

Though there have been the inevitable exceptions, in general medical men and women have a long tradition of criticising the teaching and conduct of economists and politicians when they consider these detrimental to the health of those in their care. In 1832, government appointed a Select Committee to consider the implications of Michael Sadler's Bill to limit the hours of child labour in mills to 10 per day from age nine years. Many prominent medical men were called as expert witnesses, including Sir Astley Cooper of St Thomas' and Guy's Hospitals. All challenged the ethics of the factory system and the utterances of economists such as Nassau Senior who claimed that employers made their profit only out of the last hour of child labour in the day. Child labour was economically valueless unless it was long and hard. J.R. Farre pulled no punches: "... the only safeguard to the State consists in opposing this principle of political economy ... whenever it trenches on vital economy ... (i)f it does (encroach on health and life span), it is guilty of homicide". Elsewhere he declared that medical men could "never assent to life being balanced against wealth" (Hamlin, 1995). Government sanctioned limitations on child labour in the Factory Act of 1833, but studiously not on grounds of child health. The Bill succeeded on the legal point that children below nine years were too young to enter freely into a contract of employment with the master.

Rudolf Virchow: pioneer in political medicine

Political medicine bases its opinions of political economy on the physical, mental and psychological health of the community served. Its practitioners would certainly claim as one of its father figures the great German medical pathologist, Rudolf Virchow. It was Virchow who declared that: "Medicine is a social science, and politics nothing else but medicine on a large scale" (Virchow, 1879, p 34). He it was also who put physicians on their mettle by declaring that they "are the natural attorneys of the poor, and the social problems should largely be solved by them" (Virchow, 1879, p 4). His grasp of the consequences of political organisation for health was what drove him to join the first revolt of the working class in Berlin in 1848.

Virchow was born to parents of very modest means in the Pomeranian city of Schivelbein in 1821. Like all Prussia, Pomerania was highly feudal at that time, ruled by the Hohenzollen family and subject to the militaristic and autocratic landholding class, the Junkers. Bad though the mortality was among the urban poor of Britain in those years, it was even worse in rural Prussia. As a young doctor attached to a military hospital in Berlin, Virchow was sent in 1847 to Upper Silesia by the Prussian Minister for Medical Affairs to investigate an epidemic of famine and typhus. The 19 days he spent there were to shape his thinking permanently. In 1901, the year before his death, he wrote: "In analysing the causes of the (Silesian) epidemic I became convinced that the worst were the consequences of social evils, and that these evils could be fought only by way of deep going social reforms ... I want once more to recall to memory that it is unavoidable to relate practical medicine and political legislation ..."

(Ackerknecht, 1981, p 31). His report was remarkable for recommending neither drugs nor diet, but education, prosperity and democratic freedom as the primary remedies. In calling for a strong focus on the relief of unemployment and a shift of taxes off the poor, Virchow was making a clear statement on the association of income and wealth with health and life expectancy. For him, mass diseases were sociological phenomena, and therefore medicine was unavoidably a social science. Doctors who concerned themselves with mass diseases and the health of the population had to be committed to political activity if they wished to make progress. Virchow lived in an age when many other doctors shared his views, in France, Britain and in Germany, but he is perhaps the best remembered.

Political medicine in America

Many American doctors subscribed not only to Virchow's views on the link between poverty and ill health but also to those of the economist Henry George (see Chapter Thirteen) on poverty and monopolisation of Rent. Hence for them the connection between the political economy of Rent and the prevalence of ill health was obvious. One such doctor was William Crawford Gorgas of Mobile, Alabama. Gorgas embarked upon a medical career in the army after graduation in 1879, finding himself Chief Sanitary Officer in Havana during the short period of US military rule over Cuba between 1898 and 1902. In those days yellow fever was a scourge throughout the Caribbean and Central America, and Gorgas' eradication of the disease in Havana received world-wide acclaim. About 1,000 miles to the south of Cuba lay Panama, where in 1889 yellow fever had been partially responsible for the collapse of Ferdinand de Lesseps' attempt to construct a canal across the isthmus between Balboa and Cristobal. In 1903 the US acquired a perpetual lease on the Canal Zone and moved in 6,000 American labourers to launch its own attempt to complete the canal. Gorgas accepted responsibility for the Canal Zone as he had in Havana, and with equal success.

The Panama Canal opened in 1914, and in March of that year Gorgas was promoted to Surgeon General of the US army. Six months later he was in Cincinnati to address a businessmen's club. He told his audience that should he once again go to a community such as Cuba or Panama, and he was allowed to choose one sanitary measure, he would select a rise in income of labouring families. Furthermore, he believed that the best way to achieve this end, and to promote the health of the public, was for governments to collect Rent. Gorgas said: "When the great valleys of the Amazon and of the Congo are occupied ... more food will be produced in these regions than is now produced in all the rest of the inhabited world. But unless we can so change our economic laws ... mankind will not be greatly benefited. I hope and believe that as this change in population comes about the (collection of Rent) will have caused such changes in our economic condition that wealth will be fairly distributed." His short speech was published with a Forward commending his views signed by 11 prominent medical men including the President of the American Medical Association, the President of the Alumni Association of the College of Physicians and Surgeons, New York, and the Shattuck Professor of Pathology at Harvard University (Gorgas, 1915).

'Causes' of death

Those following Virchow's quest for social and political 'risk factors' for illness and premature death know that all too often the completed death certificate is a 'sanitised' version of reality. The condition leading directly to the patient's death is what catches the eye, but it lies at the centre of a universe of causative factors. In addition to this condition there are frequently other forms of pathology which, though they did not kill the patient, nevertheless shortened life by reducing the patient's ability to cope with a major illness. Moving one step outwards into the causative universe the physician may find changes in body structure and function which played a role in the major or secondary disorders, such as a high blood cholesterol or a high blood sugar. Another step outwards and the doctor seeks causes in the patient's intimate environment: diet, smoking and drinking habits, personal hygiene and so on. This process of enquiry, looking more and more into 'deep space', can continue until, like Virchow, we enter the social realm where we discern associations between the patient's death and economic, cultural and political factors. Not surprisingly, we discover that this 'deep space' forms a common shell to the universe of many fatal diseases, each with its increasingly specific and characteristic inner shells. Socio-economic deprivation forms a nebulous part of the 'deep space' of causation of more than 60 common causes of death as stated on the death certificate.

Today, doctors have a vast array of diagnostic tools with which to classify diseases as required for certification. In fact, the method of classification and certification is the product of the use of these tools to study physical diseases. Pathology laboratories, biochemistry laboratories, radiology and nuclear medicine laboratories are routine supports to the diagnostic skills of physicians and surgeons. Their findings are used to enter on the certificate the underlying disease or injury which initiated the train of events leading directly to death. To study the 'deep space' of causation requires not the microscope, however, but the medical counterpart of the radio-telescope. This is largely uncharted territory in which what are being sought are nebulous entities rather than the discrete, solid 'planetary bodies' that are the patients and their pathologies. The demands of 'deep space' research are several. The first need is for researchers focused on their patients to 'look over their shoulder' and re-focus on what is out there. Secondly, having re-focused, a completely new set of tools for deep space research needs to be invented. Thirdly, researchers need approval to venture into this unknown. At which level of enquiry does medicine bring its quest for the understanding of disease, mental and physical, to a halt? The further into deep space the trail is followed, the more likely are politicians and economists to accuse doctors of 'losing their way'; 'veering off course'; 'going too far'; or 'getting in too deep'. Somewhere out there, nevertheless, are those forces which account for the links between socio-economic deprivation and so many fatal diseases. This is the stuff of political medicine.

In the days of the first attempts to categorise deaths according to the anatomical site of the disease or the immediately causative agent, such as 'smallpox' or 'drowning', physicians were still quite prepared to pursue their traditional practice of searching all avenues for the causes of the patient's illness. They were quite willing, for example, to regard 'privation' as a predisposing cause of the patient's poor condition, vague and 'unscientific' though this might have sounded. To note its relevance, even though the connection was poorly understood, was better than to ignore it altogether. In 1843 the medical journal *The Lancet* argued strongly that the confinement of the working class in closed apartments for long hours while they laboured lowered "the '*vis vitae*' and abridge(d) the term of man's existence" (*The Lancet*, 1843). Science has performed wonders for medicine since those days, but so all-pervasive and enduring are the effects of socio-economic deprivation that we are being forced increasingly to reconsider development of the old way of thinking about causes of ill health and death. This is not to say that our current conceptualisation of disease causation is unsound – only incomplete. Death is certainly due immediately to specific diseases but ultimately to a variety of causes which cumulatively and in combination interact to injure mind and body in many subtle and not-so-subtle ways, expressed eventually in terms of sub-health and clinical disorders of many types which are to varying degrees life-threatening. These causes tend to cluster within the domestic and working environments of poorer families.

Poor housing, a sub-standard diet, mental stresses, anxiety and depression, resort to cheap but damaging forms of relaxation as a substitute for genuinely healthy recreation and mental refreshment, exposure to pollutants, damp and cold, and occupational hazards were recognised as such causes in mid-Victorian Britain, but the more elusive causes have still to be deeply researched. One striking feature about the link between wealth and health was apparent right from the beginning, however, as mentioned earlier. Each increment in income and wealth 'buys' an increment in health. Families with semi-skilled breadwinners have better prospects for health than those with unskilled breadwinners. Similarly, skilled non-manual workers have always had a better outlook and lower premature death rate than skilled manual workers and their families. It is much more than simply 'rich' versus 'poor', as Stevenson's work was to show.

'Gone too soon': mortality and income in modern times

Medical instruction does not exist to provide individuals with an opportunity of learning how to earn a living, but in order to make possible the protection of the health of the public. (Rudulf Virchow, *Die Medizinische Reform*, 1848-49)

Working men and women tend to move up in occupational social class as they age, through promotion to jobs with better pay and, if fortunate, the purchase of property. This tendency would in itself lead to a higher death rate in social class I than lower classes, simply because the highest class would be the oldest on average. The Office for National Statistics (the descendent of the Registrar General's Office) overcomes this effect of age in the same way as did Stevenson, by calculating what is called the Standardised Mortality Ratio (SMR).

The numbers of adult males in any occupationally derived social class, and the numbers in that class belonging to each age group (15 to 24, 25 to 34 etc) are taken from the national Census. Death certificates state the last occupation of the deceased, and those issued on either side of the census are inspected to calculate the numbers of deaths by social class in the period of interest (eg 1970 to 1972). This is the *observed* number of deaths for that social class. What we now want is the number of deaths that would have been *expected* had this class experienced the same mortality rate as the general male population (the standard population). This expected number is calculated by multiplying the number of men in each age group of the class of interest by the death rate in that age group experienced by the general male population, and then summing the results across the age groups. The observed number of deaths, expressed as a percentage of the expected number, is the SMR for that class (obviously the term 'ratio' is an accepted misnomer for what is presented as a percentage). We are now in a position to compare mortality between the social classes. When the SMR is less than 100 then that class has a better

Table 2.1: Mortality experience in men of working age in England and Wales (1921-93)

	SMR by period						
Social class	1921 -23	1930 -33	1949 -53	1959 -63	1970 -72	1979 -83*	1991 -93
I	82	90	86	76	77	66	66
II	94	94	92	81	81	74	72
III⁺	95	97	101	100	99/106	93/103	100/117
IV	101	102	104	103	114	114	116
V	125	111	118	143	137	159	189
England and Wales	100	100	100	100	100	100	100

Notes:

* No data for 1981.

⁺ For 1970 onwards the SMRs are for skilled non-manual/skilled manual workers.

Source: Townsend et al (1992, p 59); Drever et al (1996). 1970-83, ages 15-64, otherwise 20-64.

survival than the standard population, and conversely when greater than 100 its survival is worse than the standard population.

Male mortality by occupationally derived social class since 1921

Stevenson's trial run around the 1911 Census produced unsatisfactory estimates of mortality by social class for reasons given in Chapter One. Revisions were therefore made to the national Census of 1921 to overcome much of the difficulty. Table 2.1, which refers to men of working age, therefore runs forward from 1921. In 1921-23, professional men experienced a death rate 18 percentage points below (better than) average, while unskilled workers had a death rate 25 points above the average. The gap between these groups was therefore 43 percentage points. Furthermore, each step up the occupational ladder was associated with a decrease in the probability of death in the years examined, a pattern which persisted across the 20th century. What surprises, however, is that in 1991-93 professional men experienced a mortality 34 points below the average, whereas men in unskilled work had a mortality 89 points above the average, a gap of 123 points. Thus, over 70 years the gap between the life expectancy of these groups has gradually widened in relative terms, particularly after 1950. In 1991-93 the death rate in unskilled men of working age was almost three times that in professional men. In 1921-23 the respective figure had been 1.5 times.

Sickness: cause or consequence of material deprivation?

Had we needed to read Table 2.1 from right to left in order to judge progress during the life of Britain's Welfare State we might have concluded that Welfare Capitalism was a distinct improvement on what had gone before. But Table 2.1 is read from left to right and the trend in SMRs is cold comfort for Britain's poor. So contrary is the pattern to what advocates of Welfare Capitalism find comprehensible that the figures have been subjected to detailed scrutiny. A major criticism has been that this series of cross-sectional analyses cannot exclude the possibility that the pattern is due to a tendency for those whose health fails prematurely to congregate in the lower occupational classes. It is not that low social status and low pay accelerate a decline in health, so the counter-argument ran, but rather that declining health impedes or reverses social advancement. The sick of the lower social classes are left behind as the healthier move up into the expanding service classes II and III. Furthermore, some of the unhealthy in higher classes are unable to sustain their position and fall in the social scale. In this way social class V acquires its high SMR (Townsend et al, 1992, p 105).

The crucial point at issue, however, is not whether it is *either* ill health that causes a fall in occupational class *or* lower occupational class that increases the risk to health. The two propositions are not mutually exclusive. Most can comprehend that ill health may reduce future occupational prospects, though nowadays this effect is much less than might be suspected. The question to be settled is whether poverty raises the chances of developing a life-threatening disease or sustaining a serious injury.

How reliable are the calculations?

The Registrar General cautioned about comparisons of cross-sectional data between the decades of the type depicted in Table 2.1. His office had to make adjustments to the occupational classification at each census, to take account of changes in the relative standing of certain occupations in the eyes of the community. Careful research has cleared alterations to classification of responsibility for the pattern in Table 2.1. Another concern related to the way occupation on the death certificate and occupation in the national census are reported by different people at different times, introducing an indeterminate amount of error. Relatives tend to elevate the prestigiousness of the deceased's occupation at death, or report a previously held occupation rather than the deceased's last full-time occupation when the former was of higher status. However, when occupations particularly prone to such effects were removed from the calculations in stages, the level of inequality by social class was amplified rather than reduced. The overall conclusion was that though class inequality in mortality had declined in the 1920s, by the 1970s it was greater than it had been in the early part of the century (Pamuk, 1985).

As the nation has moved from horsepower to nuclear power and from the ready reckoner to the computer, there has been a considerable growth of classes II, III and IV with the creation of service jobs, and, conversely, a diminishing demand for unskilled manual work. Whereas in 1911 80% of workers were in manual occupations, by 1981 the figure had fallen to about 50%. Differential rates of mobility from one class to another according to standard of health, coupled with changes in class size owing to growth of the service industries, may have contributed to contrasts in SMR by class. Only a longitudinal study in which healthy men's fortunes were tracked as they grew older could answer such criticisms.

The longitudinal study of all-cause mortality by occupational social class

Any lingering doubt about deprivation as a major cause of premature death was finally laid to rest by a study designed specifically to overcome criticisms levelled at Table 2.1. Working with the 1971 national Census, the Office for National Statistics (ONS) identified all persons born in England and Wales on four specific days in the year. At this census, people aged over 14 years had been asked whether they had had a job in the week beforehand and the nature of this employment. Those out of work for any reason, including retirement, were asked to state their last main occupation. The 6% of the population who were permanently sick or otherwise economically inactive were classified as unoccupied. This initial sample has since been updated periodically by inclusion of samples of the new-born and immigrants and exclusion of the deceased and emigrants. The study is therefore tracking anonymously the vital status of a 1% sample of the population, about 550,000 people who were clinically free of life-threatening illness at recruitment. Routine data on deaths taken anonymously from the National Health Service Central Register

Table 2.2: The ONS Longitudinal Study

Social class in 1971	SMR by period: men aged 15-64 at death			
	1976-81	1982-85	1986-89	1976-89
I	69	61	67	66
II	78	78	80	79
IIIN	103	98	85	97
IIIM	95	101	102	99
IV	109	113	112	111
V	124	136	153	134
Unoccupied	212	165	137	182
England and Wales	100	100	100	100

are linked to the longitudinal study to obtain SMRs in sequential years during follow-up. The findings summarised in Table 2.2 confirm the gradient between occupational class in 1971 and subsequent mortality in men initially in good health. They also attest to the increase in the gap between classes I and V over the period of follow-up (Harding, 1995). The SMR for the unoccupied was very high in 1976-81 because many of the permanently sick died over the first few years. British national mortality statistics and the ONS Longitudinal Study confirm the same socio-occupational contrasts in childhood (Botting, 1997), women (Harding et al, 1997), and in those of pensionable age (Hattersley, 1997).

Material possessions and premature mortality

John Kenneth Galbraith remarked: "Nothing, it must be recognised, so comprehensively denies the liberties of the individual as a total absence of money; or so impairs it as too little" (Galbraith, 1996, p 4). If access to an income is what we are mainly talking about when we refer to social class, then we are using a very rough-and-ready measure. Within each social class there is a wide range of incomes, and the ranges of adjacent classes overlap considerably. The Longitudinal Study therefore looked at not only the effect of social class on death rates, but also other indicators of financial standing including ownership of a house and a car. Social class, home-ownership and car-ownership each had something separate to say about risk of death, so that those at most risk were more clearly distinguished from those at least risk when all three characteristics were taken into account. Within each social class, possession of a car or

Table 2.3: Cause-specific SMR by occupational social class for men aged 20-64 years (1991-93)

	Social class[+]					
	I	II	IIIN	IIIM	IV	V
Stroke	70	67	96	118	125	219
Coronary heart disease	63	73	107	125	121	182
Lung cancer	45	61	87	138	132	206
Skin cancer*	136	106	106	107	91	100
Accidents	54	57	74	107	106	226
Suicide	55	63	87	96	107	225

* Malignant melanoma.

[+] I professional; II managerial/technical; IIIN skilled non-manual; IIIM skilled manual; IV partly skilled; V unskilled.

ownership of the home is associated with a longer life span (Fox and Goldblatt, 1982; Davey Smith et al, 1990; Wannamethee and Shaper, 1997).

Cause-specific mortality by occupationally derived social class

There is not one particular 'disease' responsible for these gaps in mortality between social classes. All of the major conditions listed in the International Classification of Diseases show a clear gradient with social class (Drever et al, 1997). In its declared strategy for *The Health of the Nation* (Department of Health, 1992), the Conservative government identified stroke, coronary heart disease (heart attack), lung cancer, skin cancer, accidents and suicides as priority areas. The SMRs for these causes by social class for England and Wales in 1991–93 are presented in Table 2.3. For all but skin cancer the SMRs in partly skilled men (IV) were two to three times those in professionals (I); in unskilled workers (V) three to four times those of professionals. Skin cancer or malignant melanoma, due to excessive exposure to sunlight, was the exception that proved the rule. Professionals had a higher SMR than other groups, although the absolute impact on class differences was small because this cancer caused fewer than 1,000 deaths each year in England and Wales in the 20-64 year age group.

The Longitudinal Study also provided the ability to test whether among men in employment both in 1971 and 1981, who changed occupational class in that time, mortality between 1981 and 1985 was related to the direction of change. The question was: 'Were men who "moved down" in poorer health as a group than those who "moved up"?' Those who crossed class boundaries in either direction had SMRs similarly intermediate to the classes of origin and destination. Thus while mortality of class-mobile men appeared to have been influenced both by where they came from and where they went to, there was no evidence to suggest that those who had 'moved down' were sicker than those who had 'moved up' (Goldblatt, 1989).

Further evidence on relative deprivation and health status has been provided by the Whitehall study of civil servants. Those who took part in this prospective study were carefully screened and given a clean bill of health at the start. Over the following 25 years death rates in this initially healthy population were much higher in the lower grades than in the higher grades of the service (van Rossum et al, 2000). Manual workers had higher death rates from every major cause of death than men in the top administrative grades, even for heart attack. The evidence is now irrefutable that relative deprivation leads to sub-health, illness and premature death. This is why the injustice in the mistreatment of Rent can no longer be ignored.

There is reason to believe that the SMR is not the best measure of social class contrasts in mortality, because it treats all deaths as if they are of equal significance, irrespective of the age of occurrence. Most, however, would accept that death is especially tragic in the young, a fact which can be captured by estimating the years of potential life lost. We cannot know the age to which an adult would have survived had not death intervened before retirement age. But we can calculate the years of *working* life lost, taking retirement age in men as 65 years and focusing only on deaths before this age. When this was done for men in England and Wales, the ratio of potential life lost in social class V relative to social class I was 2.1/1 in 1970-72, rising to 3.3/1 in 1991-93. The respective ratios when the SMR was used were smaller at 1.8/1 in 1970-72, and 2.9/1 in 1991-93 (Blane and Drever, 1988). The conclusion has to be that if we could devise a measure indicative of what matters most about social and economic stratification for health, and then relate it to an index which best captures social contrasts in health, the importance of relative deprivation for health would be more fully exposed.

A watershed for political medicine

Finally conceding the fundamental importance of social and occupational contrasts in death rates, the Conservative government set up a Working Party during the early 1990s to see what the Department of Health and the National Health Service could do about them. In 1995 Stephen Dorrell, the Secretary for Health, acknowledged the truth in a summary of the findings (Mihill, 1995):

1. Within the UK there are marked differences in death rates by occupational class, by sex, by region, and by ethnicity. These differences affect not only life expectancy but also healthy life expectancy. What the figures meant was that the life expectancy of the new-born child was seven years more when the father happened to belong to social class I than when he fell into social class V. Children of social class V were four times more likely to suffer death from accident in the home or on the road than the children of social class I.
2. Of 66 major causes of death in men, 62 were more common in social classes IV and V combined than in class I. Of 70 major causes of death in women, 64 were more common in women married to men in social classes IV and V than in those married in social class I.
3. Contrasts between classes in dietary, smoking or drinking habits could explain no more than one third of the observed difference in coronary heart disease death rates.

Stephen Dorrell stressed that "overall, health is improving in all regions of the country and across all social groups". So it is, and unless the nation's economy, science and technology went into a severe reverse it is difficult to see how over the long term this could be otherwise. Mr Dorrell's remark sidestepped the central message of the SMRs, which is that average figures for the population can conceal a plethora of unpalatable facts. The report stressed: "An important way of achieving *The Health of the Nation* targets is to improve the health of the least healthy groups, (bringing it) closer to the levels attained by the most healthy groups". Two comments are called for in response. First, narrowing this most fundamental of gaps has *always* been a major aim of public health and the Welfare State. Secondly, the Welfare State can improve the nation's health not only by narrowing the gaps but also, at least in theory, by assisting families to move up into a healthier social class with a lower SMR. This latter point is discussed in detail in Chapter Five.

Alternative classifications of occupation and cause-specific mortality

As in Edwardian times, social empathy, which is the power and willingness to identify with others, continues to rest on displays of material resources, lifestyle and manners. So the Cambridge scale, devised by sociologists, classifies occupations according to the material resources, lifestyles and social advantages that they carry with them or foster (Prandy, 1990). When, in *The Health and Lifestyles Survey* (Cox et al, 1993) of British men and women, individuals were categorised by occupation according to both the Registrar General's and the Cambridge methods, death rates from coronary heart disease were related even more powerfully to the latter than the former scale (Chandola, 1998). The high rates of death in the least advantaged groups on the Cambridge scale were hardly affected by allowance for group differences in age, smoking habit, alcohol intake, levels of exercise and diet. Thus occupationally attached social advantages are major determinants of risk of death from coronary heart disease.

Party political affiliation, Rent and death rates

The government has detailed statistics on home-ownership and car-ownership by family, and researchers continue to show how these indices of income and wealth are related to mortality in the same manner as occupational class (Smith and Harding, 1997). By contrast, the government collects no data on income specifically as Rent, so relations between health and possession of Rent cannot be tested directly. However, those with Rent tend to vote for the party of the property-owning classes, while those without Rent tend not to vote in this way, if they vote at all. One study examined the associations between voting patterns, indices of social deprivation and mortality by electoral constituency in England and Wales, using data for the general elections of 1983, 1987 and 1992 (Davey Smith and Dorling, 1996). There were strikingly powerful associations between the SMR for a constituency and its percentage of Conservative voters (an inverse association – the more Conservatives, the lower the mortality) and Labour voters (a direct association). So strong were these associations that the correlation coefficients are presented in Table 2.4 (0 represents no association; +1.0 or −1.0 indicates a perfect relation).

Professor Peter Townsend devised a score based on car-ownership, unemployment rate, overcrowded housing and housing tenure to reflect

Table 2.4: Correlations between the strength of political party support and SMR by constituency in England and Wales

Election	Men	Women	Overall
		Correlation coefficient[+]	
1983			
Conservative	−0.81	−0.65	−0.76
Labour	0.79	0.67	0.76
Liberal*	−0.52	−0.42	−0.49
1987			
Conservative	−0.80	−0.64	−0.75
Labour	0.80	0.68	0.77
Liberal*	−0.54	−0.45	−0.52
1992			
Conservative	−0.79	−0.61	−0.74
Labour	0.75	0.63	0.73
Liberal*	−0.53	−0.42	−0.50

Notes:

[+] All statistically significant at $p<0.0001$.

*Liberal Party, Social Democratic Party, the Alliance and Liberal Democratic votes combined.

the level of material wealth. The score given to a constituency was strongly associated with its voting pattern, in the expected way. Nevertheless, when the score was taken into account, voting pattern remained independently associated with the SMR for the constituency. In other words, there was more to Conservative voters as a group that was protective for health than was captured by the number of cars they possessed, or by whether they were in work, or by whether they owned their home. This is not surprising, for there is unlikely to be any stronger link with allegiance to the Conservative Party than the privilege of Rentholding through land-ownership and the receipt of dividends. After taking account of social class and car-ownership, owner occupation remains uniformly associated with a lower SMR in men and women of working age (Smith and Harding, 1997). In an examination of equity in housing and life expectancy in the early 1990s, a fall in equity from £15,000 to £5,000 was associated with a loss of 100 days of life (*The Daily Telegraph*, 5 January, 1996). What we want to know, however, is the loss of life associated with no equity in housing at all.

Britain's Welfare State struggles to overcome the very same preternatural forces that energise party politics. We can liken its institutions to a fleet on its perpetual voyage of relief, tacking valiantly against the shifting winds that blow from Westminster, sometimes this way, sometimes that, its admiral constantly amazed at the ever growing need for more canvas and tonnage. Not so long ago the rough sleeper was a rare sight in Britain. Nowadays, on any one night there are up to 2,000 without a roof in England and Wales, 600 of them in Central London. Exceptionally vulnerable long before they come to the attention of the charities and government's Rough Sleepers Unit, pneumonia, drug poisoning and suicide claim the life of one of these 600 every five days. The life expectancy of the rough sleeper is no better than that of England's rural population of 1840, about 42 years (*The Lancet*, 1843, p 661). In Bangladesh today, average life expectancy is 58 years (World Health Organization, 1996). Small wonder at the uproar in late 1999 when Louise Casey, head of the Rough Sleepers Unit, chastised the charities for increasing the comforts of the streets by distributing sleeping bags and mugs of soup (*The Observer*, 14 November, 1999), thereby thwarting, she believed, her efforts to clear the cities of the homeless without shelter.

Deprivation of income and poor health – a world-wide phenomenon

Social inequities in health, lifespan, Rent and wealth exist wherever the economic treatment of Land, Capital and Labour is similar to that in England and Wales. The Scottish Office noted: "Throughout the western developed world (and even more acutely in the Third World) health varies according to socio-economic standing and wealth. Scotland is no exception" (Scottish Office 1992). In one study, even when allowing for social class differences in age, smoking habit, body fatness, blood cholesterol, blood pressure and other relevant characteristics, Scottish men and women in the manual occupational classes were more than twice as likely to have coronary heart disease than those in non-manual occupations (Woodward et al, 1990). Scotland has a problem with AIDS and HIV, where between a third to one half of cases arise from sharing needles for injection of drugs (McKeganey, 1994). Drug abusers are predominantly the young of socially and economically impoverished families, living mostly in inner-city housing estates with high rates of unemployment. One study found that only 4% of victims had a regular source of income. This problem is not Scotland's alone. Both HIV and AIDS are likely to become increasingly concentrated among the disadvantaged around the world (Mann et al, 1993).

On the European continent, contrasts in death rates between the social classes are found wherever they are sought. Generally the overall premature mortality in the manual classes is 30 to 40% above that in the non-manual classes. However, the mix of diseases contributing to the higher death rates in the families of manual workers differs from one population to the next. For example, accidents and violent deaths account for only 10% of the manual excess mortality in Italy, but 33% in Portugal. Most probably these findings reflect national differences in contrasts between the classes in the mix of potentially harmful environmental and cultural factors. Alcohol would not be expected to be a major cause of disease in the poor, relative to the rich, in a country where it is very costly and access to bootleg liquor is difficult. Where alcohol is cheap and plentiful, however, its associated diseases, accidents and injuries may then make a major contribution to class contrasts in health and life expectancy. Throughout Europe the under-privileged appear to be more exposed than the over-privileged to factors which damage health, though what those factors might be, their relative importance, and the way the several sectors in society cope with them are clearly far from uniform (Kunst et al, 1998).

The same 'health and wealth' phenomenon is well recognised in the US. Working with a national sample of adults aged 25 years to 74 years, the Centers for Disease Control and Prevention in Atlanta estimated the proportion of deaths associated with poverty between 1973 and 1991. Poverty was defined in terms of monetary income and family size. In 1973 there were approaching 87,000 deaths in the US associated with living below the poverty line (74 per 100,000 of the population). In 1991 the figure had risen to 91,000 deaths (82 per 100,000 of the population). These figures mean that about 6% of all adult deaths in the US are attributable to impoverishment (Hahn et al, 1995).

Another American study (Lynch et al, 1997) collected information on incomes in 1965, 1974 and 1983 for adults in Alameda County, California. The purpose was to examine the cumulative effects of economic hardship on those alive in 1994, by which time the median age of the 1,100 participants still available was 65 years. The more the occasions when income had fallen to below 200% of the official federal level of poverty, the greater was the decline in physical, cognitive, psychological and social functioning. The investigators found little evidence for episodes of illness as a cause of economic hardship. The harder had life been economically, the less equipped was the subject to deal with the adversities of old age.

In the developing world, where socio-economic contrasts often exceed those in the developed nations, gaps in health and life expectancy between classes can be particularly marked. In Sao Paulo State, Brazil, for example, the standardised mortality for professionals and business managers was found to be 38% below the population average, while for unskilled manual workers it was 130% above the average. In England and Wales in 1981, about 40% of deaths of men of working age occurred in the lowest 30% of the population ranked by social class; in Sao Paulo more like 50% of deaths occurred in the bottom 30% (Duncan et al, 1995).

But one need not travel to the developing world to find such stark contrasts. In New York's Central Harlem, where almost all citizens are black and 41% were living below the government's poverty line in 1980, death rates for women aged 25 to 34 years were more than six times those of American white women of that age. Similar findings applied for men aged 35 to 44 years. Like London's homeless, a man aged 40 years in Harlem has a poorer chance of survival than a man of the same age in Bangladesh (McCord and Freeman, 1990). In terms of poverty and ill health, Harlem and similar pockets of deprivation blight America's cities. The way in which social deprivation and human humiliation of the magnitude experienced in the South Bronx and Harlem brush against the skirts of affluent Manhattan is a deeply troubling testimony to political and social shortcomings in one of the wealthiest cities in the world. In few places would political medicine condemn political economy so thoroughly for its discordance with political morality. Here the power of Rent and the consequences of its privatisation are on full display for all who travel along say, Fifth Avenue, between Central Park South and Martin Luther King Boulevard.

Life expectancy in the OECD: the distribution of wealth is more important than the average

Among developed nations there is at best only a weak relation between gross national product and the population's average life expectancy (Maxwell, 1981). This lack of association has been confirmed in an analysis of gross domestic product per capita (adjusted to standardise for the purchasing power of the currencies) and life expectancy in the 23 members of the Organisation of Economic Co-operation and Development (OECD), which includes Australia, Canada, the Netherlands, the UK and the US. National average life expectancy in these affluent populations had little connection with national average income and purchasing power, though *within* these countries individual or class life expectancy was clearly associated with class income relative to the national average (Wilkinson, 1992).

In the US, the degree of income inequality and mortality have been examined within each state. The greater the income inequality, the greater the death rate and the less the average life expectancy. In New York State, for example, where the less well off half of the population received about 18% of all household income, the age-adjusted death rate for the entire community was about 86 per 10,000. In Wyoming, the respective figures were almost 22% of total household income and approximately 80 per 10,000. This relation was unaffected by the state's median income level. The conclusions were: "Variations between states in the inequality of the distribution of income are significantly associated with variations between states in a large number of health outcomes and social indicators and with mortality trends. These differences parallel relative investments in human and social capital. Economic policies that influence income and wealth inequality may have an important impact on the health of countries" (Kaplan et al, 1996).

Another American study published in 1996 concluded: "Variations between states in inequality of income were associated with increased mortality from several causes. The size of the gap between the wealthy and less well off – as distinct from the absolute standard of living enjoyed by the poor – seems to matter (for the mortality rate in the state) in its own right. The findings suggest that policies that deal with the growing inequities in income distribution may have an important impact on the health of the population" (Kennedy et al, 1996). The message coming through is that societies which tolerate a wide distribution of what wealth and income they create do themselves more harm than those that ensure less inequality. Nations that minimise such inequalities in future by ensuring that Rent is used for public purposes rather than private gain will therefore be doing themselves a great favour if, as professed in England, the health of the nation is of primary concern. Societies which tolerate large gaps in income between richer and poorer suffer self-inflicted sub-optimal health (Wilkinson, 1996).

In summary, where there is income inequality there is inequality in health such that the poorer have the weaker life chances. It follows that a political economy which acquiesces in an inequitable distribution of income and wealth owing to its treatment of Rent is culpable of inflicting an unjustifiable loss of life on those classes that suffer this inequity. But privatisation of Rent does not only create under-privilege and deprivation directly. By encouraging speculation in the land market and by forcing governments to tax wages and interest, the privatisation of Rent creates unemployment, as described in Chapter Three.

THREE

Rent and the dysfunctional economy

In a world in which material and social circumstances are such powerful determinants of health and lifespan, it behoves us to ensure that the political economy we accept generates wealth efficiently and distributes this wealth in a manner consistent with fairness and the common good. For if the political economy countenances otherwise, to accommodate privilege, then it stands accused of placing the lives of the disadvantaged at unnecessary risk. People who suffer poverty and inequity will lose years of life, not through any fault of their own, but because of the nature of the society into which they were born.

To search for serious inefficiencies and inequities in the economic system, this chapter reviews the fundamentals of income, its distribution in Capitalist societies, and what happens to this distribution when Capitalism becomes Welfare Capitalism as currently structured. In the search for inequities, a major source is soon revealed in the treatment of Rent. In the search for inefficiency the damaging effects of taxation are exposed. The distribution of income is revealed to be grossly inequitable and Welfare Capitalism a poor defence for the health of those who are disadvantaged.

The nature of Rent

There are many causes of impoverishment, unemployment and premature death, but to resolve those that governments have sought to solve, and which have their basis in the political economy and the law, there is a pressing need to understand Rent. What follows is not simply a recantation of elementary economics, but a framework which needs to be grasped by any ordinary citizen who has a genuine concern for the health of society and the standards of political economy.

Land, labour, capital and wealth – everyday and economic distinctions

The ordinary meanings of land, labour, capital, wealth, wages, interest and rent are inadequate for our purposes, being either too narrow or vague. In order to make headway and understand these clearly, the terms must be defined more satisfactorily than in the dictionary.

Inevitably, in acquisitive societies wealth is synonymous with riches, but here Wealth has a rather different and highly specific meaning. Wealth consists of all materials provided by nature which have been modified by exertion and ingenuity so as to satisfy human needs and desires. In this sense even a stick sharpened to form a primitive tool is a form of Wealth. Three primary and mutually exclusive ingredients go into the economic mix that produces Wealth: namely Land, Labour and Capital. These three factors, put together in a seemingly infinite variety of ways, produce innumerable finished products and services for the benefit of mankind.

By land we generally mean a stretch of ground or countryside, as opposed to the atmosphere and seas. In the present context, however, Land is not merely our farms, parks, moors and woodlands. Its forms are not even exhausted when we include our housing estates, industrial estates, landed estates, docklands and city centres. Land in the sense used here encompasses all opportunities, forces and materials provided by nature, whether under, on or above the surface. It therefore *includes* the seas and atmosphere (even the jet lanes at 33,000 feet). Note well, however, that this is not the legal definition of land (discussed in Part II). Labour includes all human physical and mental exertion devoted to the productive processes in the economy.

The process of production is nowadays subdivided into so many separate occupations that, though each represents a distinct step on the road to the finished products, or in the facilitation of this process, the great majority of adults have lost all sense of the 'application' of Labour to Land in the economy. Yet this application is as much there now as ever (otherwise nothing would be created and mankind would not survive). By this application the nation's Wealth is produced, some for consumption, some for recreation and pleasure, and some to further the generation of Wealth. It is the last that is the nation's Capital. Very importantly, all *improvements* to land in the furtherance of productivity are species of Capital. Although part of commercial real estate, they are not Land in the economic sense.

Landholders, labourers and capitalists

Wealth produced is shared as income going to the three productive factors. Labour takes Wages and Capital takes Interest, while Rent becomes identified with Land. Thus as used here, Wages are far more than the daily or weekly payments made by employers to employees for service; Interest is not money paid for money lent; Rent is not synonymous with money paid to landlords by tenants. Rather, they are more abstract forms of income as defined, mutually exclusive and together account for all Wealth created. This much was understood by the classical economists of the late 18th century and 19th centuries. They saw of course that one and the same person could earn income as labourer, capitalist and landholder, but the fact was that some had inherited the privileges of landholding and others had accumulated great wealth in personal capital, while the majority depended entirely on what income they could get for their labour. Furthermore, capitalists and landholders were those to whom the great majority were forced to look for the opportunity to work; for Labour cannot produce without making application to Land assisted by Capital. This economic dependency of labourers placed considerable social and economic power in the hands of landholders and capitalists, even though they had not been democratically elected to such a position by ordinary labouring families.

Despite its vast powerhouses of industry, technology and finance, Britain's economy remains utterly dependent for its creation of Wealth on the cooperative application of Labour and Capital to Land. We are not describing the rustic economy of yesteryear. What follows is even more relevant for the future of Welfare Capitalism and our big cities than it ever was for the rural village of the 19th century.

The creation of Rent

Of the three forms of income going to the factors of production, Rent is by far the most neglected and yet the most intriguing, intellectually challenging and elusive. The very obscurity of Rent represents a profound but unappreciated source of power in the hands of its holders. Rent is the quintessential ingredient of Britain's political economy, ancient and modern. First described by Dr James Anderson of Edinburgh in 1777, it was the highly polished presentation of the concept by David Ricardo through which Rent came to be more generally understood. In his *Principles of political economy and taxation*, published in 1817, Ricardo struggled to convey the essential properties of Rent without resort to mathematical formulae or economic jargon. He wanted to set down his opinions on "the principles of Rent, Profit and Wages", especially when they "differ(ed) from the great authority of Adam Smith, Malthus etc" (Sraffa and Dobb, 1951, p xiii).

In order to explain Rent and its significance for modern Welfare Capitalism, we need to set up a simple model. We have our three mutually exclusive factors of production, Land, Labour and Capital, the output of Wealth, and the distribution of this Wealth in Rent, Wages and Interest. We need to fix the productive properties of our units of Labour and Capital while allowing the productivity of Land for modern economic activities to differ between sites. Let us speak of orders of Land, from prime sites down to seventh quality sites (and below). Let us also hypothesise that we have identical workers each with identical resources of Capital. Being identical, all units of Labour command an identical Wage in the common Labour market in which they operate, and all units of Capital command an identical return as Interest in their own market. We are now ready to begin working Land, and naturally we gravitate towards prime sites.

On each prime site, our 'standard' Labour with 'standard' Capital produces a standard number of units. It does not matter what these units are in our hypothetical model, except that they command a price in the market, which goes to pay Wages and Interest. To keep the model simple, let Labour take a fixed amount, just enough for subsistence in a modern economy (it does not matter what this actually amounts to for present purposes). After taking subsistence Wages, the nett productivity goes therefore as Interest to Capital; let us say this Interest is 10 units. So we have:

Site	Interest	Nett productivity*
Prime quality	10	10

* Subsistence wages have been taken from the gross product.

If our standard worker is, say, a homesteader, producing with his own Labour and Capital on the prime site he occupies, it would not matter whether he chooses to credit this nett product of 10 units as an addition to his subsistence Wages, or to Interest on his Capital, or even to Rent for the Land which he pays to himself: whichever way, the worker is 10 units better off. This is not the position in which most of us find ourselves today, however.

Over time our standard workers increase in number and their Capital grows commensurately. Prime sites are eventually completely occupied, so newcomers have to avail themselves of sites of second quality. On these sites our standard Labour with standard Capital can produce only nine units nett after subsistence Wages have been taken, and these nine units go as Interest. Because second order sites produce one unit less than prime units, the cost of production per unit, counted in terms of Labour and Capital inputs, is slightly higher than on prime sites. However, in a freely competitive market under stable conditions, the Wages going to a standard input of Labour, the Interest going to a standard unit of Capital, and the price obtained for a standard unit produced, are constant in their respective markets, whatever site they are applied to or produced on. Thus our standard Labour takes the same subsistence Wage on both sites and the standard Capital must take nine units nett both on prime sites and second order sites. *This leaves one unit of production unspoken for on each prime site, a 'surplus' or economic bonus called economic rent, hereafter termed more simply Rent.* So now we have:

Site	A Rent	B Interest	C Nett productivity
Prime quality	1	9	10
Second quality	0	9	9

Our population of workers thrives, multiplies and continues to accumulate Capital. The time comes when new arrivals must open up third quality sites to productivity, on which the nett Interest (on the standard subsistence Wage) is only eight units. By the same principle, Interest going to standard Capital on second quality and prime sites is now reduced to eight units in the Capital market. Hence Rent on prime order sites rises to two units of production, and on second quality sites to one unit:

Site	A Rent	B Interest	C Nett productivity
Prime quality	2	8	10
Second quality	1	8	9
Third quality	0	8	8

We need not follow this process as fourth and inferior quality sites are brought into the economy. Suffice to say that there comes a point when the price of units produced on inferior sites, and which therefore

Table 3.1: Rent, Interest and nett productivity: the basic model

Site	A Rent	B Interest	C Nett productivity
Prime quality	6	4	10
Second quality	5	4	9
Third quality	4	4	8
Fourth quality	3	4	7
Fifth quality	2	4	6
Sixth quality	1	4	5
Seventh quality	0	4	4
Totals	21	28	49 units

determines the price of units produced on all sites, matches the demand in the market. Consumers will pay no more. Let us say this point is reached on sites of seventh quality which produce four units nett. The units are too expensive in terms of inputs of Labour and Capital when less than four are produced by our standard Labour with its standard Capital. Units would then be left on the shelves until by some means demand was raised or supply fell back. So we have a distribution of income as shown in Table 3.1, remembering that Labour is taking a subsistence Wage out of gross productivity.

Our standard workers, with their standard units of Capital and their standard inputs of Labour, have produced 49 units nett. On account of the way the market operates, however, only 28 units have gone to Interest while 21 have gone to Rent under the conditions of our model. Note also how the proportion of nett productivity going to Rent rises as the economy grows. When the economy had brought in only prime and second quality sites, this proportion was 1/19, or about 5%. By the time seventh quality land is taken completely into production, the proportion going as Rent has increased to 21/49, or 43%. Columns A and B in Table 3.1 show just how differently Rent and Interest behave in a free market economy.

Rent, the economic margin and prices

Table 3.1 also shows that the proportion of nett productivity going to Interest is determined by the number of units produced on sites at the margin of the economy, on which no surplus is generated as Rent. The price of units is therefore determined by the amount of Labour and Capital needed to produce those at the margin (in our example, the four units on seventh quality sites). No Rent is created at this level, so Rent can never feature in the price of commodities, no matter what the quality of the site on which they are produced.

Rent and urbanisation

Economic growth is not simply a sprawl from prime sites outwards, as the presentation of our model might suggest. Growth also occurs by raising the density of economic activity on sites already in production, as in our towns and cities. In other words, having taken development to the extensive (horizontal) margin, we can now take it to its intensive margin. This is where the 'law of diminishing returns' enters into our model. It was David Ricardo's friend and intellectual adversary, Thomas Malthus, who developed the concept (first propounded by Anne Robert Jacques Turgot) that Labour and Capital could not be laid out in increasing amount "without diminishing return" (Malthus, 1821, p 137n). Let a second standard labourer with his standard Capital move on to a prime site. The mere presence of a productive worker already on site means that for the second worker the site cannot have a productivity identical to that for one standard labourer plus Capital. Let us say that for the second input of Labour and Capital the prime site behaves as a second quality site, generating for this additional input only nine units nett. Still, the same economic forces apply. The second worker's Capital receives four units in its market, leaving five units to take total Rent on the prime site to 11 units. All prime sites are eventually occupied by second workers, so newcomers move on to second quality sites where their Labour generates eight units after subsistence wages. This process continues until all sites capable of bearing two standard labourers with their standard Capital are so occupied (Table 3.2). For second workers, sites of sixth quality are marginal, rather than seventh quality sites. Thirteen workers produce 88 units of productivity nett, 36 units going to Rent and 52 units to Interest.

One can imagine this process of additional workers continuing until we have the maximum number on the seven types of site, each producing four units of Interest. Table 3.3 shows that at 'saturation' there are 28 standard workers with their standard Capital producing 168 units nett of subsistence, 56 (33.3%) of these units going to Rent and 112 (66.6%) going to Interest. This is how Rent grows with urbanisation.

Table 3.2: Rent, Interest and nett productivity: two standard workers with standard Capital per site

Site	A Rent	B Interest	C Nett productivity
Prime quality	6 + 5	4 + 4	10 + 9
Second quality	5 + 4	4 + 4	9 + 8
Third quality	4 + 3	4 + 4	8 + 7
Fourth quality	3 + 2	4 + 4	7 + 6
Fifth quality	2 + 1	4 + 4	6 + 5
Sixth quality	1 + 0	4 + 4	5 + 4
Seventh quality	0	4	4
Totals	21 + 15	28 + 24	49 + 39 units

Table 3.3: Economic activity taken to the extensive and intensive margins of economic productivity

Site	A Rent	B Interest	C Nett productivity	D Workers on site
Prime quality	21	28	49	7
Second quality	15	24	39	6
Third quality	10	20	30	5
Fourth quality	6	16	22	4
Fifth quality	3	12	15	3
Sixth quality	1	8	9	2
Seventh quality	0	4	4	1
Totals	56	112	168	28

Rent – communal or privatised?

What society does with Rent is its responsibility. In considering its decision, however, a crucial point to appreciate is that Rent arises not because of any superior talents or qualities of Labour and Capital applied to Land, but because of the application of Labour and Capital to sites of variable quality. Growth in population and Capital, combined with the demand of the market, enables society to bring sites of poorer productivity into the economy. Rent on better sites is the indirect product of economic activity on poorer sites, and labourers applying standard inputs of Labour and Capital to prime sites have no greater entitlement to the Rent of those sites than workers applying identical inputs to marginal Land. Should identical workers exchange places, then self-evidently Rent and the economy would be undisturbed.

Society would be right to conclude that Rent belongs to no one in particular; rather it conforms naturally to a communal income. Governments, at least in theory, having equal regard for all citizens, Rent becomes the obvious source of public revenue. Unless, however, the State is careful to secure the national Rent for social purposes, a most dismal alternative emerges all too easily, the result of opportunism. Rent neglected by the State falls prey to the holders of Land who claim it for themselves, either merging it with Interest and Wages into the commercial rent they charge their tenants, or 'paying' it to themselves as an imputed income when they occupy the site, or including its total value over 15 to 20 years in the sale price (the origin of this practice is discussed in Chapter Seven). Those seizing Rent enrich themselves with an unearned form of income at the expense of those with no access to Rent. Even worse, they deprive the dependants of the producers: the old, the infirm, the young, the pregnant mother and others who, because of their constitution, fall outside the productive economy, and are of no value in the Labour market.

When this morally inferior alternative becomes sanctioned by custom and law, society has created a gross inequity in the distribution of its income and Wealth. Two great and unnatural classes emerge: the over-privileged and the under-privileged. The social consequences are unnatural, especially the gap between the two classes in their life expectancy. This form of political economy in which Rent is in the exclusive possession of a private monopoly in Land is the system into which Ricardo was born, in which he operated, and which he described so well (monopoly in land arises because each site is unique and non-reproducible). It is the one that remains in England and all other national economies of similar form, the growth of Capitalism, the partial dissolution of the landed aristocracy and the emergence of the urbanised middle classes notwithstanding.

Rent in profits and dividends

When productive Land is scarce relative to Labour and Capital, and landholders, whether large or small, have title to Rent of the sites they possess, inequity reigns. There are, however, some other points of interest to note at this stage. First, the landholder, though taking the surplus income, has no economic power to determine the Rent, which is a by-product of the state of the productive sector of the economy. Nevertheless in real life the private landholder has the political power to speculate in Rent, trying to obtain more than the state of the economy justifies. Secondly, Rent-takers do not necessarily declare themselves or even know themselves to be Rentholders. In today's complex industrial economy many investors have no appreciation of the extent to which they derive unearned income from Rent. Much of what is called 'interest', profit or dividend is a variable mixture of true Interest and Rent, though in business economics the distinction is held not to matter. For a government seeking to advance from pure Capitalism to Welfare Capitalism, however, the distinction is crucial. In our model (Table 3.1) there are 21 units of Wealth generated by the indivisible and collective effort of the workforce. This Wealth has been appropriated, albeit legitimately under current laws, by private Rentholders, often unknowingly because no effort whatsoever is required on their part. There is no logical refutation of this analysis. An economics for true Welfare Capitalism is very different from an economics of Business Capitalism. The former depends on Rent for social purposes, while the latter takes Rent for private interest.

Rent in an increasingly sophisticated economy

Table 3.1 describes a simple and unprogressive economic state. Supply and demand are in equilibrium and 49 units are produced nett in each unit of time. The cycle of production is replicated in all future units of time in this model, but not in the real world. Labour is restless, ambitious and discontented. Ingenuity, invention and entrepreneurship turn a stable state into a metastable state, in which progress is constant but indiscernable on a day-to-day basis. In fact, the economy is growing in every manner and dimension. Labour increases in number and raises its level of skills and ability. Capital accumulates, improves in efficiency and becomes increasingly diversified. The productive margin of Land, meaning Land in the three-dimensional sense, shifts ever more from the centre. Soon, today's standards are things of the past. But let us say that our unit of production is unchanged: only the way it is produced changes. Our new standard input of Labour with its improved standard input of Capital now produces 12 units nett on prime sites after improved subsistence wages have been paid. Technological advances mean that the margin of economic activity now extends to sites of tenth quality, where our standard Labour and Capital produce three units nett. The cost per unit in Labour and Capital is therefore raised but remains affordable in the wealthier economy. This economic sophistication automatically raises Rent as shown

Table 3.4: Growth of Rent in an increasingly sophisticated economy

Site	A Rent	B Interest	C Nett productivity
Prime quality	9	3	12
Second quality	8	3	11
Third quality	7	3	10
Fourth quality	6	3	9
Fifth quality	5	3	8
Sixth quality	4	3	7
Seventh quality	3	3	6
Eighth quality	2	3	5
Ninth quality	1	3	4
Tenth quality	0	3	3
Totals	45	30	75

in Table 3.4. In comparison with Table 3.1, Interest has risen from 28 to 30 units, nett productivity has increased by 53% from 49 units to 75 units, and Rent has risen spectacularly by 114%, from 21 units to 45 units.

Speculation in privatised Rent and economic recession

Our economy is booming, yet in the real world this will not last. Expansion turns into recession, with nett productivity falling. The standard explanation for this phenomenon is that managers and owners of Capital suffer a collective loss of confidence. Economists talk of panic spreading through the business community like a contagion. But what is there in Tables 3.3 or 3.4 to create fear and trepidation? The answer is nothing at all, but then these tables do not model the real economy properly. Only when we introduce the speculative rentholding monopoly can we appreciate what happens.

Because the market is far from perfect, landholders and tenants have only a crude sense of what the economy is generating as Rent. When land is placed on the open market, the purpose is to assess what labourers, capitalists or other landholders will pay for the economic advantages afforded by the site were it in an undeveloped state (all developments, it will be recalled, are species of Capital). Statistically, the best estimate of the Rent would be the average of a random sample of bids. The landholder, however, is never interested in the average, but only in the highest. Hence the market's site valuation is perpetually biased towards an over-estimation

Table 3.5: Speculation in Rent and destabilisation of the economy

Site	A Rent	B Interest	C Nett productivity
Prime quality	9.3	2.7	12
Second quality	8.3	2.7	11
Third quality	7.3	2.7	10
Fourth quality	6.3	2.7	9
Fifth quality	5.3	2.7	8
Sixth quality	4.3	2.7	7
Seventh quality	3.3	2.7	6
Eighth quality	2.3	2.7	5
Ninth quality	1.3	2.7	4
Tenth quality	0.3	2.7	3
Totals	48	27	75

of Rent, especially when the economy is expanding and Labour and Capital compete heavily for a fixed supply of sites. Furthermore, fearing that a premature sale or commercial renting agreement might mean the loss of an even more lucrative offer, landholders can create artificial shortages by temporarily holding sites off the market. A holder with no private vested interest in Rent, ideally the State, would test the market objectively to arrive at a best estimate of true value before collecting what was due, unlike the private holder who ignores all but the highest and (by definition) biased offer.

What economists describe as a contagion of 'collapse of confidence' is more like the disabling after-effect of an infectious epidemic rather than the febrile episode itself. The insensitivity of the market, and the constant desire of Rentholders to force unearned income to its maximum, mean that in an expanding economy Rent soars beyond that which productivity justifies. A good economy may be on course to deliver 48 units as Rent next year rather than the 45 it delivers this year, but Rentholders want the three extra units immediately if they can get them. This is the real contagion, the febrile desire to 'get rich quick' and not be left behind in the speculative market in Rent. Since expansion of the productive margin of Land takes more time to achieve than any other economic activity, in all but the most long term of senses Land is in fixed supply. Thus speculating Rentholders can create an artificial shortage by holding sites off the high-demand market. Let us say that they take 10% of what otherwise would go to Interest, giving Table 3.5.

Table 3.6: New 'steady economic state' after recession

Site	A Rent	B Interest	C Nett productivity
Prime quality	8	3	11
Second quality	7	3	10
Third quality	6	3	9
Fourth quality	5	3	8
Fifth quality	4	3	7
Sixth quality	3	3	6
Seventh quality	2	3	5
Eighth quality	1	3	4
Ninth quality	0	3	3
Totals	36	27	63

Income has been taken from the productive sector into the unproductive sector. Table 3.5 is unstable because without increased productivity, the cost of units in Labour and Capital exceeds that commensurate with demand, and goods remain unsold. In this situation a damaging decline occurs in the amount of Interest that can be set aside for re-investment in Capital. Gross and nett productivity must therefore fall back until the economy re-stabilises. This is recession. The new 'steady-state' is as shown in Table 3.6.

Production on all sites has fallen back, irrespective of quality. Land of tenth quality has fallen right out of the economy, with consequent unemployment and collapse of business. Nett productivity is only 84% of that in the boom years, and Rent has fallen back by 25%, but the return as Wages and Interest is once more acceptable.

To recapitulate, when the commercial sale price of Land (which is Rent capitalised over, say, 15 years), Rent bundled into 'profit' and the element of Rent in commercial rent overshoot the true economic value, Rentholders are pre-empting an expansion of the economy by taking next year's assumed Rent prematurely. If the holder takes next year's Rent today then, in a dynamic economy, working Capital is left with last year's Interest. As the private economy grows at an increasing pace the market speculates in Rent, putting a damper on the return to the productive sectors, Labour and Capital. As Rent lurches onwards and upwards, returns as Interest and Wages falter and then fall back. The economy then enters the down phase of its productive cycle, or a recession, in which Labour and Capital on the lowest quality (marginal) sites are the first to experience part-time work, unemployment and bankruptcy.

Do not be misled into believing that marginal Land is somewhere out in the swamp: marginal sites exist even on intensively developed land in the City of London, as Table 3.3 indicates. Only when Rent falls back and the relations of Interest and Wages to supply and demand return to equilibrium (Table 3.6) does the collapse bottom out and recovery become feasible. Tables 3.1 to 3.6 show that if, as present day economists and governments do every day, we merge columns A and B and pay attention only to the totals in column C, all sense is lost as to what Rent is doing relative to Interest and Wages. The opportunity to explain cyclical unemployment and the deterioration in health which follows in its wake (see Chapter Four) is thereby denied. This is economic obscurantism – accepted practice in Business Capitalism but opposed to the enlightenment sought by Welfare Capitalism.

The expansion of Land in production

Our development of Table 3.1 showed how Rent theoretically increases as a proportion of total income in a growing economy. This safe proposition, though never proven or refuted for lack of adequate data, was nevertheless denied vehemently by those who argued that technological advances such as improved transportation would reduce inequalities in the productivity of sites and thereby drive down Rent. Also, the law of diminishing returns would be offset by diversification of Labour and Capital, thereby weakening the intensive gradient on heavily developed prime sites in the cities. These arguments, collected together as Ricardo's Paradox, were true up to a point, but overlooked the fact that science and technology increase the volume of Land (nature's gifts being in three dimensions) brought into the productive economy.

Agricultural and veterinary sciences, civil engineering and other technological advances move out the boundaries of production horizontally (land reclamation), upwards (into the air space) and downwards (excavation). Technological and scientific progress can tend to decrease the volume of Land in production by intensifying productive capacity of sites (eg new seed varieties could lead to a reduction of cultivated farmland), but with growth of population and raised demand the nett effect of development is volume expansion rather than retraction. Thus while the differential productivity of sites in our model may be reduced to less than one unit, more and more sites of differential quality enter the economy. The nett productivity of Land of seventh quality would no longer be four units but seven units if differential productivity

Table 3.7: Growth of Rent when inequalities of productive capacity between sites are reduced in a technologically sophisticated economy

Site	Rent		Interest		Nett productivity	
	A	**A'**	**B**	**B'**	**C**	**C'**
Prime quality	6.0	7.0	4	4	10.0	11.0
Second quality	5.5	6.5	4	4	9.5	10.5
Third quality	5.0	6.0	4	4	9.0	10.0
Fourth quality	4.5	5.5	4	4	8.5	9.5
Fifth quality	4.0	5.0	4	4	8.0	9.0
Sixth quality	3.5	4.5	4	4	7.5	8.5
Seventh quality	3.0	4.0	4	4	7.0	8.0
Eighth quality	2.5	3.5	4	4	6.5	7.5
⋮	⋮	⋮	⋮	⋮	⋮	⋮
Thirteenth quality	0	1.0	4	4	4.0	5.0
Fourteenth quality		0.5		4		4.5
Fifteenth quality		0		4		4.0
Totals	39.0	52.5	52	60	91.0	112.5

were reduced to half a unit, and the margin would now extend to Land of thirteenth quality, as shown in Table 3.7, column C.

Technological progress which diminishes the gradient of nett productivity will at the same time permit a far greater productivity of Labour and Capital on a much increased number of sites, raising total nett productivity in our model from 49 units (Table 3.1) to 91 units (Table 3.7, column C) as the high-rise buildings go up. Total Rent (column A) and Interest (column B) both rise, but their percentage shares of nett productivity are unchanged from Table 3.1, 43% and 57% respectively. If, however, technological progress also raises nett productivity on prime sites, then our model comes to resemble Canary Wharf in London's East End, with nett productivity rising to 112.5 units (C'), total Interest to 60 units (B') and Rent to 52.5 units (A'). Note, however, that in this case, despite technology decreasing the gradient of nett productivity, Rent as a percentage of total nett productivity rises almost to 47. There is no 'Ricardo's Paradox'. Technological improvements open distant sites to more intensive production as we build ever higher and to a denser capacity without risks to health and safety. Productivity is raised on all sites, irrespective of quality.

The Rent of idle land

One more property of Rent needs emphasis. The Rent that can be
obtained by the landholder of a prime site depends, not upon the Labour
and Capital that is expended on that site, but on the input of productive
Labour and Capital on sites of inferior quality. If our seven standard
labourers with their standard inputs of Labour and Capital are forced off
the prime site they occupy in our intensively developed economy (Table
3.3), the Rent value of this unoccupied prime site remains undisturbed at
21 units, even though no units of productivity are actually being created.
Rent represents not what is necessarily realised, but the price the productive
sector judges worth paying to gain the economic advantages that make
the site prime in quality. In effect, the holder of a site kept in an
unproductive state holds an imputed Rent, for the landholder still possesses
the ability to enjoy the site (even if he neglects to do so) for which others
would need to pay Rent. The fact is reflected in the reality that the
unworked site would still sell at a price which represents the anticipated
future Rent capitalised over 15 or 20 years. As Patrick Dove put it in his
The elements of political science: "... if in the heart of London a space of 20
acres had been enclosed by a high wall at the time of the Norman
Conquest, and if no man had ever touched that portion of soil, or ever
seen it from that time to this, it would, if let by auction, produce an
enormously high rent. Hampstead Heath ... in the immediate vicinity
of London, would ... let for an enormous Rent, which ... in nowise
depends upon any labour or capital hitherto expended on the Heath"
(Dove, 1854, p 283). Thus the landholder has no fear of depressing the
Rent simply by leaving the site idle. Rent exists for the landlord whether
or not the land is occupied by owner or tenant, the proof being that he
can sell it. The landlord of an idle site from whom Rent is requested by
the State will have to find this from other productive sources, or bring
the site into the productive economy.

Rent and the domestic economy

Housework and parenting are generally thought of as separate from the
wider economy, for the fallacious reason that market forces and the price
mechanism do not apply. It goes without saying, however, that they are
essential for Wealth creation and the health of the nation. Wealth consists
of all materials provided by nature which have been modified by exertion
and ingenuity to satisfy human needs and desires. Child-rearing quite

obviously fits this definition – a labour of love and devotion from the moment of conception to the age of full maturity. This process requires Land, Labour and Capital, and the law of Rent holds true.

Let us speak of orders of Land suited to the nurturing of the family. Let us also hypothesise that we have not identical workers but identical families with identical resources of Capital. In our model only Land varies in quality. We now commence family life, and naturally families gravitate towards prime sites. Let us say that for standard inputs of Labour and Capital the quality of child-rearing and family life on these sites merits a score of 10 units. The population flourishes and the number of families grows, so that eventually all prime sites are occupied and newcomers must avail themselves of sites of second quality. Here, for the same inputs, the standard family can attain a standard of child-rearing and family life equal only to a score of nine (educational facilities, recreational opportunities, the pleasantness of the environment are of second quality only). We can proceed in this way until some families can find only sites of marginal value on which the score for child-rearing and family life is four. Scores below four, on sub-marginal sites, are below the threshold of acceptability in a modern society.

Scores above the marginal value of four convert into Rent, which represents what families are willing and able to pay for the opportunities afforded by the site for child-rearing and family life. Their ability to pay depends upon the family income coming in as Wages, Interest and Rent from the non-domestic economy. Tenant families pay Rent to their landlord in the commercial rent turned over. Those families that are 'owner-occupiers' will have paid about 15 years' worth of the assessed annual value of the Rent to the previous owner in the purchase price. After 15 years they enjoy Rent as an imputed income going to themselves as outright landholders. Families who are in effect part-owners and part-tenants for purposes of Rent, because they are buying on a mortgage or legal charge, pay part of this Rent to the lender as they return the principal borrowed, and retain the remainder as an imputed income (see Chapter Six). Obviously, Rent of a domestic site increases as technological improvements in the surrounding region raise 'productivity' (ie the standard of child-rearing) on all sites (akin to Table 3.4): improvements often provided by the taxpayer. Speculation in Rent in the housing sector sends pulses racing as house prices rise, only to bring tears when, sooner or later, they collapse.

Table 3.8: The acute effect of taxation of the productive sector

Site	A Rent	B Interest after tax	Tax	C Nett productivity
Prime quality	6	3.2	0.8	10
Second quality	5	3.2	0.8	9
Third quality	4	3.2	0.8	8
Fourth quality	3	3.2	0.8	7
Fifth quality	2	3.2	0.8	6
Sixth quality	1	3.2	0.8	5
Seventh quality	0	3.2	0.8	4
Totals	21	22.4	5.6	49

Taxation in lieu of Rent

We can now fully appreciate that Rent is a publicly created income which has come to be identified with the value of productive land, including that set aside for the domestic economy. As such, it belongs in the public domain rather than figuring as unearned income in private pockets. However, not even thinking to collect Rent for social purposes, successive administrations have left Rent in the private sector and imposed taxes on Wages and Interest to finance the modern Welfare State. Governments do this to some extent 'in the dark', for the lack of intelligence about the behaviour of Rent means that they cannot know the full consequences of what they do. To illustrate how the economy responds to taxes on Wages and Interest, let us return to our simple model of the operation of Rent in the free market economy. Let us say that government imposes a tax of 20% on productivity after Wages and Rent have been paid, which in our model is taken as Interest.

The imposition of 'dead-weight' taxes

Recall that our standard market will not pay the price of units when our standard input of Labour and Capital yields less than four units nett for the effort. Any attempt to generate Labour's subsistence Wage and an acceptable level of Interest on the Capital would then mean asking for more than what less than four units could fetch on the market, a price beyond and inconsistent with the level of demand. We now need a new column in Table 3.1, to produce Table 3.8, showing the tax at 20% of nett income (after payment of 'subsistence' wages).

This model is clearly not viable, because the defined conditions of the

Table 3.9: The 'steady economic state' to accommodate taxation

Site	A Rent	B Interest after tax	Tax	C Nett productivity
Prime quality	5	4	I	10
Second quality	4	4	I	9
Third quality	3	4	I	8
Fourth quality	2	4	I	7
Fifth quality	I	4	I	6
Sixth quality	0	4	I	5
Totals	15	24	6	45

economy yield only 3.2 units of Interest nett for standard inputs of Labour and Capital. Production on marginal sites of seventh quality therefore goes to the wall. So sites of sixth quality yielding five units now represent the economic margin in the metastable state, as shown in Table 3.9.

Taxation of Interest at 20% diverts six units of a total of 45 units (over 13%) of nett output to the exchequer, but at what cost to the economy? First, nett productivity declines by more than 8% from 49 units to 45 units as businesses on sites of seventh quality fail, offices, workshops and factories fall idle, and the workforce resorts to unemployment benefit. Nett Interest falls from 28 units before the introduction of taxation (Table 3.1) to 24 units. These effects of income tax are called 'deadweight' by economists, the result of inefficiencies created by taxation of the productive sector. But Rent going to holders of Land from prime to marginal sixth quality, which remains in the productive sector, falls by six units from 21 to 15. Obviously, therefore, the tax falls ultimately on Rent even though imposed initially on Interest. Some of the tax received has to be spent softening the blow to families previously supported by their own Labour on sites of seventh quality, for example through income support. Yet had the exchequer decided to collect Rent directly, instead of indirectly and unwittingly by taxing the productive sector, there would have been no damage to the economy, and no need for income support.

Tax breaks go to Rent

Now let government be selective as to where it imposes its tax. Let us say it attempts to stimulate forestry by giving this industry a tax break of all six units, mimicking what the government attempted to do in the Budget of 1988. In this scenario Table 3.1 remains valid as a model for forestry, while for all other economic activity Table 3.9 applies. Therefore we compare these tables. Marginal land is now turned over to forestry and Rent (and therefore selling price) of forestry lands already in production increases (a windfall for the landholder). There are four units more produced in forestry than before, but six units of wealth have been sunk in land values, a gift from the exchequer. Facts bear out our theoretical model. Sir Richard Body, farmer and Conservative member of parliament, reported that between 1946 and 1982 governments subsidised British agriculture to the tune of £40 billion. In the same period, agricultural land values increased by the same £40 billion (Body, 1982, pp 20-32). None of these features of the behaviour of the economy and its responses to government intervention are fully discernible if, as is the standard practice, Rent and Interest are merged for business purposes as profit.

'Welfare taxes' as Welfare's dead-weight

Crucially, the economic impact of taxation on Wages and Interest is exactly the same when it is imposed to fund the Welfare State. The 'seventh quality' sites that fall out of the productive economy into the non-productive Welfare sector are in real life the deprived neighbourhoods with high rates of unemployment so admirably described by the Social Exclusion Unit (2000), peppered with collapsed business enterprises, large and small. Government collected six units for Welfare purposes, but society lost four units of production in our particular model. Add to this the expense of the social dislocation with raised levels of petty crime, increased levels of mental and physical illness, family breakdown, the expense of means-testing applicants for Welfare, and the costs of Welfare administration, and the best intentions of government are more or less reduced to rubble: little more than increased economic inefficiency. This policy sits oddly with fairness and efficiency.

'Enterprise' zoning

Now, having exacerbated a bad situation, let government attempt to alleviate the damage in the worst areas by creating (let's call them) enterprise zones to regenerate employment. In these zones taxes on Interest are removed, so we move back to Table 3.1. We therefore put back four units of productivity, but privatised Rent rises by six units! Interest rises by four units from 24 to 28, improving the local economy, it is true, but too much of the tax subsidy has gone into increases in Rent and therefore the commercial rents and land prices demanded by landlords. Just as taxes on productivity ultimately come out of Rent, so subsidies to productivity ultimately end as Rent. Even worse, the tax break creates an artificially high demand for sites in the enterprise zone. Speculating landholders, always holding out for the highest offer on a sale price or commercial rent, force the Rent to overshoot.

The blinkered focus on 'Interest' and Wages

The economic and social effects of privatised Rent are the same, no matter how far advanced is the division of Labour and Capital among different classes and occupations, or how complicated the tax system on Wages and Interest. In our model our worker keeps the system simple by being both labourer and capitalist, holding wages constant at a fixed level adequate for subsistence. Nett productivity after deduction of subsistence Wages and Rent is therefore Interest. But let us return to when we had two workers (standard units of Labour) per site with their standard amounts of Capital, producing on a prime site (Table 3.2). They generated 19 units nett and the landholder took 11 units. Now let us introduce a division of Labour by making one worker responsible for the eight units of Interest on their Capital. Both labourers still work, but one manages the Capital while the other, relieved of this responsibility, puts effort into producing with this Capital. There now arises the question of a fair division of these eight units between the keeper of the Capital and the labourer. The difficulties in deciding what is fair and just are the stuff of industrial relations. So focused are they on the important issues that arise, however, that the underlying and fundamental effects of Rent on what they have to share is completely lost. Indeed, so forgotten is Rent that governments, unions and employers' organisations seek the origins of low pay, unemployment and cyclical recession entirely within the roles played by Labour and Capital. This fault is inevitable in an economic system which insists in treating Rent as though it were Interest, and lumps the two together as profit.

Taxation and unemployment

In the real world, Labour exists these days on more than a 'physiological' subsistence Wage owing to the power of the electoral franchise and the Labour unions. Also, Rentholders, capitalists and employers tend to be one and the same. Let us now assume that standard Labour has raised its

Table 3.10: The battle between employer and employee

Site	A Rent	+	B Interest	=	profit	Wages above subsistence after tax	Wages tax	C Nett productivity
Prime quality	3	+	4	=	7	1.5	1.5	10
Second quality	2	+	4	=	6	1.5	1.5	9
Third quality	1	+	4	=	5	1.5	1.5	8
Fourth quality	0	+	4	=	4	1.5	1.5	7
Totals	6	+	16	=	22	6.0	6.0	34

Wage to three units above subsistence, at the inevitable expense of Rent, in which case we have Table 3.10 when Wages above subsistence are taxed at 50% and Interest is untaxed.

By comparing Tables 3.10 and 3.1 we see that the Rentholder-capitalist-employer is unhappy because profits have fallen by the extent that Rent has decreased (15 units), Interest has decreased (by 12 units) and Wages have increased (by 12 units). Labour is unhappy because taxes have severely reduced the disposable income fought for (from 12 units to 6 units) and created unemployment. Nett productivity has fallen by 30% as Land below fourth quality has fallen beneath the productive margin. We now have another battle royal in which Rentholder-capitalist-employer and employee struggle to minimise their losses. Labour, if powerful owing to, say, effective unionism, will demand an increase in real Wages to offset the impact of taxes, handing the burden to the Rentholder-capitalist-employer. To the extent that Labour succeeds in raising Wages, Rent will be reduced and there will be further marginal unemployment (only by raising productivity can Labour take increased Wages without forcing marginal Land out of economic viability, for on marginal sites the funds must come from Interest, and hence from Interest on identical Capital on all sites). The employer will attempt to lower Labour costs by reducing the workforce and increasing the productivity of workers remaining in employment by raising the ratio of Capital to Labour, thereby shifting income from Wages to Interest. The result – further unemployment with resort to Welfare. A study sponsored by the Centre of Economic Policy Research suggested that this is exactly what has happened in Europe. Opening with the declaration that "There is no doubt that the most pressing economic problem in Europe today is the apparently endless surge in unemployment" (Daveri and Tabellini, 1997, p 2), the report concluded that the rise of almost 9.5% in the rate of effective Labour taxes between 1965 and 1991 accounted for a 4% rise in unemployment in the European Union. The authors also noted that despite high Labour taxes, unemployment had remained low in Scandinavia where the workforce is well organised, and suggested that this result may have been owing to the public sector having expanded, thereby offsetting the effects of the private employers' actions (Daveri and Tabellini, 1997, p 35).

Now let us suppose that taxes are imposed on Interest, and that Labour is unorganised. The Rentholder-capitalist-employer is again affected by loss of Rent and Interest, and uses the power of an employer to impose a reduction of Wages on Labour to transfer some of the loss. The result is resort to Welfare subsidies, perhaps as the working family tax credit. This dead-weight effect of taxation on the productive sector is quantified for the UK in Chapter Seven.

Economic graduation of labour and capital

Of course, not only Land is of graduated economic quality: so also are Labour and Capital. Wages and Interest are likewise graduated, and governments impose graduated taxation with the highest incomes paying most. The outcome is a graduated series of margins of economic activity, rather like contour lines on an economic map. The margins of productive activity for the most heavily taxed sectors with high incomes are the innermost contours on relatively high quality Land, while those for the lightly taxed, low income sectors lie on relatively low quality Land. In a modern complex economy in which there is much economic interaction due to specialisation, taxation on one sector is bound to have knock-on effects in other sectors. Hence unemployment at the margin of top quality Labour and Capital due to heavy taxation will create secondary unemployment in the lower income bands.

Privatised Rent and social class

There is no difficulty in demonstrating the strong association that persists between Dr Stevenson's occupational social classes and privatised Rent going to those enjoying land-ownership or investment incomes as commercial rents and dividends. Table 3.11 has been adapted from the 1988 General Household Survey (Office of Population Censuses and Surveys, 1988, p 242). First, of the economically inactive group (group 8), mainly the retired, about half are owner-occupiers and the other half are not. There could be no clearer distinction between the 'have Rent' and the 'have not Rent'. Secondly, the proportion of owner-occupiers

Table 3.11: Household tenure by socio-economic group of head of household

	Socio-economic group %[+]							
	1	2	3	4	5	6	7	8
Owner-occupied:								
outright	15.1	13.0	13.5	14.7	11.9	12.3	9.8	40.5
with mortgage	75.5	74.0	68.0	57.5	58.2	41.1	16.4	7.3
Rented:								
with occupation	3.6	3.8	2.1	2.4	1.3	4.2	13.5	0.8
local authority	0	5.3	7.3	15.9	22.1	36.7	53.3	40.6
other	5.9	3.9	9.0	9.4	6.4	5.6	7.0	11.5
Total %	100	100	100	100	100	100	100	100

[+] 1 professional; 2 employers/managers; 3 intermediate non-manual; 4 junior non-manual; 5 skilled manual; 6 semi-skilled manual; 7 unskilled manual; 8 economically inactive. Armed forces, full-time students and permanently unemployed are excluded.

declines steadily and that housed by the State through the local authority increases as socio-economic status shifts from professional (group 1) to unskilled manual (group 7). Any subsidies going to those in local authority accommodation will be derived from taxes on Wages and Interest (including the tax on buildings in the local rate). What would be most interesting is an analysis of mortality by social class where class is defined according to possession of Rent (unearned income). The working class would be those whose sole source of income was earned Wages; the middle classes would have a little Rent; the upper middle classes rather more; and the cream of society the most. This fundamental distinction of what separates one social group from another is surely, even today, more meaningful than secondary characteristics such as gross income, where it is banked and how it is spent.

Land for housing accounts for about two thirds of site values in Britain (Richards, 1989, table 19): thus Table 3.11 illustrates starkly how inequitably Rent is distributed. Yet the reality is far worse for several reasons. Land sites owner-occupied by the professional and managerial families are much more valuable and attract far more Rent than the sites of groups 2 to 7. Added to this, investment income as commercial rents and dividends is far more unequally distributed than income earned from Labour. Among families paying income tax, the 5% with the highest earnings receive 45% of all rents and 52% of all dividends (*Survey of Personal Incomes*, 1987, tables 4 and 15). Rent, a major source of income so inequitably distributed, must play a major role in the perpetuation of inequitable class differences in health and life expectancy associated with relative material deprivation. Each unit increment in Rent, like income from any other source, will buy an increment of health. Similarly each unit decrement of Rent imposed on the materially deprived must increase their vulnerability to disease and premature death. This is the inequitable force in the Welfare State, the privatised Rent of vitality: the deadly legacy.

The State, the citizen and ownership of Rent

Political economy and political medicine

Men and women embark upon the creation of political society when they agree to surrender their natural powers and erect a common authority to settle disputes, reconcile competing interests and punish offenders. They accept government to bring order into their lives, recognising that the capacity for achievement by a properly ordered society far exceeds the sum of their individual capacities. When left to their own powers, men and women veer too much towards self-regard, bringing conflict and confusion. Governments are therefore granted powers which affect all dimensions of the human condition: economic, social, physical and psychological. A prime function of political economy is to examine the economic and social aspects of government performance: how wealth and income are generated and distributed within society under various political systems. This is much, much more than mere academic exercise. Every action (or inaction) of government in the economic sphere has consequences for the physical and mental health of society, while the physical and mental health of all sectors of society is of profound importance for the health of the economy. In linking the generation and distribution of wealth and income to health and lifespan, as modern research is doing more than ever before, we are witnessing the growth of a discipline unfamiliar to most people. Political medicine is the embryonic partner of political economy, focusing not on the distribution of wealth and income under diverse political systems, but the distribution of health and life expectancy under those same systems. There are hundreds of books on political economy, but none published under the title of 'political medicine'.

The discipline of political medicine, as the term is used here, is not to be mistaken for medical politics (how the profession is governed and regulated) or health politics. Health politics covers lobbying activities and legislation concerning such matters as abortion, quarantine, smoking in public places, drug abuse, the employment of medical and nursing staff, the relations between the public and private sectors of health care, funding of medical research and so on. Political medicine judges the health consequences not of health policy, but of political and economic policy. Political economy and political medicine are inter-related sub-disciplines of politics itself. The correct conjunction of political economy and political medicine depends crucially upon their mutual observance of an overarching political morality that is clear about what distinguishes inequalities from inequities. Small wonder that Adam Smith published his *The theory of moral sentiments* (1759) 17 years before *An inquiry into the nature and causes of the wealth of nations* (1776). For Smith to have approached what he regarded as two parts of a greater whole in reverse order would have been a logical absurdity.

Political morality and the institution of private property

Political morality, a set of principles stating what by moral consensus are the ethical goals of government, describes what *ought to be*. Good government pays equal regard to the Welfare of all citizens, thereby ensuring equal consideration, and equal expression of that consideration, for the health of all. In short, when it comes to health there can morally be no such thing as a second-class citizen. Political medicine, recognising the strong dependency of health on wealth, provides, with its statistics on sickness and death rates within the various divisions of society, the means to judge the degree of incongruence of political economy with political morality. Life being what it is, that some individuals enjoy better health and a longer life than others, amounts only to a truism. Consciences are troubled, however, when society is confronted with the unsettling reality that length of life is inextricably bound up with class, income and wealth. To what extent is the political system, through its influence on the distribution of income and wealth, the agent responsible for the reduced prospects for health and longevity among the under-privileged? In ensuring that the political economy creates no inequitous deprivation and poverty the guiding principle must be 'render unto Caesar those things that are Caesar's'. The Biblical commandment, 'thou shalt not steal', justifies the institution of property, but neither saying helps us to decide what justifies ownership. How do we discriminate between what is and what is not Caesar's, so that we can recognise stealing when it occurs?

The claim to ownership originates with mental or physical Labour. Labour put into anything gives a right to say 'this is mine'. If there is only the Labour of one individual then there is private ownership. If there is Labour of more than one, then there is some form of joint ownership. If there is pooled Labour on a public and indivisible scale, then there is public ownership. The status quo persists until the owner transfers what is owned either by exchange (eg sale in the open market) or gift. In political economy this rule translates into 'income and wealth created in the private domain belongs in the private domain and equally, what has been created in the public domain belongs in the public domain'. This is not to say that what belongs originally in the private domain cannot morally find its way into the public domain either by private sale or lease or gift. Similarly, what originally has been created in the public domain can morally find its way into private hands by sale at a fair price, rent or gift by a public agency. No greater conflict with morality arises in the sphere of political economy, however, than when what is rightfully private is *appropriated* by the public domain, or conversely when what is rightfully public is *appropriated* by the private domain.

The early medieval concept of landed wealth and government

Rent today is public property sequestered into private ownership, an arrangement that would have offended early medieval morality. There was a time when Land and Rent were seen for what they truly are, long before economics was shaped into a recognisable discipline. St Thomas Aquinas (1226-74), reflecting on political society, considered that: "The control of one over another who remains free, can take place when the former directs the latter to his own good or to the common good ... there could be no social life for many persons living together unless one of their number were set in authority for the common good.... Secondly, if there were one man more wise and righteous than the rest, it would have been wrong if such gifts were not exercised on behalf of the rest" (Aquinas, 1959, p 105). From such thoughts arose the concept that the society man creates by using his reason and powers of self-restraint is analogous to a living organism. In this system of order each member plays an assigned role in harmony with the rest of society. So arises a differentiated hierarchy in which persons are in one sense equal but given greater and lesser roles to play in the ordered society whose government all submit to for the common good.

Christian theologians of the 13th century, schooled by Thomas Aquinas, viewed medieval social order as a divine institution arising naturally from the gift of reason given to man. This social order was as pre-ordained as the order displayed by the movements of the moon, the stars and the planets. Furthermore, men undertaking great responsibilities needed not only the allegiance of those for whom they laboured, but also the resources to achieve what was expected of the offices they held. Thus there was divine logic in the fact that great men held great riches and little men were poor. Importantly, however, holding landed wealth was an honour tied to onerous responsibilities to the State, *not* an endowment for personal indulgence or frivolous use. Great men were entrusted with vast estates of land because in a world where communication was difficult and travel hazardous, there was no other way for government to function but to parcel out the State between those who governed. But no one was entitled to hold more landed property than would support his station, and the Rent of that land was held in trust for the State. Land-ownership in the modern sense simply was not recognised.

Thomas Aquinas was canonised in 1323, and in 1567 Pope Pius V placed him among the great Latin fathers of the Catholic Church. His beliefs about the hierarchical order of society and the hierarchical distribution of land and wealth to support this order were not published as a complete work, however, until 1787 (possibly intended as an antidote to the threat of revolution in France), by which time Church and State had long since come to regard land and Rent as species of private property. A modern edition was produced by Leo XIII in 1882, after he had directed that St Thomas Aquinas' teaching should form the theological basis of the Catholic Church. The explanation for the timing was simple – the Church's intellectual response to the rising demands of the Socialists. Alarmed by the continuing rise of Socialist parties, in 1891 Leo XIII issued his encyclical *Rerum Novarum*, in which he said: "To the State the interests of all are equal, whether high or low. The poor are members of the national community equal with the rich; they are real component parts, living parts, which make up, through the family, the living body, ... It would be irrational to neglect one portion of the citizens and to favour another..." (cited in George, 1947, p 115).

This pronouncement could have come straight from the mouth of Thomas Aquinas, but Aquinas had spoken for an age six centuries earlier. Those were not yet the days when Rent was a marketable commodity like any other goods or services. So when the Pope declared in his encyclical that 'what is bought with rightful property is rightful property',

St Thomas might have turned in his grave at such an unqualified use of his 13th century teaching. He would not have sanctioned the 19th century private market in Rent, for Rent was the revenue of State. Buying and selling does nothing but transfer ownership. If what is bargained for and sold has been appropriated, as has Rent, then mere transfer of title alters nothing fundamental. Under Capitalism as practised, even Welfare Capitalism, Rent which belongs rightfully in public ownership has been taken into the private domain for private profit without due compensation. How this came about is described in Part II, but it is this appropriation which distorts the political economy and creates many of the conditions which State Welfare systems seek to alleviate. Yet the powers of restitution inherent in Welfare systems are no match for the distortionary forces creating need and, even worse, the Welfare processes adopted by modern governments are self-defeating because they exacerbate the distortions.

For the common good

For those who can perceive 'Rent' and thus recognise its relevance for modern problems, the failure of great men to acknowledge what confronts them, or admit its significance, is most baffling. Political morality calls for individual respect and service to society, and public respect and service to the individual. First, there is the service of the individual to the family, but not at the cost of dis-service to neighbouring families. Then comes service to the neighbourhood, but not at the cost of dis-service to the wider community. Taking what rightfully belongs to the wider community for the benefit of the local community, the family or the individual is quite simply wrong. And if, as is the case with Rent, the current political economy and the law condone just this, both being burdened and distorted by institutional arrangements made by men long dead for circumstances that no longer exist, then political economy and the law must put their houses in order.

The obsolescent practice of unthinkingly privatising what is public property is a dead hand of history, but one with the grip of rigor mortis on the public purse, public Welfare and the health of the nation. The monopolisation of Rent denies many thousands of families enjoyment of a share of the publicly created portion of the national income that settles in the value of land sites around the country. By holding publicly created revenue out of government's hands, the people's government is denied the opportunity of treating all families equitably. It exacerbates the situation by forcing government to collect a portion of private income (Wages and Interest) in lieu of Rent for social purposes, thereby further distorting the distribution of income by inflicting injury on those dependant on marginal economic activity. The resultant unemployment and social disruption force government to spend a large proportion of what has been collected in alleviating the damage inflicted on society by its own policies.

Those who hold Rent, essentially the upper and middle classes, unwittingly are responsible for much of what they bemoan in the Welfare State. It is they who have to free the economy of its distortions, thereby revitalising productive activity and permitting a more equitable distribution of the increased Wealth generated. Access to unearned income in the form of Rent is, however, to this day the basis of social class distinctions. What is being asked, by return of Rent to the public domain, is therefore nothing less than an expansion of a common class for the common good, at the expense of the hierarchical system the nation has inherited from former times. This is not to deny that there will be inequalities of wealth and income in this great common class. But such inequalities as exist will be based upon just returns for the value of individual effort contributed to the wealth-producing process. There will always be a need for a Welfare system to care for those affected by the vicissitudes of life, but these vicissitudes will be met largely, perhaps entirely, out of Rent reserved for social purposes. As matters stand at present, some gain more than their fair share of publicly created wealth and income at the expense of others, simply because they own Rent, not appreciating the consequences of deprivation of income for health and length of life of others.

But for how long have calls been made to live according to our common origin (as against birthright) and our common destiny, for the common good! The plea has ebbed and flowed down the ages with the constancy of the tide upon a cliff of granite, and with similar effect. Here is Charles Dickens, for example, writing for a time when diseases were believed to spread with the sickening miasma emanating from the thousands of tons of filth and excrement that fouled the towns and cities of his day:

> Those who study the physical sciences, and bring them to bear upon the health of Man, tell us that if the noxious particles that rise from vitiated air were palpable to the sight, we should see them lowering in a dense black cloud above such haunts (slums), and rolling slowly on to corrupt the better portions of a town. But if the moral pestilence that rises with them, and in the eternal laws of outraged Nature, is inseparable from them, could be made discernible too, how terrible the revelation!

Then should we see depravity, impiety, drunkenness, theft, murder, and a long train of nameless sins against the natural affections and repulsions of mankind, overhanging the devoted spots, and creeping on, to blight the innocent and spread contagion among the pure. Then should we see how the same poisoned fountains that flow into our hospitals and lazar- houses, inundate the jails, and make the convict-ships swim deep, and roll across the seas, and over-run vast continents with crime. Then should we stand appalled to know, that where we generate disease to strike our children down and entail itself on unborn generations, there also we breed, by the same certain process, infancy that knows no innocence, youth without modesty or shame, maturity that is mature in nothing but in suffering and guilt, blasted old age that is a scandal on the form we bear. Unnatural humanity! When we shall gather grapes from thorns, and figs from thistles; when fields of grain shall spring up from the offal in the bye-ways of our wicked cities, and roses bloom in the fat churchyards that they cherish; then we may look for natural humanity and find it growing from such seed.

Oh for a good spirit who would take the house-tops off, with a more potent and benignant hand than the lame demon in the tale, and show a Christian people what dark shapes issue from amidst their homes, to swell the retinue of the Destroying Angel as he moves forth among them! For only one night's view of the pale phantoms rising from the scenes of our too-long neglect; and from the thick and sullen air when Vice and Fever propagate together, raining the tremendous social retributions which are ever pouring down, and ever coming thicker! Bright and blest the morning that should rise on such a night; for men, delayed no more by stumbling-blocks of their own making, which are but specks of dust upon the path between them and eternity, would then apply themselves, like creatures of one common origin, owing one duty to the Father of one family, and tending to one common end, to make the world a better place! (Dickens, 1950, pp 647-8)

To clear the cities of dung and pollution is progress. To discover bacteria is progress. But for men and women to apply themselves as creatures of one common origin and make the world a better place, the global abuse of Rent, its unnatural disbursement as over-privilege, must be rectified. That indeed would eclipse all else that we are pleased to call advance.

FOUR

Sickening unemployment

The mistreatment of Rent causes unemployment, an unmitigated catastrophe for the health and fabric of families and their communities. Even the threat of joblessness is enough to have adverse effects on mental and physical health, as illustrated by a study in the British civil service (Ferrie et al, 1995). In the 1980s men and women in the civil service were examined for a large medical survey. The Property Services Agency entered the study in 1986, the year that the Conservative administration, through the Treasury Efficiency Unit, published its document *Using private enterprise in government*. By late 1988 plans had been laid to privatise the work of the Agency. Twelve months later, during the debate on the Property Services Agency Bill in parliament, significant staff cuts were predicted. In 1989, beginning with the Agency, researchers sent a health questionnaire to all civil servants. Apprehensions about job losses in the Agency were largely fulfilled by 1994, by which time 43% of its staff recruited into the study either had been made redundant or had opted for early retirement. Half the remainder were worried that a similar fate awaited them.

When first seen in 1986 the staff of the Agency had been in marginally better health than their fellows in other offices. They smoked less, drank less and took more exercise. By 1989 the picture had changed, especially men. Health had deteriorated more in the Agency staff than in other departments, even though their health-related behaviour such as smoking was no worse than elsewhere. Job insecurity was creating a state of sub-health which, as other studies have shown, can progress to actual illness when unemployment arrives. Similar findings have been reported prior to closure of factories (Grayson, 1985).

Unemployment and mental health

In 1985, when Britain's unemployed totalled more than three million, the *British Medical Journal* published a series of articles entitled 'Occupationless health' (Smith, 1985). These were the years when words such as 'underclass' and 'stakeholder' increased in currency as joblessness among the young reached alarming proportions. The series focused on eight longitudinal studies in all of which loss of gainful employment was followed by a deterioration in mental health and re-employment by recovery. One of these studies had been conducted among school leavers in Leeds (Banks and Jackson, 1982). While still in school, those unknowingly destined for unemployment were of similar mental health to those headed for a job. Subsequently, however, their paths diverged. The unemployed suffered a reduction in mental health while the employed actually improved in this respect.

Only an investigation the size of the Longitudinal Study of the Office for National Statistics could have the power to demonstrate an effect of unemployment on a rare event like suicide, but such an effect was found. The standardised mortality ratio (SMR – see Chapter Two) for suicide in men and women of working age indicated a risk in the unemployed two to three times that in the general population (Bethune, 1997).

Unemployment and medical care

Another British study, the household panel study (Weich and Lewis, 1998), tested whether unemployment gave rise to common mental problems such as anxiety and depression. Financial strain stood out as a cause of these symptoms, and the state of unemployment, which perpetuated such strain, impeded recovery. Not surprisingly, with the National Health Service providing care free at the point of need, the effects of unemployment fill doctors' waiting rooms (Yuen and Balarajan, 1989) and hospital beds (Campbell et al, 1991). Without such a service, however, physicians can lose business in a recession, as happened, for example, in Michigan in the US in the early 1980s. Many of the more than 10% of American workers unemployed at that time lost their medical insurance with their job. Private medical insurance being beyond their pocket when they needed it most, the unemployed forsook a doctor's opinion in order to cover financial commitments such as the rent. Waiting rooms stood empty and some doctors left for more affluent areas (Frey, 1982).

Unemployment and lifespan

Some of the most reliable data on the effects of unemployment on health and lifespan have come from the Longitudinal Study of the Office for National Statistics (Moser et al, 1987; 1990). A detailed analysis of the findings up to 1992 has been conducted for men and women of working age in 1981 (Bethune, 1997). The definition of unemployment, seeking work or waiting to start work in the week before the national Census of 1981 fitted 9.4% of men and 4.1% of women. Those unable to work at that time because of temporary or permanent illness were excluded from the analysis. The SMR for the employed over subsequent years was better than the national average at 84 in men and 80 in women, while for the unemployed the respective figures were considerably worse at 132 and 133. The temporary and permanently sick had SMRs of at least 250 (SMR for the general community is 100 by definition).

The unemployed were crowded into the lower occupational classes, 21% of men in social class V looking for work as compared with about 3% in social class I. Nevertheless, in all social classes the death rate was higher in the unemployed than the employed. When the researchers looked further back to the employment record at the census of 1971, the SMR for men who were employed both in 1971 and 1981 was found to be 83. For those working in one period but not in the other the SMR was 127, and for men unemployed on both occasions 194. Similar findings have been observed in Finland (Martikainen and Valkonen, 1996).

The Longitudinal Study has dispelled any doubt that unemployment leads to an increased risk of sickness and premature death, a fact emphasised by another British study conducted in 24 towns (Morris et al, 1994). Middle-aged men were recruited between 1978 and 1980, and each man's employment record was noted for the five years before examination and the five years afterwards. For the purposes of this investigation all who had experienced unemployment in the period prior to recruitment were excluded from the analysis. Of the 6,191 men who had been in continuous employment before entry, 71% remained in employment over the next five years, 6% fell out of work prematurely because of illness, 15% became unemployed for reasons other than ill health, and 8% retired prematurely while in good health.

Details of the medical history, smoking habits and alcohol intake had been recorded on recruitment, which meant that the effects of these characteristics on risk of death in each group could be allowed for before proceeding to look for effects of unemployment and premature retirement. Men who became unemployed for reasons unrelated to health had a death rate almost 50% higher than the regularly employed, while for men retiring on grounds other than health the mortality was 86% higher. Thus here also, unexpected and premature loss of work increased the risk of death in men who had been given a clean bill of health while still in work. Even the death rate from cancer was raised in the unemployed, puzzling the investigators who could not understand why unemployment should have such an effect when smoking habits had been taken into account. However, puzzlement may simply reflect our limited understanding of what triggers cancer.

As the *British Medical Journal* put it: "Unemployment is far too important an issue to be left to economists" (Smith, 1985). Here was political medicine speaking out. Faced in 1995 with the highest level of unemployment in Canada for about 50 years, the *Canadian Medical Association Journal* carried a review of the medical evidence (Jin et al, 1995) similar to that of its British counterpart. This updated analysis came to essentially the same conclusions. Unemployment strikes at health, particularly in the mentally and physically vulnerable.

Instability of income and life expectancy

When Mikhail Gorbachev became General Secretary of the Communist Party of the USSR in 1985 he assumed responsibility for an ailing economy. Economic growth in the Russia of the 1980s was less than half of what it had been in the 1960s. Gorbachev's answer was *glasnost* and *perestroika* as he struggled to democratise and modernise the nation. Despite a surfeit of advice from Western bankers, economists and governments, his country continued to stagger from one economic or political crisis to the next throughout the 1990s, most notably the collapse of Communism in 1991. In mid-August 1998, gross domestic product having fallen by almost 5% over the previous year and real incomes by 8%, the rouble was suddenly drastically devalued. Throughout, the toll on life was tremendous.

For more than 70 years, unemployment of able-bodied persons of working age had been a criminal offence in the USSR. Joblessness was so alien to the national psyche that the economic crisis produced far less unemployment than would have similar disasters in Western Europe or the US. Employers and employees struggled to maintain some kind of working relationship. Workers in the public and business sectors took reduced wages, worked short-time, and even received late payment. Some enterprises collapsed but the overall outcome was increased labour turnover rather than soaring unemployment. In 1994, for example, new recruitments amounted to 21% of the workforce (Parker and Layard, 1996, pp 111-15). Thus when examining the Russian experience it made sense to look at the health effects of income insecurity in terms of labour turnover rather than outright unemployment.

In 1987, life expectancy for Russia's male new-born was 64.9 years, but by 1996 it had fallen by 8% to 59.8 years. For female new-born the fall was less marked, from 74.6 to 72.5 years. There were noticeable regional differences, however, some parts faring better than others (Jozan and Prokorskas, 1997). These contrasting experiences have been explored by relating the regional fall in life expectancy to social indicators and economic factors (Walberg et al, 1998). Labour turnover was expressed as the sum of job losses and job gains per 1,000 employees in medium and large enterprises in 1993 and 1994. Trends in household income were obtained from large surveys. Equity in the distribution of income was expressed by the Robin Hood index; that is, the share of the total income that needs to be transferred from the wealthier half to the poorer half to leave each with equal shares. Trends in crime rates were used as a gauge of social cohesion.

Regional falls in life expectancy were related most strongly to the increase in labour turnover. Lesser but still impressive associations were found between the magnitude of the fall and the rise in crime. When the crime figures were omitted from the analysis, then the Robin Hood index assumed more significance as a predictor of loss of life. The more the job insecurity, the greater the disparity between the incomes of richer and poorer, the greater the rise in crime, and the wealthier the region experiencing these changes, then the greater the increase in risk of premature death. Much of this loss of life was due to accidents, injuries, violence, alcohol-related illness and heart disease.

An association between mortality and instability of income has also been found in the US (McDonough et al, 1997). In the American panel study of income dynamics a national sample of households and individuals was interviewed in 1968 and re-visited yearly thereafter. In 1989 more than half of the surviving participants were still taking part. For analysis, a series of overlapping 10 year intervals of follow-up was constructed. Then in each decade several economic and demographic characteristics were measured over the first five years and related to mortality in the subsequent five years. Among the economic indices were several designed to capture income instability. One such index was based on a loss of 50% of income or more from one year to the next. When families with low incomes (less than $20,000), middle incomes and high incomes ($70,000 or more) were each divided into those experiencing no income instability as defined, and those who had at least one 50% fall in a five year period, the researchers arrived at six categories. A strong and inverse relation between level of income and premature mortality was clearly seen, but on top of this income instability also had a major effect on mortality, especially in middle income families. In families with stable incomes the premature death rate in the middle income band was almost 50% higher than in those with high incomes. In families experiencing one or more sudden and serious losses of income, mortality in the middle income band was more than twice that of the wealthiest families. Neither health status at the start of the study, nor age, nor ethnicity had any appreciable influence on these findings.

In February 1998, Secretary of State for Health Frank Dobson presented to parliament the Green Paper *Our healthier nation: A contract for health* (Department of Health, 1998). The document openly declared: "Poor people are ill more often and die sooner. To tackle these fundamental inequalities we must concentrate attention and resources on the areas most affected by air pollution, poverty, low wages, unemployment, poor housing, crime and disorder, which can make people ill both in body and mind." On unemployment it was unequivocal:"Losing his job doubles the chances of a middle-aged man dying within the next five years" (Department of Health, 1998, p 17). There would appear to be a *prima facie* case against unemployment on both health and economic grounds: the cost in associated ill health and crime must be enormous. The social security Budget in the UK, much of it to offset the ill effects of low pay and unemployment, was then "the equivalent of almost £80 every week for every household in the country" (Department of Social Security, 1998, p 11). No wonder therefore that the Labour administration in it's *A new contract for welfare* declared "work for those who can" (Department of Social Security, 1998, p iii). "Being in work is good for your health", said the government (Department of Health, 1998, p 17), and economists would not disagree. John Kenneth Galbraith said "the first requirement is that there be ample employment and income opportunity, not enforced inactivity" (Galbraith, 1996, pp 27-8).

Unemployment and inflation – the poor on the horns of an artificial dilemma

While those working for the 'Welfare' arm of Welfare Capitalism are quite adamant when they say 'the less unemployment the better', the guardians of the 'Capitalism' arm speak less assuredly. In 1998, the Bank of England declared: "the earnings data suggested that unemployment was well below the rate compatible with stable inflation. In that case it was probable that unemployment would have to rise to hit the inflation target" (Bank of England, 1998, para 25). When the Bank and the Treasury talk of 'rise', they think in terms of hundreds of thousands of unemployed men and women. The government's advisors calculated that 500,000 workers would need to feel the hard times of unemployment in order to restrain price rises. Indeed, even Galbraith accepts that there cannot be full employment and stable prices at the same time in the market economy as we know it. He believes the best that can be done is to compensate the unemployed in some way and offset the effects of moderate inflation which he regards as inevitable. But the Welfare in Welfare Capitalism is poor compensation for the toll taken on the health of this half million and their dependants. Many of the studies linking unemployment to premature death were undertaken during the 1970s and 1980s, when social security and unemployment benefit as percentages of national income stood at record levels.

Governments, bankers and businessmen have all been remarkably influenced by a single work which Milton Freidman described as 'deservedly celebrated as an important and original contribution'. The article, published in 1958, must be one of the most thumbed and annotated of all to emanate from the London School of Economics in recent times. Supported by a grant from the Ford Foundation, A.W. Phillips of that School and the Australian National University set about plotting the annual unemployment rate against the rate of change in wage levels (a guide to inflation) for each year between 1861 and 1957 (Phillips, 1958). The result took the shape of a curve, seeming to say that when unemployment was very low the rate of increase in wages was marked. As unemployment increased, however, wage inflation receded. At rates of joblessness of 5% or higher wages remained relatively stable from one year to the next. The message seemed clear: "if ... demand were kept at a value which would maintain stable wage rates the associated level of unemployment would be about 5.5%" (Philips, 1958, p 299).

Phillips stressed that his findings were tentative and called for more research. Certainly much of the data was suspect. Before 1911, the main sources of information on unemployment were confined to the records of the trade unions for their members, many of which gave their figures to the Labour Department of the Board of Trade. Only since 1948 has universal national insurance provided a single series of unemployment statistics. The visual impression of a curve depended essentially on data for three clearly aberrant years. Between 1871 and 1873 unemployment figures were close to 1% and wage rises 5 to 9% each year, never to be equalled again in the 97 years examined. These exceptional years were not discussed, but it is perhaps relevant that 1871 was the year of the

Trade Union Act, giving unions legal recognition for the first time, with protection of their strike funds. These aberrant years certainly gave an impression that the effect of almost full employment on the rate of change of wage rates is more serious than is probably the reality. Whether curve or straight line, however, the central message appeared unchanged. The relation was used for a time to justify toleration of inflation as the price to pay for a low unemployment rate. This policy was condemned by Milton Friedman, who argued that in the long run the Labour force would learn to anticipate inflation and the trade unions would demand compensation in the wage packet rather than accept the reduction in real wages that inflation had caused. Friedman undertook the additional work called for by Phillips, taking theory one notch further. He claimed that for any set of economic conditions there was a unique or 'natural' rate of unemployment. At this rate wage rates were stable, but the unemployment rate was resistant to reduction by fiscal or monetary expansionist policies of the type advocated by Maynard Keynes, designed to raise the demand for goods and services (Friedman, 1968). In fact it was James Callaghan who announced the formal break with Keynesianism at the Labour Party conference in 1976 when he was Prime Minister.

'Supply-side' economic measures were now tried, as advocated by Friedman. Taxes were to be cut to encourage productive effort through higher rewards, while the growth in the money supply was to be held constant to check inflation. Control of the money supply demanded retraction of the public sector, announced Sir Keith Joseph. The nation seemed to be reverting to the pre-Keynesian era of the 1920s, when the Treasury held that State borrowing and raised expenditure would produce only marginal gains in employment rates at best. By 1986, cut-backs in public expenditure to levels last seen in the mid-1970s had produced a general deterioration in public services. In some parts of the country there were reports of schoolchildren needing to share textbooks. Yet in the same year the unemployment rate stood at close to 12%, not seen since 1939. The 1986 Report of the Archbishop of Canterbury's Commission on the Urban Priority Areas, *Faith in the city*, found Britain to present 'an elaborate picture of inequality'. It was Sir Keith Joseph who declared that 'monetarism is not enough'.

For those who trace the roots of unemployment largely to the original privatisation of Rent and the superimposition of taxes on Wages and Interest, as described in Chapter Three, Friedman's natural rate of unemployment was 'natural' only in the sense that it was natural for the lame to limp. By 'natural' Friedman did not mean to imply 'in harmony with the natural order' but in 'harmony with the order of the Capitalist economy as practised'.

How far from this elusive natural rate of unemployment politicians are prepared to veer, and how much inflation they are prepared to accept, is largely a matter of fashion. Not so long ago, governments preferred to err on the side of low unemployment and face up to inflation. In 1998 it was a very different story. On 3rd June, Chancellor of the Exchequer Gordon Brown wrote to the Governor of the Bank of England, reminding him of the Bank's responsibilities under the new Bank of England Act (Bank of England, 1998, para 25):

> a. to maintain price stability, and
>
> b. *subject to that*, to support the economic policy of Her Majesty's government, including its objectives for growth and employment [author's italics]

There could be no clearer statement that, unlike in former years, employment policy took second place to inflation policy. Yet this order of priority was not Brown's to claim, having been resurrected by Sir Keith Joseph in a speech delivered in Preston in September 1974. Inflation, then at 17%, was 'threatening to destroy society' and the fear of unemployment had to be overcome. New Labour has picked up the banner previously held aloft by the Conservatives and enshrined its emblazoning in law. In October 1999 figures were released showing a fall in unemployment, plus a rise of 5.4% in pay to the growing service sector during the previous year. The Chancellor's response was immediately to issue a stern caution against 'paying ourselves more than we earn'. So while 'ample employment' remains in theory the first requirement, in reality the market is not able to deliver anything close to this goal. Indeed the practitioners of Business Capitalism dismally acquiesce to rising unemployment at times, over-ruling the niceness of Welfare.

The Labour administration talks of the three ages of Welfare: the first age – stopping outright destitution; the second age – alleviating poverty; and the third (modern) age – preventing poverty. Their 'third way' will take Britain into this third age, by promoting opportunity instead of dependence: opportunities to work created through education, training and other support (Department of Social Security, 1998, p 2). But in the way of all markets, improving the quality of the workforce supplied will not have significant effects on demand for Labour during a downturn of the economy. A more meaningful way of viewing the three ages and three ways is from the standpoint of an evolving and maturing political economy. The first age – belief in the primacy of one factor of production only, Capital; the second age – concern only for two factors, Capital versus Labour; the third (future) age – a balanced consideration of all three factors of production: Capital, Labour and Land.

Human nature, the shackles of history, ingrained ways of conceptualising the world around us, long-established laws, and the extreme inertia built into the almost immovable institutional structure of the economy mean that there are strict limits to what we can realistically expect to achieve by way of reform; so the argument runs. However, it is mythical to argue that a much better state of society and its political economy than we now know is not achievable; it is not the case that conservatism necessarily rules completely in economic affairs. For far too long, businessmen – capitalists have told us that there is no other way but theirs, and so we remain stuck in the second age, drawn by the currents into a political vortex, coaxed and coddled with mellifluous rhetoric. In October 1998, a time of economic turbulence which the President of the New York Federal Reserve fallaciously described as "the most serious financial crisis since World War Two", *The Economist* pleaded that there was no call for serious questioning of the system it has consistently promoted ever since the days of the Corn Laws. What its columns advised were 'smaller, useful things that would actually help': Japan must legislate to improve its banking system; other Asian countries must show 'creative thinking' and the 'political will' needed to 'restructure their domestic debt'; Capital markets must be made 'safer' by increasing transparency, with standardisations and coordination of the rules of bank capital (*The Economist*, 10-16 October, 1998, pp 15-16). Underneath all of this special pleading is an insatiable desire to strengthen the market in privatised Rent, rather than acknowledge its destructive behaviour in a global economy.

FIVE

The palliation of penury: socialised education, health and security since 1921

Give currency to reason, improve the moral code of society,
and the theory of one generation will be the practice of the next.
(Thomas Love Peacock [1785-1866] *Melincourt*)

Rent represents the surplus in the national income after the rewards to private citizens for their Labour and use of private Capital have been drawn individually or corporately. As such, Rent cannot justifiably be taken by one sector of the community to the denial of another, for Rent is a return for the collective and indivisible effort of society as a whole. It expresses the reality that the total productivity of the economy far exceeds the sum of the output of its separate parts. For society to benefit from this collective surplus, government has a moral responsibility to gather in the Rent for the benefit of the governed. Rent is a social revenue for social purposes.

What 'ought to be' and what 'is' are not the same. Part II describes the historical processes whereby Rent has been sequestered from the public domain into the private domain, where it constitutes the principle benefit and privilege secured as a legal right within that bundle wrapped in red tape and euphemistically termed land. Land is far, far more than the earth beneath our feet. The advantages gained by that sector with powerful interests in land, at the expense of those whose interest is weak or non-existent, represent the inequitable portion in the entrenched gaps between the materially over-privileged and under-privileged tied to social class differences in health and lifespan. This distortion in the distribution of Rent, more than any other distortion, has been and remains the foundation on which is constructed social class in Britain and many other nations. Access to unearned income, not earned income, is much of what class is all about. Rent in private hands is unearned income, and because this distorted distribution is enshrined in the law of the land, so class is enshrined in that same law. In this most fundamental way the law conflicts with political morality.

Rent being held out of the public domain, governments have been forced to take part of Wages and Interest as revenue for the Welfare needs of the materially under-privileged. This approach is self-defeating, however, for taxation of the productive sector of the economy serves as a dead-weight, most damaging at the margins of the economy. Taxation places in further jeopardy the livelihood of the most insecure and, paradoxically, adds to the need for Welfare. The desire of those with Rent to inflate their over-privileged status generates yet further powerful anti-economic forces. Their speculation throws the economy into reverse gear every time it seems to be making good progress, causing unemployment and bankruptcies to soar. Yet government and its advisers are baffled as to why impoverishment and social exclusion are worsening, especially among those who are of no value to the Labour market, despite rising expenditure on social security.

The Welfare State was constructed to combat the five giant evils of Want, Disease, Ignorance, Squalor and Idleness. Lest there are any who read what follows as an attempt to belittle or deride this institution, let it be said here and now that nothing could be further from the truth. The prime objective is not to dismantle the Welfare State, but to dismantle the system which forces so many able and willing families on to Welfare. The nobility of spirit expressed in the collective solidarity that is national insurance is self-evident, as is the humanity of a system which seeks to protect those who cannot protect themselves against certain consequences of market forces within Capitalism. But when a Labour administration led by Tony Blair claims that it is embarking upon the 'third age' of Welfare – preventing poverty rather than alleviating it – then it needs to show that it recognises the Evil Giant behind the giant evils, which is the appropriation of Rent. Governments cannot claim to be truly moving from the second age of Welfare into the third age without effectively replacing the policies of palliation with those of prevention. Only by looking through Welfare Capitalism, rather than at its reflection, is the mistreatment of Rent clearly exposed as a prime cause of much that Welfare seeks to redress.

The following review of 20th century campaigns to alleviate unemployment and low pay shows the extraordinary lengths to which reforming governments have gone to reign in those five giant evils, only to end up with the gap between under-privilege and over-privilege as wide as ever. Education is considered because so much faith has been placed on the defeat of Ignorance. Health is considered because our primary concern is with social class differences in morbidity and mortality. Social security during working life is reviewed because involuntary unemployment and low income originating from the privatisation of Rent are prime sources of Idleness and Want. Housing policy is examined because Squalor is a major reason for mental and physical sub-health and ill health, and privatisation of Rent is a major cause of the unaffordability of decent housing for the under-privileged. Of obvious importance though they are, child allowances and old age pensions are not reviewed in detail because inequitable material deprivation at these times of life is the direct outcome of deprivation in the adult working years.

Education

In the mythical perfect market economy described in textbooks of economics, there are perfect consumers, perfect producers and perfect market conditions. Perfect consumers are gifted with a perfect knowledge of the market, perfectly equipped mentally and psychologically to interpret this information correctly, and completely free to act rationally so as to maximise benefits in a manner commensurate with their differing incomes. But who amongst us can make perfect judgements on such matters as private health insurance, education for our children, or the best holiday on offer? We frequently turn to brokers and experts, but how perfect is their advice? John Stuart Mill, though a proponent of laissez-faire, recognised such flaws in the free market economy and was willing to tolerate government intervention in such circumstances. As he put it: "Letting alone, in short, should be the general practice: every departure from it, unless required by some great good, is a certain evil" (Mill, 1876, p 573). He further asked: "But if the workman is generally the best selector of means, can it be affirmed with the same universality, that the consumer, or person served, is the most competent judge of the end? Is the buyer always qualified to judge of the commodity? If not, the presumption in favour of the competition of the market does not apply to the case; and if the commodity be one in the quality of which society has much at stake, the balance of advantages may be in favour of some mode and degree of intervention, by the authorised representatives of the collective interest of the State" (Mill, 1876, p 575).

To overcome this serious flaw in the market system, Mill advocated universal state education. The uneducated cannot judge perfectly what they need in the way of education or judge the abilities of the teacher.

Government, guided by experts, may err in individual cases, but must be able to do better in general. Mill went so far as to grant government the right to impose on parents a legal obligation to arrange for their children's elementary education. In return, the State was obliged to ensure universal access to instruction, irrespective of ability to pay.

Self-evidently also, access to the middle and higher occupational classes has become dependent increasingly on a formal background education and attainment of the necessary qualifications and skills. However, even an elementary education cannot be paid for in full from the wages of the lowest paid. Hence the provision of an education at the expense of the State was deemed eminently justifiable because it would raise standards of poor people both as producers and consumers, and at least in theory would increase their prospects of upward social mobility and an increased lifespan. Universal education to a common standard was expected to reduce inequalities of opportunity, hence inequalities of income and wealth, and hence inequalities in health and life expectancy.

Education is obviously of fundamental importance, and John Stuart Mill was not alone as its strong advocate. Even today, many casual observers and serious students believe that the problems of the lower social classes can be rectified by improved education, including health education. Once the lower social classes learn to function more effectively in society, their troubles will be over, so the argument runs. Education is seen as the key to upward mobility for those who are relatively impoverished, hastening the demise of poverty and the ill health that goes with it.

Mill noted how in his day the demarcations between grades of Labour were almost equivalent to an hereditary caste. Those who entered specific occupations were recruited essentially from the children of those already employed there, or in employments of the same 'social estimation'. Advocates of the laissez-faire competitive market were dismayed at "the limitations imposed by social circumstances on the free competition of labour" (Goldthorpe, 1987, p 4). Late-Victorian society was, in other words, essentially closed by the class system, and inequalities of opportunity and condition were very marked. In order that this rigid hierarchical structure with its impenetrable social barriers should give way to egalitarianism, class-consciousness needed a dose of enlightenment, the task of a persuasive education.

The advent of State education

Mill, who sat as a Radical in parliament between 1865 and 1868, lived to witness the right of every child to an elementary education secured in 1870 during Gladstone's first administration. The Education Act of that year is associated with the Bradford woollen manufacturer, William Edward Forster, whose surveys in four cities had revealed that less than 10% of citizens had received any schooling. Clearly, voluntary schools and church schools were doing not nearly enough. Forster, as Vice President of Education, shifted State involvement in public education from simple subsidy of existing voluntary schools to the supplementation of the voluntary system with the school board system. The boards were empowered to establish elementary schools, financed out of a local education rate together with central grants. Gladstone's second Liberal administration of 1880 took a further step with Mundella's Education Act, making attendance at school compulsory between ages five and 10. Fees were about threepence (3d) per week, but boards had the power to remit these for poor families.

The need for board inspectors was virtually abolished by the Fee Grant Act of 1891, which made free elementary education the norm in many parts of the country. Once State elementary schooling was free, paupers' children could leave the Poor Law schools and sit alongside other children in the State schools.

Up to 1890, a school's entitlement to central subsidy was tied to its attainment in reading, writing and arithmetic, tested by examination. This system caused schools to focus heavily on these basics, to the neglect of a broader education, so the system was abolished in that year. Educators were from then on free in theory to concentrate on more advanced curricula. The next major move came in 1900, when the school leaving age was raised from 10 years to 12 years. These extra two years could not be filled simply with more reading, writing and arithmetic, but a test case instigated by Robert Morant of the Board of Education (the Cockerton judgement of 1901) held that the London School Board had no right in law to offer more advanced courses. The result of this crisis was Balfour's Education Act of the following year. School boards were abolished. The multi-purpose county councils and county borough councils were empowered to provide elementary and secondary education, while non-county boroughs with populations of at least 10,000 and urban district councils serving at least 20,000 were responsible for elementary education.

Lord John Russell had a longstanding interest in education, having raised the central grant to elementary schools in 1839. In February 1870 he made a powerful speech in favour of Forster's Education Bill. Russell strongly advocated the introduction of the Bible, but accompanied by purely undenominational teaching. The *Saturday Review* claimed the proposal was absurd, but the great majority of school boards adopted Russell's idea. All did not go smoothly, however. By 1900, local effort had still not secured a complete national system of elementary education, and there was simmering sectarian discontent. What caused Lloyd George difficulty as a Radical Welsh backbencher was that part of Balfour's Act which provided funds from local rates to support denominational schools. In return the religious schools were to accept supervision by the local education committee to ensure standards. In 1901 about 54% of the elementary school population in England and Wales, or about 2.5 million children under 12 years of age, attended about 5,700 board schools run by 2,500 locally elected boards. But 46% were in voluntary schools and about one million Non-conformist children belonged to parishes where the only school was Anglican. This difficulty had been side-stepped by a 'conscience clause', giving parents the right to remove their children from religious instruction. Nevertheless, the large Non-conformist majority in Wales objected to their rates supporting Anglicanism, and Lloyd George in opposition was expected to fight their corner. The issue rumbled on to cause the Conservative government considerable trouble up to its downfall in late 1905.

State education and social fluidity

Between 1921 and 1991 Britain's population grew by 31% from 44 million to almost 58 million. With this expansion came massive advances in economic performance, growth of the Welfare State, and major changes in the occupational structure of the population. In 1921 about 77% of jobs were manual, but by 1971 the percentage had fallen to 62% (Routh, 1980, pp 6-7) (Table 5.1), and by 1981, 52% (Routh, 1987, p 38). In 1980, according to the national Census, the percentage of the male working population in the skilled manual class had increased to 37, while the respective figures for semi-skilled occupations and unskilled occupations were 17% and about 7% (Office of Population Censuses and Surveys, 1984, p xvii). By the time of the 1991 national census the percentages of 'economically active' men classified as semi-skilled and unskilled had dropped further to about 15 and five, respectively (Office of Population Censuses and Surveys, 1992, p 417). The trend during this century has

Table 5.1: Percentage of male working population by occupational class in Great Britain

	1911	1921	1931	1951	1971
Higher professional	1.3	1.4	1.5	2.6	4.9
Lower professional	1.6	2.0	2.0	3.2	6.0
Employers, administrators, managers	11.7	12.0	12.2	12.5	16.0
Clerical workers	5.5	5.4	5.5	6.4	6.4
Foremen, inspectors, supervisors	1.8	1.9	2.0	3.3	5.0
Skilled manual	33.0	32.3	30.0	30.4	29.1
Semi-skilled manual	33.6	28.3	28.9	27.9	20.8
Unskilled	11.6	16.7	17.9	13.8	11.9
Employers/self-employed	10.8	10.9	9.6	8.6	9.3
Employees	89.2	89.0	89.1	91.4	90.8

therefore been a steady decline in the proportion of men in manual occupations, balanced by expansion in the professional and middle classes. Women, particularly married women, have increasingly moved out of the home, many taking lower-paid work in the non-manual sector.

These changes in occupational structure obviously call for education but do not in themselves require a Welfare State and publicly funded education, though of course public education may have accelerated the pace of change. They are what one would expect as society progressed from the pocket ready-reckoner to the laptop computer, and from candlelight to nuclear power. Mechanisation, automation, computerisation, the replacement of muscle power by the combustion engine, these and more have displaced the manual worker and encouraged the growth of the service industries. Universal education was intended to 'level the playing field' to some extent, enabling those with a family background of manual work to compete more effectively for the expanding opportunities in the non-manual sector. In other words, while the economic goal of education policy was to improve national competitive efficiency, the Welfare goal was the relative improvement in the prospects of lower social classes. Those on the lowest rung of the economic ladder should have been given 'a leg up' by universal education.

To what extent has State education contributed to the diminution in social class V? The question is important, for if education policy under Welfare Capitalism has promoted the prospects of upward social mobility for the children of the old working classes, as intended, then it will have improved their prospects for health and longevity, even though the gaps in lifespan between class I and the smaller class V have remained essentially undisturbed.

Without doubt, the most thorough study of social mobility in Britain is that undertaken by the Social Mobility Group at Nuffield College in Oxford (Goldthorpe, 1987). The data were collected in 1972 from men aged 20 to 64 years resident in England and Wales. They were a population sample drawn from the electoral register, and 82% participated. A seven category classification provided a relatively sophisticated differentiation of occupational function and employment status. Class I were the higher paid professionals. Class II were lower grade professionals and higher grade technicians, often carrying 'staff' status, with salaries generally below those of class I. Class III were 'rank-and-file' service employees or 'white collar' force. Class IV comprised small proprietors, smallholders and self-employed artisans with incomes covering a wide range but less secure than a salary. Class V were 'blue collar elite' lower grade technicians and supervisors of the 'working' classes VI and VII. Class VI were skilled manual workers, and class VII semi-skilled and unskilled manual workers and agricultural workers.

The survey related the status of the father when his son was aged 14 years to that of the son at three stages of his own working life – on entry into adult work, 10 years further on, and at his 'maturity of working life'. While only about 7 % of fathers were in class I, almost 14% of their sons were at this level. The sons in class I were from all social backgrounds, but slightly more than 25% had a father in class I. Thus self-recruitment into class I was more than three times greater than had all sons possessed an equal chance of obtaining a class I occupation (Goldthorpe, 1987, p 44). Furthermore, had Class I been defined more narrowly, say to include only the top 5% of occupations rather than the top 14% as constructed for the analysis, then mobility into class I would have been much less and 'self-recruitment' almost certainly much higher.

There was, of course, considerable occupational mobility during working life. Only about 30% of men of class I and class II origins went straight into these classes on starting work; but of those who did not, half eventually returned there through career promotions. On the other hand, 75% of working class sons took a 'working class' first job, and about one in three of these moved into intermediate or higher positions over time. The relevant question was to what extent intragenerational and intergenerational upward mobility were simply due to opportunities created by advances in technology and growth of the service industries, and how much could be credited to the 'leg up' effect of State education as part of Welfare. The data showed clearly that economic advancement had certainly created a demand for recruitment from all social backgrounds into the growing service class. This expansion of class I and class II jobs not only strengthened intergenerational stability in these classes (the son of a class I or class II father had an improved chance of finding work at the father's level), but also opened 'new doors' for the sons of working class fathers. However, analysis of relative mobility rates of the different occupational classes into the service classes and into the working classes gave no reason to believe that the Welfare State and universal State education had broken down class barriers and 'opened up' society to any significant extent. If education was teaching 'openness', society did not seem to be learning.

Take, for example, men born between 1908 and 1917. The likelihood of those who were the sons of class I and class II fathers finding themselves in class I and class II at the maturation of their working life was almost four times higher than that of the sons of class VI and class VII fathers. Compare this with the condition of men born between 1938 and 1947, educated after Richard Austen (Rab) Butler's Education Act of 1944 (free State education for all up to at least 15 years of age from 1947). The respective figure was about three and a half, though this was probably an underestimate because many men of class I and class II parental origins had not yet achieved their 'mature' occupational status when the data were collected in 1972. Now let us examine what the data said about what was happening at the other end of the social scale. For men born between 1908 and 1917, the probability of the son of a class VI or class VII father being himself in class VI or class VII at his occupational maturity was three and a third times greater than that of the son of a class I or class II father. For men born a generation later in 1938 to 1947, the respective figure was not three and a third, but a little more than four and a half (Goldthorpe, 1987, p 76).

These figures 'go against the grain' of the Welfare State. Had State education fulfilled its Welfare role and given the sons of classes VI and VII a leg up, then its expansion after 1944 should have improved the relative chances of social advancement for class VI/VII sons born in 1938 to 1947 as compared with those born in 1908 to 1917. This did not happen. The Welfare State's provision of education must therefore have been impotent to overcome older entrenched forces in society that prevented the doors of opportunity opening more welcomingly to those outside, even though it placed more better educated and 'presentable' candidates at the threshold.

Goldthorpe and colleagues concluded that policies designed to improve equalities of opportunity had not been accompanied by improvements in equality of 'condition'. 'Social fluidity' had not changed so as to create a more open society. 'Immigrants', whether domestic or from overseas, are taken into a social class only as and when the economy demands, and not because of any evolving sense of greater fairness or true motivation to seek out and get rid of social inequities. The size of the old working class has been reduced by economic advancement with attendant education, but contrary to intention the diminution was not accelerated by State education.

Education and social attitudes

'Positive discrimination' is never voluntary: privilege and prejudice do not defer to education by the State. Haralambos and Holborn (1990, pp 228-53) have reviewed a range of viewpoints on the role of education. There were those, such as Emile Durkheim, who stressed the importance of the transmission of society's values through teaching and example, by inculcating 'social solidarity' from an early age. Within this shell of social cohesion, personalities develop and skills are acquired which equip the child for effective participation in a complex industrial society. The difficulty from this perspective is that education systems subserve the social system in which they are located, and therefore just as easily perpetuate a 'closed' society as an 'open' society, as they manifestly did in the past and to some extent still do. In 1999, 8% of students at Oxford and Cambridge universities were from working class homes. In the new universities such as Glamorgan, Thames Valley and Wolverhampton, the respective figures ranged between 35 and 45% (Carvel, 1999).

Those who view modern society as a 'free-for-all', competitive and aggressive, hold that education should prepare its pupils accordingly. Status, admiration and rewards are based on worth in the market place, and they argue that an individualistic, competitive ethos in schools prepares children for just such a life in adulthood. Again, such viewpoints reinforce the current social order, 'warts and all'. Schools may try to create models of 'equality of opportunity' in the classroom but have to accept that beyond the playground society is busily perpetuating age-old inequitable inequalities of condition: inequalities which the pupils bring with them into school. What enlightened and well-meaning teachers teach, and what everyday life teaches, are by no means the same.

Many educationists, recognising that it is society rather than the schoolroom or playing field that transmits values and acts as a proving ground, stress the role of education in developing individual full potential and a rounded personality. Individuals, with individual personalities, are then better equipped to examine the values and norms of their society in a critical and more 'Liberal' manner, with, in consequence, improved chances of reform for the better. Education *per se* does not break down class barriers; only the enlightened can accomplish that task.

To overcome the phenomenon of inequitable impoverishment of wealth and health, society does not need to educate the impoverished: it needs to educate itself. Those classes and neighbourhoods that are not impoverished perceive the faults creating impoverishment as being rooted in impoverished classes and neighbourhoods, while in reality they are the consequences of ethnocentric forces which operate throughout society, one effect of which is to distort perceptions. Programmes designed to treat these consequences, focused exclusively on the poor, such as the designation of 'education priority areas' to pump resources into 'dysfunctional regions', are well-meaning but misconceived. The physician who treats a dysfunctional heart, without recognising that the cause lies not within the heart but in a diseased thyroid gland, can never hope to cure the patient; so it is with programmes of a Welfare nature designed to alleviate the symptoms and pathology of poverty. It seems odd at first that an endocrinologist should hold the key to a disease of the heart, that is until human physiology is fully understood. So also it seems odd that a key to impoverishment, ill health and a reduction in lifespan should be located in Rent reform, that is until the fundamentals of the political economy are grasped.

Taxation for State education

State education has been immensely popular. As Table 5.2 shows, total spending by the taxpayer on the system increased more than 40-fold between 1918 and 1993. Some of this increase reflects the growth of population, but total spending per head of population under 15 years of age (ignoring the increase in school leaving age to 16 in 1972) increased by 50-fold, because this age group numbered 10,700,000 in 1991 but 12,300,000 in 1921. As a proportion of the national income (nett national product at factor cost), expenditure on education more than doubled in response to Fisher's Education Act of 1918, but further growth was very slow during most of the 1920s and 1930s, and fell back during the Second World War to levels of the early 1920s. Following the introduction and development of the post-war system of comprehensive free education up

Table 5.2: State expenditure on education, UK 1918-93 (in '1993 pounds')[1]

Year	Total (millions)	Per head of population under 15 years	As % of national income[2]	Notes
1918	809.5	64	1.11	Fisher's Education Act. School leaving age raised to 14 yrs. Abolition of elementary school fees. Continuation classes for those over 14 years.
1922	1,458.7	120	2.33	The Geddes 'Axe'. Education cuts including cancellation of continuation classes.
1938	2,574.9	229	2.72	5.8% of 18 year olds enter full-time education beyond 14 years.
1944	2,316.4	205	1.76	Butler's Education Act. Comprehensive National Education System. Free education for all up to 15 years of age. Free school meals, milk, transport.
1947	3,815.6	338	2.75	School leaving age raised to 15 years from 1st April.
1963	12,076.7	963	5.78	The Robbins Report. All capable of benefiting from higher education should be entitled to it.
1972	21,595.0	1,637	7.83	School leaving age raised to 16 years.
1976	25,362.0	2,042	7.84	Education Act. Local Authorities to submit plans for comprehensive education.
1980	26,481.3	2,273	7.44	85% of state schools are comprehensive. Education Act. Abolition of local authority requirement to submit plans for comprehensive schools.
1988	30,254.5	2,759	6.39	Education Reform Act (Kenneth Baker). Schools right to opt for grant-maintained status. Parental right to select child's school. National curriculum.
1993	33,929.0	3,196	7.00	

[1] Newman, O. and Foster, A. (1995) *Value of the pound. Prices and incomes in Britain 1900-1993*, New York: Gale Research International, p 305.

[2] Nett national product at factor cost. Estimates of A. R. Prest, 1870-1946 in Mitchell, B.R. (1962) *Abstract of British historical statistics*, Cambridge: Cambridge University Press, p 368. More recent estimates are those of the Central Statistical Office.

to 15 years of age, expenditure as a proportion of national income almost trebled between 1947 and 1976. From then onwards, however, this process went into decline until 1990. As a proportion of national income, spending on State education increased by a little more than six fold between 1918 and 1993.

Health education

Universal education could improve the health of the poor by encouraging a healthful lifestyle. Certainly those charged with the health of society have no doubts about the value of education for future physical and mental well-being. Children who do well at school and stay on to college or university tend to make healthier choices as adults than those of the same social background who do less well educationally; for example their diet is better, they smoke less and they take more exercise (Wadsworth, 1991). In an American longitudinal survey (House et al, 1994) of a sample of about 3,600 men and women aged 25 years or older, the level of education and the level of income both had something separate to say about health and physical mobility at any given age in working life, especially in the middle-aged. The more education received before adulthood, the better was health and physical mobility in adulthood, even after allowance for income. Rates of disorders such as high blood pressure and heart disease found at a particular age in the least educated group were not seen in the most educated group until perhaps 20 years later. Those with the least education are as a group the most exposed to adverse biological, social and financial stresses and are the least equipped to deal with them. Thus a good education goes a long way towards a good and healthy life within each social class, but set in the British social milieu manifestly cannot close the gaps in health between the occupational social classes.

Health

Impoverishment is most life-threatening when sickness intervenes and the power to hold house and home together is thereby critically diminished. Perhaps this is why the humaneness of the National Health Service makes it the most cherished aspect of Britain's Welfare State. Before the mid-1970s, expenditure on State education always exceeded that on the National Health Service; from then on the order has been reversed. In 1921 a little under 1% of the national income was spent by government on health; in 1993 the figure was more than 9%, an 11 fold increase over 72 years. The respective percentages for education were about 2 and 7, representing a three-and-a-third-fold rise. The difference is accounted for partly, but by no means entirely, by the ageing of an expanding population.

Inter-war development of the health services

In many respects, the National Health Service of 1948 was shaped many years earlier by the Consultative Council on Medical and Allied Services appointed by the first Minister of Health, then Dr Christopher Addison, under the chairmanship of the future Lord Dawson, as part of national reconstruction after 1918 (Ministry of Health, 1920). The system proposed five types of service: domiciliary, primary health centres, district general hospitals, special institutions for fevers, tropical diseases and so on, and the teaching hospitals. The primary health centres would have been the forerunner of the modern group general practice, funding for which eventually followed the massive protest by general practitioners over their status and pay within the National Health Service in 1965. One of the reasons why primary care centres did not evolve in the 1920s was that general practitioners feared that they would threaten their independence, making them employees of the local authorities.

In the event, nothing was done to implement these proposals owing to the state of the economy in the 1920s. General practitioners continued to be paid either through private insurance, or on a fee for service basis, or through the fledgling system of National Health Insurance. Hospital beds continued to be offered through 54 Poor Law infirmaries, more than 700 local authority hospitals, and the voluntary hospitals (which received grants-in-aid from central government at times of financial crisis). The Poor Law infirmaries were so strapped for cash in those years that some boards of guardians resorted to circulating general practitioners with an offer to receive cases at fixed weekly rates of payment as non-Poor Law patients (Ministry of Health, 1921). Some entrepreneurial specialisation also developed in these infirmaries, such as the separate provision of beds for children at Booth Hall in Manchester and Alder Hey in Liverpool. Poor Law dispensaries continued to provide a service for families through the relieving officer, and in 1929 local authorities were empowered to take over these services and incorporate them with the municipal hospitals. Figures gathered from the annual reports of the Ministry of Health (1920-30) and Board of Trade (1932) indicate that

Table 5.3: State expenditure on health, UK 1919-62 (in '1993 pounds')[1]

Year	Total (millions)[2]	Per head of population	As % of national income[3]	Notes
1919	397.0	9.1	0.49	Ministry of Health established. Dr Christopher Addison first Minister of Health.
1921	436.8	9.9	0.82	174,000 public hospital beds, 87,000 voluntary hospital beds.
1929	843.2	18.5	1.08	Local Government Act. Local authorities empowered to convert Poor Law infirmaries to municipal hospitals.
1938	1,480.8	31.2	1.56	176,000 public hospital beds.
1942	1,172.5	24.3	0.98	1st December: Beveridge Report declares that reform of social security must be accompanied by a National Health Service.
1946	1,846.6	37.5	1.45	November: Aneurin Bevan's National Health Service Act. Universal service, free at point of need. Nationalisation of hospitals.
1948	4,949.5	99.8	3.52	5th July. National Health Service launched.
1950	7,418.6	148.3	5.09	Health services costing more than expected.
1951	7,378.5	146.9	4.81	Introduction of charges for dentures and spectacles. Bevan, Harold Wilson and John Freeman resigned from Labour government.
1952	6,680.7	132.4	4.51	Conservatives introduce one shilling prescription charge. Massive pay award to general practitioners. Minister of Health loses seat in Cabinet.
1953	6,541.3	129.0	4.30	Peter Thorneycroft begins to raise payment of the service from national insurance rather than income tax.
1956	7,322.0	142.3	4.39	Claude Guillebaud's Report, based on work of Brian Abel-Smith, notes the fall in spending on health as a percentage of gross national product.
1959	8,114.0	155.4	4.51	Mental Health Act. Beginning of 'care in the community for mentally ill'.
1960	9,141.1	174.2	4.75	Prescription charges raised to two shillings per item. 22% of health expenditure now met by charges and national insurance.
1962	9,460.7	178.5	4.69	Hospital building plan. £500 million earmarked for renewal.

Notes to Table 5.3

[1] Newman, O. and Foster, A. (1995) *Prices and Incomes in Britain, 1900-1993*, New York: Gale Research International, p 305.

[2] Early health service expenditures include local authority hospitals, mental hospitals, medical and related benefits, public health expenses (excluding sewage and refuse disposal), including maternity and child welfare. Statutory sick pay from 1983 and statutory maternity pay from 1987. Data derived from Ministry of Health, *Local Government Financial Statistics, England and Wales. Part I: Poor Relief.* London, HMSO, 1920-1937; Board of Trade. *Statistical Abstract for the United Kingdom.* London, HMSO, 1920-1937 (various years of publication up to 1939); Central Statistical Office, *Annual Abstract of Statistics.* London HMSO, various years up to 1996.

[3] Nett national income at factor cost.

state expenditure on health grew slowly over this period to reach just over 1% of national income by 1929 (see Table 5.3).

Only 2,000 public hospital beds were added to the national stock between 1921 and 1938. A report from the Hospital Almoners Association disclosed that in 1939 conditions almost everywhere could only be described as poor, more so in the North than in the South. Specialist services were generally in short supply, and the costs charged to the non-insured made them think twice about 'running up a doctor's bill', with consequent delay in diagnosis and treatment (Pater, 1981, p 19). Here it is worth repeating what *The Lancet* said in 1942: "Even before the war, there were voices crying in the wilderness that all was not well with the medical services. The burden of their cries was that preventable diseases were not being prevented; that the chances of avoiding death in infancy, in childbirth, from tuberculosis, and from rheumatic carditis were much greater among the rich than the poor; that for most of the population such financial burdens were added to the burdens of ill health as to discourage early treatment; that the standards of treatment available in different places and institutions, and among different social classes, varied enormously; and that the annual income of those who cared for the sick ranged from £40 plus keep and laundry paid to the probationer nurse to the £40,000 earned by the successful surgeon" (*The Lancet*, 1942). In 1939, a married woman had no access to free medical attention unless she was pregnant or had recently given birth. Pupils came under the care of the school medical inspector. Health standards in many families were very low, and the plight of many elderly people was pitiable.

York: a case study of health services development, 1900-38

Seebohm Rowntree reviewed the development of health services in York between 1900 and 1938 (Rowntree, 1941, pp 281-303). In 1900 the city's health department employed nine persons, including the ambulance driver and the disinfecting agent; in 1938 there were more than 50 full-time employees and 18 part-time workers. In 1908 the education committee established a school clinic with a full-time school medical inspector, and over the years the service became so developed that by 1938 every scholar received what medical, surgical, dental and ophthalmic services there were to offer. A voluntary antenatal and infants clinic was taken over by the department and a corporation maternity hospital opened in 1921. In all, by 1938 there was a hospital maintained almost entirely by voluntary subscription, an old Poor Law infirmary maintained by the local authority, a mental hospital, a tuberculosis sanatorium, a maternity hospital, a hospital for infectious diseases, and various clinics and dispensaries.

In 1899 more than 10,000 workers in the city saved for times of sickness through friendly societies and sick clubs, and almost 2,000 more received sickness benefit through Trade Union schemes. Then in 1911 came the National Health Insurance scheme. By 1938 all workers earning not more than £250 annually were compulsorily insured against sickness. Men paid in 4½d and women 4¼d each week, with their employers adding similar amounts and the State about a quarter of the total cost. For this the insured received free medical attention and treatment. Men received 15 shillings (15s) weekly when sick and off work, and women 12s. After 26 weeks these benefits were reduced to 7s 6d and 6s weekly, respectively. The 46,000 insured workers could choose from 44 'panel' doctors and take their prescriptions to 41 chemists. Most workers supplemented this State support by continuing to contribute to a friendly society.

Over this period the general death rate fell by one third, and mortality in infancy by two thirds. Much of this improvement was due to higher standards of drainage, sanitation, water quality, and food and milk hygiene. Consequently by 1938 the population was ageing noticeably and the prevalence of chronic degenerative diseases was rising. Rowntree stressed, however, that poor families in York still lacked the income needed to provide the necessities for full physical health, no matter how careful they were. In families with the equivalent of a disposable income of £2.3s 6d a week or less (after rent), the annual death rate, standardised for age and sex, was 135 per 10,000 in 1935–1936. For those with a disposable income after rent of £2.13s 6d or more the death rate was 38% less, at 84 per 10,000.

Rowntree concluded: "It now remains for us (I hope in a period much shorter than 40 years!) to bring the death rate in classes A and B (the poorest) down to that of classes D and E (the better-off of the working class)." To achieve this goal: "First and most important, the income of classes A and B must be raised, and second, the health services must be still further developed, especially those concerned with the prevention rather than the cure of disease" (Rowntree, 1941, pp 296-303). He recognised that the 'curative' nature of the forthcoming National Health Service would offer little prospect of a significant impact on the health gap between richer and poorer: first and foremost the wealth gap had to be closed.

Preparations for the National Health Service

Plans for comprehensive medical health care evolved over the years between 1939 and 1948. In December 1942 the Beveridge Report was published with its famous 'assumption B', that there would be a comprehensive health service available to all and divorced from any requirement for insurance contributions. The White Paper of 1944 on the universal health service was clear: "The government want to ensure that in future every man and woman and child can rely on getting all the advice and treatment and care which they may need in matters of health; that what they get shall be the best medical and other facilities available; that their getting them shall not depend on whether they can pay for them, or any other factor irrelevant to the real need – the real need being to bring the country's full resources to bear upon reducing ill health and promoting good health in all its citizens" (Ministry of Health and Department of Health for Scotland, 1944).

Taxation for the National Health Service

Financing the National Health Service was planned only partly through National Health Insurance (soon to become simply National Insurance), anticipated at about £36 million (about 25% of the total), with the Exchequer contributing about £103 million and local taxes (the property rate) about £6 million (Pater, 1981, p 115). These estimates proved hopelessly unrealistic, mainly because nobody had recognised the pent-

Table 5.4: State expenditure on health, UK 1964-91 (in '1993 pounds')[1]

Year	Total (millions)[2]	Per head of population	As % of national income[3]	Notes
1964	10,830.9	202.3	4.91	Labour abolishes prescription charges.
1965	11,612.2	215.7	5.08	General practitioners threatened mass resignation from health service. Big pay rise and beginning of financial support for group practices.
1968	13,419.4	245.4	5.46	Labour re-introduces prescription charges with many exemptions. Department of Health and Social Security established, with minister in Cabinet.
1973	19,160.0	345.7	6.21	Regional differences in spending on health service found to be as large as in 1948 (E Trent, £15 per head; NE Thames, £25 per head).
1974	23,263.9	420.0	7.36	British Medical Association demands £500 million to 'save the National Health Service'. More than two million with private health insurance.*
1975	26,050.2	470.7	7.77	Annual 2% rise in expenditure estimated as needed to cover medical advances, population ageing and development of neglected areas. Consultants and junior hospital doctors in prolonged dispute with government.
1979	26,646.5	482.9	7.39	Royal Commission finds too many levels of administration. Area health authorities abolished.
1980	29,760.8	539.8	8.36	Black Report on inequalities in health. Minister declares he wants private health insurance taken out by 20% of population to ease State health expenditure.
1982	29,319.4	530.9	8.46	Beginning of 'efficiency drive'. Beds and wards start to close at end of financial year. Margaret Thatcher; 'The National Health Service is safe with us.'
1983	29,987.9	541.6	8.17	Roy Griffiths of Sainsbury supermarkets recruited to report on management in the health service. Administrators begin to move over to line management system.
1986	31,458.7	564.0	7.70	First closure of a mental hospital.
1987	33,750.7	603.6	7.73	Health service owes £400 million to creditors. Abolition of free eye tests and free dental checks.
1988	36,891.5	658.1	7.79	Health service review by ministers. Ideas of hospital trusts and general practice fund-holding evolve for creation of 'internal market' to improve efficiency.
1991	41,283.0	731.1	8.83	Kenneth Clarke launches review reforms.
1993	44,893.0	791.2	9.26	

Notes for Table 5.4

* Sir Keith Joseph's re-organisation of the National Health Service, aimed at reducing splits between hospital, local authority and general practitioner services. Creation of fourteen regional health authorities, ninety area health authorities, and two hundred district management teams.
For footnotes 1, 2, 3 see Table 5.3.

up need for medical attention. In 1948 expenditure was £334 million at current prices, rather than £145 million, and the difference had to be raised by the Exchequer. Not until 1960 did national insurance approach the intended quarter of total health expenditure.

Governments appear never to have recovered from the shock of the unanticipated expenditure on the health service following the National Health Service Act of 1946. The service began in July 1948. When in 1953 expenditure stood at about 4.5% of national income, an alarmed Conservative administration asked the economist Claude Guillebaud, nephew to Alfred Marshall (see Chapter Thirteen), to consider how 'rising charge' on the Exchequer might be avoided. His small committee consisted of a chemist, an industrialist, a Trade Union nominee and a former Permanent Secretary to the Ministry of Health. Lacking current experience in health affairs, the group was forced to rely on the guidance and advice of expert witnesses. Work in the field of social accounting was passed on to another economist, Brian Abel-Smith, with Richard Titmuss as consultant, under the National Institute of Economic and Social Research. Their memorandum to Guillebaud noted that health expenditure had actually declined as a proportion of national income since 1949. This observation, added to the fact that capital investment in the health service was very low, led the Guillebaud Committee to recommend more expenditure rather than less (Webster, 1988, pp 204-11). Over the next two decades spending on the National Health Service increased steadily (Tables 5.3 and 5.4), despite government attempts to staunch the flow. Significantly, however, in 1973 regional differences in the distribution of this expenditure were still marked, with the poorer North receiving less than the richer South (Timmins, 1996, p 342).

Another leap in health service expenditure accompanied Sir Keith Joseph's re-organisation of administration in the early 1970s, reaching almost 7.5% of national income by 1974 (Table 5.4). Government spending on health per head of population continued to rise up to the pronouncement of the Black Report on Inequalities in Health in 1980 (Townsend et al, 1992). A peak of 8.5% of national expenditure was achieved in 1981, during Margaret Thatcher's first Conservative administration.

Professor Sir Douglas Black, Professor Jerry Morris, Dr Cyril Smith and Professor Peter Townsend rightly argued that the sources of the inequalities in health which they had explored on behalf of the Labour government fell largely outside the scope of the National Health Service. Their 37 recommendations covered not only the health service but also the level of child benefit, maternity grants, infant care allowances, school meals, local authority provision of housing and other ways to assist poorer families (Townsend et al, 1992). The Conservative administration calculated that the additional bill to the taxpayer would exceed £2,000 million a year (over 1% of national income) and considered such an amount to be unrealistic.

As it happened, Labour and Conservative administrations both concluded that the nation was simply not earning enough to meet such expenses – that Labour costs were too high relative to productivity, and expenditure on the Welfare State had to be contained. The Conservative administrations of the 1980s sought to improve 'productivity' and efficiency within the National Health Service, calling in Roy Griffiths of the Sainsbury food empire for advice. A complete re-organisation of management and 'internally competitive markets' were the solutions offered, plus increased charges at the point of need and encouragement of 'customers' to opt instead for private health insurance. The problem for the government was the inability of private health care to deliver as much per pound as the public service, a fact most unpalatable for an administration which viewed the Welfare State as a reason for poor economic performance. The public knew this, and any attempt to limit services offered through the National Health Service was certain to create an adverse reaction. When the average premium for private health insurance increased by 60% between 1981 and 1983, at a time when the retail price index increased only by 14%, the government realised that advocacy of the private system would simply throw the burden off the taxpayer and on to the employer. In order to avoid unpopularity, the government continued to raise expenditure on health, though holding it as a proportion of national income for a time. By 1993, health expenditure was running at more than 9% of national income.

The old rule of thumb, that a 2% increase annually (as a proportion of the previous year's expenditure in real terms) was needed simply to keep up with medical advances, an ageing population and attention to the 'Cinderella' services, remained as true as ever. From the perspective of 'health and wealth' however, it also remained true that a service designed to provide universal treatment of sickness cannot hope to make any significant impact on the reduced life expectancy of poorer families. Basically, there is within the system little in the way of a timely and consistent redistribution of wealth to younger families in deprivation to prevent the premature onset of sub-health and ill health.

Social security

Social security is designed to provide poorer families with additional income in times of need. What counts, however, is not simply the level to which this additional income brings the recipient relative to the national average. Negative effects of potential importance are: adverse psychological, emotional and physical effects of a confirmation of dependency and marginalisation in a society which admires economic independence, affluence and the display of wealth while equating poverty with failure; the response of prices to this re-distribution as they affect poorer families; and adverse economic consequences for poor families of the appropriation of additional revenue from the productive sector to support the system. Taxation for social security damages the economy as surely as taxation for any other purpose, and for this reason has paradoxical effects on the nation's health, as described in Chapter Three.

The jaded economic view of unemployment

The curse of the current economic system is unemployment. We are not discussing here the short periods of unemployment between leaving one job and starting another, nor the unemployment of temporary sickness in persons who can expect a full recovery. We are talking of mass unemployment with national rates of above 10% of the workforce, as occurred consistently between the First and Second World Wars, during the 1980s, again in the early 1990s, and which as sure as 'eggs are eggs' will re-appear at some future date. With mass unemployment there is long term unemployment, reaching the horrific figure of 45% of all unemployed people in 1994. As already discussed (see Chapter Four), this curse has come to be accepted by politicians and economists as an unavoidable evil inextricably harboured within what is otherwise the best of economic systems that man has devised. Recurring mass unemployment is the cross Capitalism has to bear. Such resignation reflects how jaded our economic philosophy has become with experience.

In 1936, John Maynard Keynes wrote that unemployment is "the outstanding fault of the system in which we live.... It is certain that the world will not much longer tolerate the unemployment which, apart from brief intervals of excitement, is associated with present-day capitalistic individualism" (cited in Fraser, 1984, p 198). Keynes mistakenly thought he had given the world a practical way of overcoming the problem, and an explanation for its occurrence. The long period of low unemployment after the Second World War persuaded many that the fault had indeed been corrected, but when unemployment started to rise in the early 1970s and inflation hit an annual rate of 17%, Keynesian doctrine was abandoned. Socialists thought they had the answer when they advocated public ownership of the means of production, but Labour governments proved as powerless as Conservative, James Callaghan having to struggle with an unemployment rate in the late 1970s not seen since before the Second World War.

Students of economics learn that the trade cycle or business cycle has four phases: slump (or depression), recovery, boom and deflation. It is unthinkable, and it has never happened, that the cycle does not run to completion, though the duration of each phase varies from one cycle to the next. The dogma is that recessions are associated with pessimistic expectations and hence little investment, cutbacks in production and unemployment. In the recovery there is more optimism as consumer demand picks up and Labour and Capital are brought back into production. This leads into a boom where there is clearly over-optimism and speculative activity, because, as sure as 'night follows day', deflation follows. Governments, banks and economists try to manage the cycle to cushion its worst effects, but cannot prevent it. One popular theory is that during a recovery, increasing investment generates income, and an increasing income stimulates further investment, this going on until there is full employment. Thereafter, the rise in real income starts to decelerate, leading to a deceleration of investment, and onward into the deflationary phase. These periodicities can be altered in detailed form by 'random' economic events such as a war or a balance of payments crisis, but the fundamental form continues on its own cyclical way.

The most sophisticated of mathematical models have been produced to fit the phenomena, but they remain descriptive rather than explanatory. The repertoire of those given the job of management of the economy is restricted to manipulation of interest rates on capital, control of wages in the public sector, shifts in taxation of wages and interest, and government borrowing for public expenditure to raise demand. The importance of the markets in land and Rent (see Chapter Three) never even enters consciousness, or so it would seem.

Table 5.5: Unemployment insurance (UI) and poor relief (PR) (in '1993 pounds', various years)

Year	Total (millions)	Per head of population*	As % of national income	Notes
1921 UI	695.0	23.7	1.31	Proof of 'seeking work' required for entitlement to unemployment benefit without national insurance cover.
PR	394.4	8.9	0.74	
1927 UI	759.7	24.8	1.03	Report of Blanesburgh Committee. Unemployment Insurance Act.
PR	922.0	20.4	1.25	
1929 UI	996.9	32.1	1.28	Local Government Act. Public assistance committees to manage poor relief.
PR	765.6	16.8	0.98	
1932 UI	2,500.0	79.2	3.30	Report of Holman Gregory Commission
PR	856.2	18.5	1.13	
1934 UI	2,168.4	68.3	2.55	Unemployment Insurance Act. Central Unemployment Assistance Board established.
PR	998.6	21.4	1.17	
1936 UI	1,824.0	57.1	1.96	Agricultural workers brought into the National Unemployment Insurance Scheme.
PR	1,088.9	23.1	1.17	
1939 UI	1,695.0	52.6	1.68	Outbreak of war.
PR	838.1	17.6	0.83	
1948 UI	349.1	10.5	0.25	Launch of the modern welfare state. Marshall Plan aid received from US.
PR	743.3	15.0	0.53	
1951 UI	218.0	6.5	0.14	Full employment defined as more than 97% in work (Gaitskill).
PR	995.3	19.8	0.65	
1965 UI	438.6	12.7	0.19	New Ministry of Social Security. Attempt to remove discretionary element to supplementary benefits and emphasise rights and entitlements.
PR	2,180.3	40.5	0.95	Move away from Beveridge flat rate of benefit to earnings-related benefits.
1967 UI	958.1	27.7	0.41	Introduction of means-testing local rate rebates and local authority rent rebates.
PR	3,201.6	58.9	1.36	

Table 5.5: Unemployment insurance (UI) and poor relief (PR) (in '1993 pounds', various years) (continued)

Year		Total (millions)	Per head of population*	As % of national income	Notes
1970	UI	1,026.4	29.5	0.40	Introduction of means-tested Family Income Supplement (compared with income
	PR	3,907.9	70.8	1.53	supplements to poor families in early 19th century under Poor Law). Only 60% take-up. The 'poverty trap'.
1971	UI	1,497.2	43.0	0.56	Start of long-term rise in post-war unemployment rate.
	PR	4,576.4	82.4	1.71	
1973	UI	940.5	26.9	0.30	Two-tier system of lower benefits to the unemployed and temporarily sick and
	PR	4,538.2	81.9	1.47	higher longer term benefits to the disabled. Further disruption of flat-rate benefits.
1974	UI	1,056.1	30.2	0.33	Sir Keith Joseph denounces Keynesian policy.
	PR	5,069.8	91.5	1.60	
1975	UI	1,868.4	53.3	0.56	Margaret Thatcher declares that UK had gone too far in attempts to promote
	PR	6,121.1	110.6	1.83	'equality'.
1982	UI	2,604.6	73.2	0.75	Unemployment reaches three million.
	PR	12,768.0	231.2	3.69	Unemployment and other benefits become taxable.
1988	UI	1,538.1	42.3	0.32	Major restructuring of benefit system with shift to more means-testing
	PR	14,933.0	266.4	3.15	(eg family credit)
1989	UI	971.0	26.6	0.20	Norman Tebbit tells unemployed to 'get on their bikes' and look for work like his
	PR	14,754.9	262.6	2.99	father.
1991	UI	1,773.3	48.3	0.38	Norman Lamont – 'unemployment is a price worth paying to beat inflation'.
	PR	19,324.4	342.2	4.13	
1993	UI	1,689.6	45.7	0.35	More than 30% of unemployed had been out of work for at least a year.
	PR	25,290.0	445.7	5.22	Monetarism abandoned.

Newman, O. and Foster, A. (1995) Prices and Incomes in Britain, 1900-1993, New York: Gale Research, International, p 305.

* For UI, per head of population aged 15 to 64 years inclusive; for PR, per head of total population.

Taxation for social security, 1921-39

The figures for Table 5.5 were drawn from the Statistical Abstracts of the Board of Trade published in conjunction with the Ministry of Labour and the Registrars-General (Board of Trade, 1917-39) before the Second World War, and the Annual Statistical Abstracts of the Central Statistical Office in more recent years (Central Statistical Office, 1949-96). The table shows how unemployment insurance rose in '1993 pounds' from £23.7 per head of population aged 15 to 64 years inclusive in 1921, to almost £80 per head in 1932, falling to £52.6 in 1939. As a proportion of the national income, these figures amounted to 1.3%, 3.3% and 1.7% respectively. Poor relief in its various guises totalled £20.4 per head of the total population in 1927, or 1.3% of the national income, falling steadily thereafter as a proportion to 0.8% of national income in 1939, despite the great depression.

William Beveridge and social security, 1941-44

In 1941 there were seven government departments concerned with social security. Unemployment insurance was the responsibility of the Ministry of Labour, non-contributory old age pensions was managed by Customs and Excise, contributory old age pensions by the Ministry of Health, and supplementary pensions and forms of assistance for the long-term unemployed by the Unemployment Assistance Board. There was still a residual form of public assistance, run by local authorities and paid for out of the local rates, for the small numbers who slipped through the net of central government provisions. This was the stubborn residue of the old workhouse system, described in Chapter Eleven. The multiplicity of independent departments created many glaring anomalies. For example, the average weekly benefit for an unemployed man, his wife and two children in 1940 was 20s 6d if he was sick, 38s if he was healthy, and 42s 6d if receiving worker's compensation for occupational injury (unless his employer went bankrupt, in which case he received nothing) (Harris, 1977, pp 378-9). There had been repeated reports that many workers with large families took home more through benefit entitlements while out of work than their employers paid them in work. In other words, the age-old problem of wages in work below an income considered by the State necessary to meet the basic needs of a large family was as entrenched as ever (where it remains to this day).

This confused situation, and a return of the feeling that a country coming through war owed its citizens more, gave rise to calls for 'social reconstruction' after 1939. The stresses and disruption of war exposed to the glare of daylight defects in social order which had lingered in the shadows during peacetime. Memories of the awful chaos following the First World War, and the high unemployment that started soon after the Armistice, led to resolutions that this time the nation would be better prepared for the peace. In April 1941 the Minister of Reconstruction, Arthur Greenwood, suggested that a special committee be convened to examine the social insurance system. In June he announced the appointment of William Beveridge to head a Committee on Social Insurance and Allied Services. All those on the Committee were civil servants apart from Beveridge, and all were overshadowed by Beveridge's pre-planned outcome of their work, mapped out for them in his working paper 'Social insurance – general considerations'. After three decades of study Beveridge was certain about what was needed: nothing less than a fundamental overhaul of the whole system in order to align it with his own concepts, many of which were shared, of course, by many others. Above all, he strove for administrative unification and standardisation of policy. His approach was first to outline the ideal scheme, then consider the practical difficulties and the changes in the current system that would be needed (Harris, 1977, p 387). His radical approach and free-thinking style alarmed Arthur Greenwood, who after seven months withdrew the civil servants from full membership of the Committee, downgrading their status to 'adviser' (Harris, 1977, p 388). Beveridge was reduced to a sort of 'one man band'.

Beveridge strongly favoured flat-rate contributions and standardised benefits for different kinds of interruption of earnings. However, the health departments criticised the former because of its regressive effect, in proportional terms taking more from the incomes of the poorer than the wealthier. These departments felt that the time had probably come to divorce health care entirely from insurance and for the State to administer a universal health service paid for out of public funds. Beveridge accepted the need for a National Health Service to complement his system of social security, though recognising that issues relating to health were not for his Committee's consideration. He argued for child allowances, whether the breadwinner was in work or out of work, to help large families with little income. Above all, he recognised that his system of social security could never remain solvent without the maintenance of full employment. The real need of an unemployed worker is not the support of the State but decently paid work. The fear of idleness on the part of those supported by the State remained with him, but he considered that the onus was on the State to prove unwillingness to work by offering the unemployed a suitable and adequately paid job, with re-training if such were not available. (This remains a driving force in current Welfare approaches to the problem.) Yet barely a decade later, economists from Beveridge's old school were to press the belief that unless one in every 20 workers was kept back from work the State would have to grapple with inflation and the difficulties this caused for pensioners and those on fixed incomes (see Chapter Four). Instead of pulling together, the Welfare and Capitalism arms of Welfare Capitalism were working for irreconcilable objectives: the one to reduce unemployment to close to 1%, the other to hold it at 5% or whatever higher level was judged necessary to stabilise wages and prices.

Beveridge argued that employers, employees and the State all stood to benefit from protection of the workforce during bad times, in readiness for the 'good times'. Therefore, all three should contribute equally to the insurance fund. He was not in favour of the Continental system whereby contributions and benefits were graduated according to previous earnings. In Beveridge's opinion, those with higher incomes could afford private insurance to supplement the State scheme. He believed his plan would encourage thrift and responsibility.

Many people were vulnerable economically not on account of any 'interruption of earnings' but rather an enduring absence of earnings because they could not compete in the Labour market (the chronically sick, the aged, children, the handicapped, single parents with the responsibility of young children). For these sections of the community Beveridge envisaged different kinds of cash benefit, including old age pensions, disability benefit and family allowances. He wished to see provision for married women at times of special need. For those who failed to qualify for any of these benefits but who were shown by means-testing to be in need of support, there should be a residual form of public assistance. He hoped, however, that the benefits system would be sufficiently comprehensive to make such 'residual' cases few and far between. Beveridge was convinced that the nett national income was adequate to banish all forms of want that amounted to poverty through a State system for the redistribution of wealth – a universal Welfare State (though he did not like this term and preferred universal social security).

The correct level of benefit caused the Committee much headache, but there was ready acceptance that 'subsistence' in modern society amounted to more than simply staying alive. Subsistence meant the ability to conform to what society customarily expected of its citizens in the manner of dress, conduct and social intercourse. A child who receives birthday gifts is expected to give something on the birthdays of others. An adult reporting for an interview for prospective employment must appear presentable to the potential employer, and so on. The scope for disagreement here was obviously considerable, but within the context of social security as conceived, unavoidable. To look into this whole question in detail a sub-committee was organised consisting of Seebohm Rowntree (whose social surveys of York were highly regarded), a statistician, a doctor and a nutritionist. Regional variations in rent for housing posed a major problem, and Rowntree urged that benefits should consist of a flat-rate for necessities, plus the actual rent. One can almost hear the gasp of the landlord at the possibilities for *him* of such an arrangement. Beveridge came out against Rowntree's idea, but not because of the landlords' likely response. Rather, he believed that claimants should cut their coat to suit their cloth, an obviously unrealistic response to the housing problem, regional variations in rent and availability of adequate accommodation. Beveridge wanted none of the means-testing that would go with rent assessment (Harris, 1977, pp 398-9).

Then came the thorny question of affordability. There was much alarm in the Treasury at the projected expense, officials doubting whether the country could afford such a comprehensive Welfare State. Old age pensions caused much soul-searching, particularly because even in those years the increasing population of pensionable age was very noticeable. To give all pensioners an adequate allowance, even though those approaching retirement at that time would have made few contributions, seemed to be over-burdening the insurance fund. Beveridge finally accepted that pensions should be phased in, even though this would throw some pensioners on to the public assistance system which he had hoped to minimise.

All benefits were to be paid as a statutory right within a unified system administered by a single ministry, to prevent the left helping hand not knowing what the right helping hand was doing. There was no doubt about the popularity of what Beveridge was proposing among the general public: a fact which caused the government considerable disquiet, given the frequency of his broadcasts and articles on the topic (Harris, 1977, pp 419-26). The commercial insurance interest was also highly alarmed and attacked his report vigorously when it finally emerged. The major innovations were: the universal nature of the coverage, all in the workforce being covered irrespective of occupation or usual level of income; a subsistence income geared not merely to maintaining life but to living in a modern industrial society; and the standardisation of payments irrespective of the reason for 'not working'. There was an unequivocal recognition that what Beveridge was proposing added up to re-distribution of wealth from wealthier regions to poorer regions and from wealthier families to poorer families in the implicit belief that it was 'right' to do so. Universal social security would counter the 'wrongs' in the socio-economic ordering of daily affairs: wrongs which economists like Beveridge believed could not be prevented but only alleviated. Rent reformers, recognising the economic and social ills caused by privatisation of Rent, insisted that much more could be done but by now they were voices in the wilderness.

In October 1942, Sir Stafford Cripps, the new Leader of the House of Commons, told his aunt, Beatrice Webb, that the Beveridge Report was held up in Cabinet because some considered it too revoluntionary (Harris, 1977, p 419). When *Social insurance and allied services* finally appeared in December it created a sensation. Beveridge described its contents as merely a stage in a "comprehensive policy of social progress" against the "five giants on the road of reconstruction – Want, Ignorance, Squalor, Idleness and Disease". This was the 'Beveridge plan' as it was popularly called, debated enthusiastically throughout 1943. Officials were less keen. They did not believe that mass unemployment could be slain within the existing economic system. Many still held on to eugenic theories of a residual helpless and pitiful underclass which would call upon public assistance forever. The concept of subsistence was rejected in all but the vaguest of terms. Subsistence requirements differed so much from one family to the next, especially when the element of rent for housing was taken into account. The Treasury doubted that post-war Britain could afford it all, and the reality that national insurance contributions were in fact a tax on the income of Labour was not lost on its officials. In April 1943 a group of civil service officials began to consider the Beveridge Report and its implications, leading to the White Paper on social security of 1944. When things settled down Beveridge went back to what he knew to be more important than any other topic – how to secure full employment at a respectable minimum wage, and thereby real social security.

Throughout the century there had been those who believed that the faults in the economy could be removed by planning on a national scale, thereby raising national efficiency, and Beveridge had always believed in the essential wisdom of the benign and enlightened expert. He now pinned his faith on a planned economy to reduce unemployment to not more than 3%, though what would be in this plan he was not yet certain. He said to the Advisory Panel on Home Affairs in June 1942: "Although it was possible to plan attacks on Want, Disease and Ignorance, the fight against Idleness (ie unemployment) and Squalor (ie poor housing) raised vast political issues which would certainly strain national unity.... Their defeat could not be secured without, on the one hand, State planning and on the other, relaxation of Trade Union restrictions: two things which together would forfeit all the votes in the country" (Harris, 1977, p 431). Want was to be struck down by social insurance and a statutory minimum wage. Disease would be cured by a National Health Service and prevented by better housing, better nutrition and better sanitation. Ignorance would respond to a system of free and universal education with better uptake in adulthood. Idleness would be defeated by State planning to maintain full employment. Squalor needed better control of the use of land with strict controls on what industry could do, and renovation of the inner cities. The money for all of this, however, depended on a successful economy, producing wealth at more than an increase in national income of the usual 2.5% per annum, and every opportunity for each member of the workforce to put his or her mind and back into the effort, while rearing the next generation to take up the task competently when its turn came. This simply could not happen when each and every time growth accelerated, it became choked off within a few years as the economy collapsed into recession.

The explanation for this repeated economic cycle Beveridge was never to identify, but whatever it was, it was to prove the 'Achilles' heel' of his Welfare State. Startlingly, at a meeting of the Advisory Panel on Home Affairs held in July 1942, he stated his belief that unemployment, poor housing and a squalid environment could not be conquered without some form of public ownership of land and essential services (Harris, 1977, p 433). This smacked of Richard Tawney, his colleague at the London School of Economics, and it was a pity that neither saw that the public control they sought for their purposes could come not from public ownership of land but by restoration to the public of the original and natural value in Rent long since appropriated into private ownership.

Beveridge's hopes were shattered by Lionel Robbins, who countered the recommendation of Oliver Lyttleton, Minister of Production, that Beveridge should report on the employment question by saying that Beveridge "was not a genuine expert on the unemployment question" (Harris, 1977, p 434). Robbins, another professor at the London School of Economics at that time, had written widely and published seminal work on the Labour supply curve in the 1930s. His advice was probably readily acceptable to many who found Beveridge's style much too unconventional for their taste. Instead, Beveridge had to proceed outside government by chairing a small group financed by businessmen. In this group he was swayed away from the Socialist thoughts of Tawney towards the doctrine of Maynard Keynes as the solution to unemployment. With the rejection of Keynesian beliefs that was to follow, we now know that Beveridge had jumped out of the frying pan into the fire. The cost of this tragic sequence of events for Britain has been incalculable. The fault in the economic system, which Beveridge, Keynes, Tawney and Robbins failed (or did not dare) to acknowledge, continues to cost the nation very dearly indeed and leaves the man and woman in the street sceptical of the expertise of economists and politicians. The swinging pendulum of political and economic fashion is counting the time but hardly marking progress.

The price of ignoring Rent monopoly

There were those in Beveridge's private group who feared full employment, believing this would raise wages and fuel inflation because supply would not rise commensurably with increased demand. With a weaker pound the worker would be little better off, and the effects on the other aspects of the economy could be devastating. Beveridge's colleagues were in fact setting out theory which A W Phillips was soon to propose as historical fact (Phillips, 1958). However, the failure of supply to be sustained in a state of full employment arises in large measure because so much of the surplus generated goes not to Wages, Interest and investment in Capital but into growth of Land values and Rent. This creates the inefficiencies causing eventual collapse of economic activity. There is no good reason why, in a properly functioning economic system which takes full account of the role of Land, a fully employed workforce should not produce goods to meet demand. Keynes' notion that a synchronised propensity to save rather than spend leaves goods standing on the shelves has long since been abandoned. The very fact of price inflation in full employment means that most people are only too willing to spend and consume. It is not savings that act as a sink, but Rent.

Prices and incomes policies, formalised first in 1966 with the establishment of the National Board for Prices and Incomes, were attempts by government to control the power of monopoly in industry, whether private or publicly owned, and the powers of monopoly created in the

Labour market. Yet because these policies remained blind to the power of the monopoly in Rent, prices and incomes policies failed. The battles between government, the Trade Union Congress and employers raged on during the 1970s, 'pay round' after 'pay round', eventually bringing the Labour administration to its knees, but the Rent monopoly got away scot-free.

In 1979 the economy went once more into reverse. While the landholder was doing well for rents and property prices, unofficial strikes to press demands for higher pay had the Labour administration in a spin. In January, the government faced industrial disputes with local authority manual workers and health service workers, but could not agree to the wage rises demanded. Strikes in the water industry had elderly people struggling with buckets to standpipes. Health services workers and lorry drivers were threatening similar action. In February there was a walkout without notice in a children's hospital. The nation appeared to have gone mad. Tony Benn said: "When decent people become irrational, something else must be wrong if they are driven to such desperate acts" (Barnett, 1982, p 175). Reports of food shortages caused panic buying. Blaming it all on the Labour administration and the Trade Unions, the confused electorate turned their eyes once more towards the Conservatives and Margaret Thatcher, looking for salvation. The Labour government had its Operation Brisket to meet the road haulage dispute, Operation Bittern to meet the ambulance drivers' dispute, and Operation Nimrod for the water workers, but the situation was desperate. Gerald Kaufman suggested that the next Operation should be called 'Loony' (Barnett, 1982, p 171).

The Labour government was unfortunately in power just when the social and economic systems favoured by Beveridge and Tawney were collapsing. Tawney's ardent Socialism was in tatters; unemployment at more than 5% and about to soar had Beveridge's Welfare State on its knees; those who believed in nothing better than 'laissez-faire' were crowing 'we told you so'. The Trade Union movement, at its lowest level of popularity for decades, was about to have its horns drawn by Margaret Thatcher's administration. It all seemed to add up to the statement, 'everything we strove for this century in the field of social policy has culminated in disaster'. When the gravediggers went on strike the nation turned against itself in revulsion. The Trade Union Congress mistakenly saw the government and its pay policy as the enemy, when in fact the unions and the government had not the foggiest idea why their best schemes had ended in a state which had Europe and America looking on in astonishment. The best that each could do was to blame the other.

The steady rise in pressure within the great fault in Land policy had precipitated a socio-economic earthquake. The result: the Trade Unions were reduced to a shadow of what they once were; Labour jettisoned its beliefs in nationalisation and public ownership of the means of production; the Conservative Party's reward for their 18 year campaign to dismantle the Welfare State (Pierson, 1994) was a crushing defeat in the election of 1997. New Labour was born in what it was pleased to call the advent of the Third Age, leaving many to ask, 'What is this Third Age?'

'Less eligibility' in modern social security

Any attempt to catalogue the long series of departures of post-war administrations from the principles of William Beveridge would be futile. Beveridge wished for a State in which social insurance would help the family through periods of interruptions of earnings, special cash benefits would care for the aged, chronically sick, disabled, and large families, and a residual system of means-tested benefits would care for the small minority who slipped through the net. He would have been horrified to see how his principles had proved impossible for governments to live up to, though not surprised once the persistence of low pay in work and chronic unemployment were appreciated.

Beveridge flouted contemporary opinion when he stated that if a man with a family was so badly paid that he got less from wages than from benefit, then his moral duty was to apply for benefit (Harris, 1977, p 414). At the same time he was absolutely clear that what was best was a decent job with a decent wage. So ineffectually has the latter objective been tackled that an army of disadvantaged families has been forced to resort to exactly what Beveridge regarded as their moral duty. Beveridge had never envisaged benefits being paid at a higher level than that needed for subsistence in a modern economy, so he was clearly thinking of the family's moral duty when wages were below this amount. He accepted that the narrower the gap between income in work and income out of work, then the smaller the incentive to work for those with little ambition. This gap can be widened either by reducing benefits to the very lowest deemed acceptable to the social conscience, or by raising income and increasing the attractiveness of work. Real wages are of course forced down by taxes at the point of payment and the point of expenditure.

Thus income taxes can destroy incentives to work by narrowing the gap between real income in work and real income out of work.

To 'get the balance right' between benefits and wages within the constraints of the private market in Labour, successive governments have turned what was in 1948 "a book of rules which ... every NAB (National Assistance Board) officer had been able to carry around in his pocket" into "several massive volumes, so often amended and so complicated that even the staff could not understand them" (Donnison, 1982, p 43). This was light-years away from what Beveridge had envisaged. The bureaucracy was as degrading as ever, especially that going with tests of willingness to work and of real financial need. The system forces down take-up rates, and prolongs 'interruption of work' by tolerating low wages. When government accepts reductions in disposable income through income taxes and sequestration of Rent, to the point where, reluctantly, families are better off even on low benefit rates, then the system becomes part of the problem rather than part of the solution. This is precisely what has happened. Despite refinement, social security as designed can do little to create work. Instead, it tends to perpetuate unemployment by accommodating low pay and insecurity of employment within the Labour market, raising tax on the productive sector, and destroying prospects for employment at the margin of the economy, as described in Chapter Three.

When the basket of benefits available to counter the worst effects of low pay is comparatively attractive, then the lowest paid jobs go to illegal immigrants, young people not entitled to social security, and to second earners needing to raise the family income. Much of what second earners achieve is taken by a rise in the cost of rents and mortgages, as, in the competitive market for housing structured on land monopoly, the landholder captures the increased Rent. There are numerous 'two-earner' families today paying out as a proportion of total income the same as or more than the 'one-earner' family of 40 years ago in the way of rent or mortgage for the same property.

Social security and its unemployment and poverty traps

Willing workers who find unemployment benefit financially preferable to low-paid work are said to be 'trapped'. So too are those who choose to supplement a low-wage with Welfare benefits rather than accept more work or a higher wage. The traps are blamed upon a mismatch between entitlements and wages, benefits and taxes, such that any gain in income from work is offset by the attendant eligibility for taxation and reduction in benefits. All such problems remain tertiary in nature, however, to the secondary problem of low wages and insecurity of employment at the low end of the Labour market, due in turn in large measure to the primary problem of privatisation of Rent and its monopoly.

The computer has been put to work in an attempt to pay out benefits low enough to preserve work incentives by maintaining a sufficient gap between spending power in and out of employment. Nevertheless, government has had great difficulty moving some families off benefits on to wages, because their spending power in work remains no better than that out of work when taxation, loss of benefits and working expenses are taken into account. The unemployment trap, which is 'less eligibility gone wrong', arises when the spending power gained from a working wage adds up to less or hardly more than what the State offers in benefits as the minimum amount considered necessary for the maintenance of health and prevention of social isolation. The fault in the system which failed to preserve 'less eligibility' was given its name as a result of Sir Ralph Howell's persistent questions in parliament in the 1970s and early 1980s (Howell, 1976).

With taxation starting at a low level of income, some people who moved into work could discover that they had been better off when out of work with benefits untaxed. The response after 1979 was not to raise spending power when in work by raising wages or the tax threshold, but to make benefits out of work of less value. This change had been agreed among the Conservatives when in opposition during the late 1970s following discussions in the home of the Shadow Chancellor of the Exchequer, Geoffrey Howe (Timmins, 1996, pp 363-4). Benefits were raised in line with prices rather than with earnings, because prices tend to rise more slowly than earnings. The Labour administration of 1964-70 had introduced 'earnings related additions' to the benefits paid for unemployment, sickness and widowhood as a way to help skilled Labour through the transition from obsolescent industries into new technologies. These supplements were abolished by the Conservative administration in the Social Security Act of 1982. In the same year, all National Insurance benefits (except invalidity benefit) and supplementary benefit (national assistance) became reckonable for purposes of taxation. In this way low benefits tended to drift further below low earnings.

The rule of five per cent for three per cent

In only 30 years the State's enthusiasm for its post-war solution to want had turned sour. Social security, once a major achievement, was by 1980 a major problem. The primary objective of government was now to rein back the monster it believed its post-war predecessors to have created. In reality, however, little had changed between 1921 and 1979. Indeed, in the most fundamental of senses little was to change after 1979. The flaws in the political economy for which the Welfare State was meant to compensate proved too much. The cost of the Welfare system between 1922 and 1993 (excluding the Second World War) had increased more or less steadily by almost 5% per year in real terms throughout the period. The regression was:

Log_e (all services, '1993 pounds') = 0.047 (year) [SE, 0.0006] + 21.54; r = 0.995 r^2 = 0.99, where year equalled (19) 22 to 93. [SE = standard error].

National income grew over the same period by 3% per year in real terms, the relation being:

Log_e (national income, '1993 pounds') = 0.030 (year) [SE, 0.0003] + 24.20; r^2 = 0.995.

Welfare services expenditure therefore increased as a percentage of national income from a little less than 12% in 1930 to 16% in 1950, 23% in 1970 and 32% in 1990. Social security took 2.2% of national income in 1979, but 5.6% in 1993 (see Table 5.5).

Reforms to social security after 1979: 'Beveridge' in reverse

In 1984, seven million people were living on social security. Sixty per cent of adults on supplementary benefit had no change of shoes for themselves or their children, and almost the same proportion were in debt, owing on gas and electricity bills. An army of families was out there running out of money before the next benefit payment, thrown into severe difficulty because of a trivial expense about which middle class families would not think twice.

Driven by a sense of public spending out of control, Norman Fowler announced in April 1984 the biggest review of social security since the days of the Beveridge Commission (Secretary of State for Social Services,

1985). A report to government from the Policy Studies Institute noted that the rules on supplementary benefit had reached an incomprehensible 16,000. Changes in the rules and regulations for social security had been so complex that not even the experts were able to judge the effects with accuracy. The social security Budget was open-ended, vulnerable not only to recession, high unemployment, and an ageing population, but also to dramatic increases in private housing and council housing rents.

As one observer put it, in essence the Fowler report produced a set of 'cleverly designed molehills' rather than mountains (Timmins, 1996, p 401). Supplementary Benefit was converted into Income Support, providing a basic allowance for adults to which were added premiums for dependants: children, pensioners and the disabled. Family Income Supplement, the means-tested benefit designed for poor families supported by a working adult, introduced by Sir Keith Joseph during the Conservative administration of 1970-74, was converted into 'Family Credit'. Housing benefit was simplified. Previously, Family Income Supplement and Housing Benefit had been income-tested rather than means-tested, leaving the family's capital out of the equation. Now, for the first time the same means-test was applied to all three forms of benefit. The new arrangement threatened family savings, discouraging thrift. Beveridge would not have been pleased.

Between 1979 and 1994 rents demanded by local authorities increased six fold on average, and increases in the rents of housing associations were even more spectacular. For the single wage couple with two children, local authority rents took about 10% of the wage of the man on two thirds average manual earnings in 1979, but almost 20% in 1994 (Parker, 1995, p 128). Try as it might, the government was not able to lower the benefit entitlement of the non-working couple with two young children to much below three quarters of what the average male could expect to earn in manual work (Parker, 1995, pp 31-2). This was the amount they had to earn in 1994 in order to be £25 better off in work than out of work and on benefits, assuming work expenses of £10 a week (Parker, 1995, p 34). Given the official attitude towards Welfare spending, this speaks volumes for the level of pay going to unskilled labour. Those in work on less than three quarters of average earnings for manual work, and who had a wife and child, had no recourse but to turn to Welfare.

For families moving into work on low wages, there remained, however, the poverty trap. In 1994, for those in unskilled work and partly dependent on Family Credit, each additional pound earned could be expected to raise spending power by only two pence to 25 pence. Rarely, the family that managed to earn a little more could see spending power actually reduced when benefit reductions and tax increases were particularly punitive. For each means-tested benefit to which the working family was entitled there was what was called an 'applicable amount' calculated on the basis of family size, the age of the children and other considerations. Then for housing benefit, for example, 65 pence was withdrawn for every pound earned above the applicable amount, while for family credit the equivalent 'taper' was 70 pence in the pound. When it came to high earners, the Conservative argument was that tax rates of 80% or more were a disincentive to work and an encouragement to cheating the Inland Revenue or opting out by going abroad. Yet, at the bottom end of the income scale, for some odd reason the same forces were actually introduced into social security.

A word must be said about another outcome of the Fowler review, namely the Social Fund. For years, extra payments had been made to cover sudden needs, such as replacement of defective kitchen equipment or essential repairs. David Donnison was successor to Richard Titmuss at the Supplementary Benefits Commission after the latter's death in April 1973. He cited as examples one-off payments to replace "the worn out underclothes of an impoverished woman, the wear and tear inflicted by a lame man's caliper on his threadbare trousers, or the extra laundry costs of an incontinent old lady" (Donnison, 1982, p 45). Numerous dismissals of claims were taken to appeals tribunals, some even going to the higher courts as claimants demanded what they considered to be their rightful entitlements. The system was just as chaotic in 1984 when the Policy Studies Institute began the enquiry which ended up as the Fowler review of supplementary benefits. The result was conversion of discretionary extra payments into the Social Fund. One-off payments for mattresses, clothing and so on were converted into loans awarded on a discretionary basis and not, as previously, as of right. This Fund was cash-limited, meaning that local offices stopped payments, no matter how bad the personal crisis, when the cash ran out. The loan was interest free, but there were no longer any appeals tribunals to turn to on rejection, and the loan had to be paid back out of an unchanged weekly benefit entitlement, making daily living that much harder.

Taxation for Welfare services and redistribution of income in kind

In 1939 the average wage was £180 a year, and there were fewer than four million taxpayers in a working population of more than 20 million.

The Labour government therefore saw the National Health Service, education and other services as redistributing wealth in kind from the wealthier to the poorer. However, this mechanism was increasingly undermined during the 1950s. Since 1960, essentially the whole working population of Britain has been eligible to pay income tax and, through various adjustments to income bands for taxation and the tax rates applied, progressivity has been diminished. Progressivity was reduced even further with the introduction of value added tax (VAT) by a Conservative administration in 1973. In 1974 the Labour government reduced VAT from 10 to 8% on most items, and to 12.5% on luxury items. However, Joel Barnett, Chief Secretary to the Treasury in that year, considered this strategy mistaken. The yield of income tax came mostly from the average paid worker, not the rich as in earlier years. It was therefore a pretence to regard VAT as necessarily more regressive than income tax, Barnett argued, as duties and excise taxes had been in earlier years, especially when VAT was not levied on food, fuel or housing (Barnett, 1982, pp 32-3).

The Labour administration might have been reluctant to raise VAT, but not the Shadow Cabinet. The Conservatives agreed to adjust the tax to a single rate of 15% should they return to power. This increase came about in 1979, though businesses selling food, children's clothes, books, railway tickets and household fuel were left 'zero rated' (ie not only did they not charge VAT on their sales, but they reclaimed any VAT included in the price of their inputs). State education and health services were 'VAT exempt', meaning that they paid VAT on purchases in the usual way (putting up their costs), but did not add VAT to the 'added value' element which they put into their products. Because of the zero rated items, VAT was still mildly progressive; in 1985 it took about 6% of the disposable income of poor households, as compared with a little more than 7% of that of the richest fifth of families (*Economic Trends*, 1986, p 101).

As personal taxation goes, the decade 1985-95 was as topsy-turvy as any previous; perhaps more so than most. Reductions in income taxation at the point of receipt meant gains in nett income of almost 10% for the wealthiest 10% of UK households, while the poorest 20% were slightly worse off. In 1990, the government abolished local taxation based on the value of land and buildings, replacing it with a per capita Community Charge ('poll tax'). This move was immensely unpopular, forcing the government to introduce a central subsidy of the charge amounting to £140 per adult per year. To fund this change, Chancellor Norman Lamont increased VAT to 17.5%, bringing in an extra £2.7 billion per year. In

1993, VAT was extended to household fuel, this measure coming fully into force in 1995. The effect was to make the bottom 10% of households another 2% poorer, and most other households around 4% poorer. On top of it all, the Community Charge was quickly replaced by the Council Tax, a reversion to property-based local taxation. The overall effect of this turbulent decade was to increase inequality: the poorest 10% paid over 25% of their gross income in taxes, while the top 10% paid 38% (Giles and Johnson, 1994). By 1993 VAT was clearly regressive, taking 11% of the disposable income of the poorest fifth of 'non-retired' households, but only 7% of that of the richest fifth (*Economic Trends*, 1994, p 42). In that same year, the average benefit in kind provided by the National Health Service was estimated to be worth £1,359 to non-retired households in which at least 95% of gross income came in the form of cash benefits (income support, housing benefit etc), and £1,190 to those in which cash benefits comprised less than 10% of gross income. The respective figures for education were £2,079 and £1,329, the difference explained almost entirely by the greater number of people in full-time education in younger households (*Economic Trends*, 1994, p 46).

Welfare subsidy or tax credits?

Such is the state of the Welfare State that Chancellors can bring hope to the unemployed when they reverse the adverse consequences of the Welfare schemes and taxation measures of previous administrations. The point was illustrated by yet another tale of family hardship published in *The Times* on the day after Gordon Brown had announced the New Labour administration's Budget for 1998-99. The goal was not that of the founders of the Welfare State, who had introduced a taxation system to alleviate poverty. Rather, the purpose of the Budgetary reforms was to create 'a tax system that rewards enterprise and makes all work pay'. In other words, the Budget was an attempt to remove the poverty traps and unemployment traps constructed by Gordon Brown's predecessors, and which had ensnared families such as the Hills of Birkenhead.

Gary Hill had lost his job during a bout of ill health in 1990, and had not found work since then. He was taking a part-time course in mechanics in the hope of self-employment, an initiative which disqualified him from government assistance under its job seekers' allowance scheme (which replaced unemployment benefit and income support for the unemployed in October 1996). The family got by on a weekly allowance of £100 in income support and £29 in child benefit which they collected from the post office. However, because their situation entitled the family to relief from charges for water and the National Health Service, exemption from local taxes and provision of school meals, Gary estimated that he would need an earned income of at least £400 a week before tax in order to gain from being in work. The family was hoping that the Chancellor's introduction of the negative income tax system would improve their position by raising the parents' prospects in gainful employment.

The negative income tax, or tax credit, was another brainchild of the monetarist economist Milton Friedman. He had proposed that taxation should taper off to zero as low incomes were approached, and then convert to tax credits as earned incomes fell below a critical level, thereby securing a socially acceptable minimum income for all. The system was advocated in the era of Richard Nixon and operates in the US today (Galbraith, 1987, pp 271-2). Gordon Brown's 'working family tax credit' may well have helped one and a half million families on low incomes who had one working breadwinner, by alleviating some of the poverty traps and unemployment traps, but could not create work. On this account the Chancellor relieved employers of the low paid from the employers' contribution to national insurance, the tax introduced by the Act of 1946 to fund the universal Welfare State. The lost revenue was recouped by raising the tax on employers of high earners, and by increases in various excise duties. The bottom line, however, was that government spending in 1998-99 was estimated to be almost £300 billion, as compared with £290 billion in the previous financial year, an increase of 3.5%. Allowing for inflation, the burden of taxation on the productive sectors of the economy was unchanged: only its distribution had been altered somewhat. Several measures were taken to improve the efficiency of the Labour market, for example lower taxes on business corporations and employers' subsidies to encourage employment of the long-term unemployed. Nevertheless, the Chancellor was able to do what he did because the economy in general was expanding at the time. The real test of the measures would be another recession. Tax credits are not for non-working families.

Child allowances and old age pensions

"One of the reasons children make up a high proportion of those at the bottom of the income distribution is that a growing number of parents, especially lone parents, are out of work. Paid work also allows people to save for their retirement" (Department of Social Security, 1998, p 23).

Table 5.6: Retirement pensions (P) and family (child) allowance (F) (in '1993 pounds')

Year	Total (million)		Per head of population		As % national income		Notes
	P	F	P+	F†	P	F	
1921	313		132		0.6		Non-contributory pension, means-tested, for 70+ year olds, from 1.1.09 [10 shillings/week].
1925	647		232		0.9		Neville Chamberlain introduces contributory pensions to cover 65–69 year olds.
1936	1,958		498		2.1		1.8 million in occupational pension schemes.
1937	1,960		486		2.1		1925 scheme extended to previously uninsured workers.
1940	1,939		447		1.8		Qualifying age for women reduced to 60 to promote the war effort.
1945	1,945		401		1.5		Family Allowance Act. Five shillings/week for second and subsequent children from August 1946.
1946	3,044	879	614	18	2.4	0.7	13% of population pensionable. 'Old age' changed to 'retirement' pension.
1951	4,421	894	809	18	2.9	0.6	Less than seven million State pensioners.
1956	5,227	1,233	897	24	3.1	0.7	Eight million in occupational schemes.
1961	8,145	1,278	1,316	24	4.0	0.6	Introduction of graduated insurance contributions.
1965	11,260	1,255	1,697	23	4.9	0.5	Labour raised family allowances but reduces child tax allowances.
1972	14,765	1,965	1,997	35	5.4	0.7	Ten pounds Christmas bonus for pensioners.
1974	19,009	1,669	2,512	30	6.0	0.5	Basic pensions rise to £14 a couple and £10 a single person per week.
1976	20,165	1,831	2,606	33	6.2	0.6	State earnings-related pension scheme.
1977	20,344	2,546	2,600	46	6.4	0.8	Child Benefit: cash payment for all children to the mother.
1979	23,103	6,976	2,889	126	6.4	1.9	Pensions linked to price increases only, as against prices and incomes (whichever increased most) in previous years.
1985	26,680	6,908	3,137	124	6.7	1.7	Incentives to quit State earnings-related pension scheme for private pensions.
1988	28,066	6,325	3,205	113	5.9	1.3	Child benefit 'frozen' for second year in a row.
1993	32,923	6,347	3,587	112	6.8	1.3	Basic pension worth about 15% of male average earnings. Ten million pensioners.

+ Population aged 65+

† Population less than 15.

This statement, set against another in the Labour administration's publication of 1998, *A new contract for welfare*, "one in five working age households have no one in work" (Department of Social Security, 1998, p 3), explains why policies regarding retirement pensions and family allowances are not discussed here in any depth. The need for subsidies in young parenthood and old age is secondary to the underlying problem of low earned income or no earned income during what should be profitable working years. Table 5.6 shows that retirement pensions paid by the State have increased in real terms by more than 25 fold per head of the population aged 65 years or more since 1921, representing an 11 fold growth as a proportion of national income (from about 0.5% to approaching 7%). In the same period the numbers of men and women in this age group increased almost four fold.

The chequered history of child allowances

At a conference on the maintenance of children by the State, held in London's Guildhall in early 1905, concern for the health and fitness of the working classes was running high. Few, however, were enthusiastic about 'State maintenance'. The fear was that this policy would pose a threat to the family as an institution, although school meals were not regarded as dangerously obtrusive in this respect. Xenophobia and eugenics coloured the debate. Sidney Webb wrote in 1907:

> In Great Britain at this moment, when half, or perhaps two thirds of all married people are regulating their families, children are being freely born to the Irish Roman Catholics, and the Polish, Russian and German Jews, on the one hand, and to the thriftless and irresponsible – largely the casual labourers and the other denizens of the one-roomed tenements of our great cities – on the other. Twenty five per cent of our parents, as Professor Karl Pearson keeps telling us, are producing 50% of the next generation. This can hardly result in anything but national deterioration; or, as an alternative, in this country falling gradually to the Irish and the Jews.... In order that the population may be recruited from the self-controlled and foreseeing members of each class, rather than those who are feckless and improvident, we must alter the balance of remuneration in favour of the child-producing family. (Webb, 1907, pp 16-18)

In other words the English middle classes should receive child allowances and educational subsidies to help them to support larger families and thereby compete with the 'thriftless and irresponsible'. Lloyd George introduced a tax allowance for children in families on low income in 1909, and once established this was gradually increased. Separation allowances were also paid during the First World War to support the families of volunteers in the armed forces, the amount being governed by the number of children.

In November 1921, with unemployment standing at least at two million, the government was forced to add a dependants' allowance to unemployment benefit. This measure was seen by many as strengthening the case for family allowances whether or not there was a breadwinner in work (Hall et al, 1975, pp 163-4). Eleanor Rathbone and the Family Endowment Society campaigned hard during the 1920s, believing that such allowances would raise the status of motherhood and (if financed through a graduated income tax) assist in the redistribution of income to the poor. They faced the scepticism of some economists who believed that high unemployment signified over-population, those trade unionists who feared that such allowances would be used to depress the working wage, and many worried about adverse effects on parental responsibility. Then, in the 1930s, the nation was confronted by the prospect of a declining population. There were predictions that, should contemporary birth rates and death rates be sustained, then by 2030 the population would have been reduced by 90% (Charles, 1935). In response to the alarm, the government set up a Population Investigation Committee in 1936 to consider the question of family allowances. Eugenic and Imperial notions were still in the air, leading Neville Chamberlain to justify an increase in the child allowance against taxation with the remark that, "the British Empire will be crying out for more citizens of the right breed, and then we in this country shall not be able to supply the demand" (Hall et al, 1975, p 172). The first priority was to reverse the decline in population, and all classes were rallied to the cause. Even the noted Professor R.A. Fisher told the Eugenic Society in 1932 that while in theory to discourage child-rearing in working class families and encourage it among the middle classes would be a good idea, theory could not be turned into practice at that time because it would not prevent the loss of the "eugenically valuable qualities of the nation" (Hall et al, 1975, p 173). Family allowances came to be seen increasingly as in the national interest, the cause being boosted by surveys which continued to reveal high rates of under-nutrition in poor families. Government, however, dragged its heels on the matter. Outside of the House of Commons, by contrast, some such as William Beveridge held that an allowance paid to all families with children would promote child-rearing without reducing the income gap between those in and those out of work, thereby retaining the benefits of work.

The Second World War served to emphasise once again the nation's inevitable dependency on a large, healthy and skilled workforce. Economic changes precipitated by the war, leading to a strong demand for Labour, rising wages and increased rates of direct taxation, brought the income of many married men with young families into the tax bracket for the first time. Family allowances set against taxation cushioned this effect, especially among the working classes. John Maynard Keynes, in his book *How to pay for the war* (1940), proposed family allowances paid in cash rather than as tax allowances. This publication was the outcome of a series of articles in *The Times* which had provoked widespread discussion shortly after the commencement of war. Beveridge backed the call, recalling how the separation allowance of the First World War had helped to sustain the health of children in those years. By 1941 the government was committed to family allowances provided that the Beveridge Committee was in support, accepting Keynes' reasoning that, in addition to the social advantages, allowances would suppress inflationary wage demands. Indeed, family allowances were proposed by Beveridge after consultation with Keynes, and accepted by the government on the first day of the debate on his plan in February 1943. In addition to child Welfare services, there was to be a cash allowance of 5s per week starting with the second child, anticipated to cost the Exchequer less than £60 million a year.

Keynes and Hubert Henderson proposed that family allowances should be financed out of taxation of luxuries. This idea met strong opposition (in these days immediately prior to the introduction of the universal Welfare State) from the Inland Revenue on the grounds that the purpose of the income tax was not the redistribution of income (Hall et al, 1975, p 209). Government being unwilling to raise direct taxation, and pressed to support servicemen's families with improved allowances, the family allowance was therefore deferred until the end of the war. The Family Allowances Bill was debated in March 1945, during which Eleanor Rathbone, now over 70 years of age and within months of her death, fought successfully to have payments made to the mother rather than the father. Payments commenced in August 1946. Over the years, as Table 5.6 shows, the value of family allowances in '1993 pounds' increased, per head of population under 15 years of age, by about six-fold up to 1993.

They accounted for less than 1% of national income until the introduction of Child Benefit in 1977, reaching almost 2% of national income in 1979 but falling back thereafter. How stood child Welfare at the turn of the millennium? Prime Minister Tony Blair put it succinctly in a speech in March 1999: one third of Britain's children were living in 'frightening' deprivation. About the same proportion live in families without an adult in full-time employment (*The Guardian*, 19 March, 1999, p 10).

Old age pensions

In these days when women have equal citizenship to men, and increasing numbers are joining the labour force outside the home, child allowances are no longer seen as influencing their status. Neither does a decline in the population threaten the nation. What continues to cause anxiety is the thought that in an ageing population the burden of health care in old age and the costs of retirement pensions may test the Welfare State to the limit. In 1935 it was estimated that by 1975 the percentage of the population aged over 60 would have risen from 12 to 30; in fact it increased to 20% by 1981. Similarly, the percentage under 15 was anticipated to fall from 25 to seven; in fact it had hardly changed up to 1981 (Office of Population Censuses and Surveys, 1996). Duncan Sandys, recently married to Diana, daughter of Sir Winston Churchill, declared in 1937:"A declining population must inevitably involve a deterioration in the whole standard of living of our people. With a population whose numbers are declining, and where average age is rising, we shall be faced with the situation of a smaller and smaller proportion of active workers having to support an ever increasing proportion of old age" (cited in Hall et al, 1975, p 172). In fact, the national income (in '1993 pounds') per head of population aged over 64 was about £25,000 in 1937. In 1981 it was about £43,000. Nevertheless the fear remains. In its document of 1998, *New ambitions for our country,* the Labour administration declared that:"In 1953, there were 4.6 people of working age for every pensioner. Today there are 3.4 and by 2040, the ratio will have dropped to just 2.4, even allowing for equalisation (for men and women) of the retirement age" (Department of Social Security, 1998, p 14).

In his Budget speech of March 1998, Chancellor Gordon Brown raised child benefit significantly, deliberately aiming to target support at low income families with young children. There is no doubt that family allowances are seen as a way of improving financial security when bringing up children, and to "give every child a better start" (*The Times*, 18 March

1998, p 18), but the economic necessity of a large, healthy and skilled workforce to take on the nation's commitments, including those promised to elderly people, is never lost from sight.

So much for the nation's efforts to slay four of Beveridge's Giants: Ignorance, Disease, Idleness and Want. They are not to be derided or belittled. But the Welfare State was introduced primarily to reduce the wide spread of incomes, standards of health and length of life around their respective averages, which has not been achieved. Although the Welfare arm of Welfare Capitalism grew immensely after 1948, it was during this post-war period that researchers documented the impact of poverty and unemployment on health and lifespan more convincingly than ever before, publicising the growing gaps in income, wealth and health between richer and poorer. The umbrella of the Welfare State has been more than leaky. The Giant Squalor remains to be considered.

SIX

Squalor: the affordability of housing

Clearly the market cannot provide enough decent homes at prices people can afford. (David Butler, Chief Executive of the Chartered Institute of Housing, January 2000)

A major determinant of health and happiness is the affordability of decent housing. In Britain home-ownership is a prized goal, but for many little but a dream, and for others something of a myth when it is remembered that in law, those with a mortgage do not in the final analysis truly own their property (see below). For poorer families their only resort is to social housing.

When 'house prices' soar ahead of economic growth, and homeowners become excited by monthly bulletins on the size of their windfall, it is not the value of the bricks and mortar that is rising. Mass speculation on the part of Rentholders and their agents is once again fanning the flames. For a while, in the frenzied 'get rich quick' climate, inflated land prices divert billions of pounds from the productive sector. Sooner or later, the fire rages out of control. Rents rise, land is withheld from the market in expectation of higher returns, and business costs accelerate. Ever sniffing the air, the business community scents danger, at first indistinct, later unmistakable. The boom is 'peaking out', and confidence collapses as the productive economy is engulfed. Only when the conflagration is spent does the recession bottom out. Land prices then stabilise at a sustainable level, and the first shoots of recovery follow. Though seared so many times, Business Capitalism steadfastly refuses to contemplate the fact that speculation in privatised Rent is its economic tinder-box. Such speculation is the bane of housing policy.

Victorian urban development

The Britain of the 1920s inherited a housing stock that had been thrown up to meet the phenomenally rapid growth of its labouring communities during the Victorian era. Between 1801 and 1851 the population of England and Wales doubled, from just under nine million to close to 18 million. By 1921 the figure stood at almost 38 million (Registrar General, 1925, table 2). This astounding growth imposed an unprecedented demand upon an ill-equipped building industry. Extraordinary pressure was put on urban and suburban land, enriching landholders as never before, especially those with land in and around the industrial towns of the Midlands and the North. By 1851 a quarter of the population lived in 10 urban centres, and the communities of towns and cities were growing at twice the rate of the national population as people migrated from the rural areas, Scotland, Wales and Ireland. Between 1821 and 1831, Liverpool's population increased by 44% and Leeds' by more than 47%. Middle class spas and resorts such as Cheltenham and Scarborough grew at the same phenomenal rate in the first half of the 19th century (Burnett, 1986, p 10).

Houses were erected on pockets of vacant land, rear gardens and in rows inserted between or behind earlier structures. As these spaces were exhausted, the towns sought to sprawl outwards. Long terraces began to stretch across the countryside. Sometimes new towns arose. The Duke of Devonshire erected Barrow-in-Furness on his land in the middle of the 19th century. In 1829, six Quakers bought 500 acres of farmland on the banks of the River Tees, laying out Middlesbrough on a gridiron plan, its population of 154 in 1831 soaring to 40,000 by 1870. The ancient towns, however, struggled to come to terms with the old property rights fixed to the surrounding open fields. Particularly awkward were the Lammas rights of pasture, under which some townspeople had an entitlement to graze livestock on the open fields after the harvest. These were a species of property rights known in English law as *profit à prendre*: rights to go on to another's land and take something away. The landholder may have wished to sell for building purposes, but the *profit à prendre* thwarted him. The consequences for the people of Nottingham were serious (Hoskins, 1985, pp 280-9).

Nottingham, one of the most attractive towns of the 18th century, walled like Chester and York, had by 1845 been reduced to a slum. As the Health of Towns Commission heard that year: "nowhere else shall we find so large a mass of inhabitants crowded into courts, alleys and lanes as in Nottingham, and those, too, of the worst possible construction.... Some parts of Nottingham (are) so very bad as hardly to be surpassed in misery by anything to be found within the entire range of our manufacturing cities" (Hoskins, 1985, pp 280-1). To the north and south of the town, brushing against three quarters of its boundary, were nearly 1,100 acres of open fields. Those townspeople who held pasture rights steadfastly refused to permit development. Borough elections were fought over the issue, and candidates supporting development were burnt in effigy. The freeholders of the land could do nothing against the 'Cowocracy', as those with *profit à prendre* were called. Other townspeople opposed enclosure and development, because they foresaw the land sold off for speculative building without proper planning and reservation of space for public recreation. Also benefiting from the confusion were the owners of what were rapidly becoming urban slums. Demand for any piece of land within the town became so intense that landholders made fortunes in exorbitant rents and sales, as invariably happens when neighbouring land is held off the market. Streets required precious land, so mazes of courts and alleys were erected on former gardens, orchards and parks. In some areas there was one person to every six square yards of living space.

By the time a town corporation was elected by Nottingham in favour of enclosure and development, the damage was done. Not until about 1880 could a start be made to clear some of the worst slums in the country. In Leicester, by contrast, rights of common land had been lost with enclosure of its surrounding fields in the 18th century. Hence landholders were free to sell for development and Leicester expanded outwards. With abundant land available, wide streets were constructed and houses often had four rooms for a family.

The ancient fragmentation of property rights in land had serious social, political and economic consequences for the town of Stamford in Lincolnshire (Elliot, 1969). The land in dispute was the Borough waste beyond the town walls, kept vacant for purposes of defence. The waste lay in the Manor of Stamford, whose lord came from the Cecil family, but the freemen of the town had had customary pasture rights on this land for as long as anyone could recall. For the town to expand, the waste had to be developed, and this perceived need for growth had driven up its rental value by the early 1800s. The freemen started to build on the waste, and by 1828 there were about 100 scattered buildings valued at about £15,000. This development upset the Lord of the Manor, who considered that if any had a right to the fee simple of the waste it was he.

Lord Burghley, descendent of Lord High Treasurer William Cecil of Elizabethan fame, had two sons. Robert inherited Theobalds and the family estates of Hertfordshire. The elder son, Thomas, inherited the vast Burghley Park straddling Northamptonshire, Huntingdonshire and

Lincolnshire. Burghley House was near Stamford, and the perimeter of Burghley Park abutted the town limits. Thomas, Lord of the Manor of Stamford, enjoyed considerable political clout. Stamford returned two members to parliament, and the Cecils had control of voting behaviour. The Marquess of Exeter (the Cecils' title from 1801) influenced the occupiers of the town houses he owned, he had the town's six advowsons (the Manor appointed the churchmen), and he had the patronage of all tradesmen in the Borough. The Cecils owned more than half of the 12,000 acres of open field to the south of the town. As Lord of the Manor, Lord Exeter's permission was needed to procure an Act of Enclosure of these lands from parliament, but he would not give it – not until he acquired full title to the waste.

These, the years of the early 19th century, saw massive enclosures of the ancient commons and open farmlands (see Chapter Twelve). By 1817 the enclosure of parishes surrounding Stamford had been completed with that of Easton-on-the-Hill. But Exeter would not agree to enclosure of Stamford's fields until the Borough waste was his settled property. The dispute eventually forced up the Rent of surrounding land, an enclosed paddock of under two acres in Wothorpe selling for the 'extraordinary price' of £245 in 1829.

The town's freemen insisted on their customary rights. They packed the Town Council and declared that it, not Lord Exeter, held the fee simple of the waste. To advance their claim, the freemen built on parcels of the waste and even sold some to unsuspecting purchasers. As Lord of the Manor, Exeter regularly amerced (fined) the occupants through the Manor Court, calling these amercements 'rents' in the hope that they would become accepted as such.

Problems arose for the freemen with the passage of the Municipal Reform Act in 1835 (see Chapter Eleven) which abolished the ancient chartered constitutions of government in the boroughs. The Act did not make explicit what should happen to their privileges. This development weakened their case and failed to clarify who had rights to exercise on the waste. With the Rent of this land rising, neither lord nor freemen would relent, so deadlock persisted until Lord Exeter's death in 1867. The third Marquess of Exeter then abandoned this policy and allowed the Stamford Enclosure Act. Those on the waste were now allowed to convert what they held to legal freeholds on payment of a fine to the Marquess, as assessed by a valuer.

Industrialism passed Stamford by. Today it is treasured as an old and picturesque town of pearly-grey limestone – popular with tourists. Why did Stamford not turn into a congested slum like Nottingham? The answer is that owing to the dispute the main railway line was diverted to Peterborough, about 10 miles to the east. No railway meant no industry, and therefore no industrial workforce to accommodate.

Some great landlords were laying out towns with good streets, a water supply and drainage, as, for example, Sir John Ramsden of Huddersfield, or the Duke of Norfolk at Glossop. Too often, however, the landholder was simply profiteering, as in many Midlands towns where formerly substantial houses were repeatedly sub-divided and over-crowded to become what were known as 'rookeries'. Speculative builders threw up mean 'back to back' terraces and courts, niggardly with land and materials.

House building and the Victorian economy

There is little information about house building between 1800 and 1850, but what there is: "makes clear ... that building activity moved, not in step with the increasing population and social need, but in waves and cycles determined in part by external economic considerations. House building experienced two types of fluctuation – short term, averaging between five and 10 years and based on the business cycle, and long term, of 20 or more years' duration and of wider amplitude. The latter was much more evident from the 1860s onwards, and the short term more significant for the first half of the century ... peaks in 1819, 1825, 1836, 1847, troughs in 1821, 1832 and 1842" (Burnett, 1986, p 16). This pattern was clearly related to the combination of high demand for living accommodation and repeated efforts by landholders to 'cash in' by forcing up land prices and rents, bringing in the cycles of acceleration and recession.

The Royal Commission on the Poor Laws (1905-9) heard how economic depression followed peaks in house building with monotonous regularity: 1820 was a year of 'depression and revival'; in 1826 there was a 'crash' and in 1827 to 1831, 'distress'. In 1835 to 1837 there was 'urban prosperity', but in 1838 to 1842, 'universal distress'. Between 1843 and 1845 there was 'prosperity and speculation', and in later 1847 'crisis and depression' (Royal Commission on the Poor Laws and Relief of Distress, 1909, p 421). In 1876 the annual rate of house building reached 47 per 10,000 population. Then came the great depression, persisting with little relief until 1887. House building per 10,000 population fell back to 23 in 1890 before picking up to 44 in 1898. The period 1897 to 1900 was another of 'prosperity', but by 1903 there was once more 'deep distress'.

Yet extraordinarily, despite the collapse in the general economy and the decline in capital investment in these years of recession, the return to Land as Rent continued to rise steadily (Harrison, 1983, p 74).

Landlords, house jobbers and tenants

In 1848 the Statistical Society recorded the wages and rents in London's St George's-in-the-East, and the exercise was repeated by the Board of Trade in 1887 (at the end of the recession). The comparison showed that for some workers, the increase in wages over this 40 year period had gone completely on a rise in rent (Stedman Jones, 1971, p 216). The Royal Commission on Housing of the Working Classes, meeting in 1885, heard that in those hard times rents were rising dramatically even though food prices were falling and wages were stationary. Landholders of inner-city slums were generally separated from the tenant by the small leaseholder, often a small businessman with sufficient capital to acquire a lease on a piece of land. He then sub-let to another, known as a 'house jobber' or 'knacker', who made a quick profit on the tail-end of a lease by over-crowding and charging extortionate rents. The profit was often very large because the ground rent going to the original landlord having the freehold might amount only to a small fraction of the tenant's rent. For example, Lord Northampton had leased land in Clerkenwell for £20 a year. The leaseholding 'jobber' had on that land a house, sub-divided and over-crowded, on which he collected £100 annually in rents while allowing the property to decay. Of course defaulting tenants often did a moonlight flit, and firms of carters hired out their equipment especially for this purpose. Such activities were only aggravated by the Small Tenements Recovery Act of 1838, giving the landlord summary powers of eviction for non-payment of rent.

Taxes and house prices in the 19th century

Further distortion of the housing market was imposed by the government's habit of taxing almost everything that could be sold. Excises on bricks, timber, stone, slates and tiles were estimated in 1850 to add £20 to the basic cost of £40 for the ordinary cottage (Burnett, 1986, p 21). Then there was the window tax, by 1850 criticised for restricting light and ventilation, and therefore replaced by a tax on inhabited houses in 1851, at a loss to the Exchequer of more than £1 million a year. The brick tax was also repealed in 1850 at a further loss of revenue of about £500,000 annually.

First local experiments with public housing

Many towns became alarmed at the degeneration of the urban environment. Liverpool designed its first building by laws between 1842 and 1846, panicking speculative landholders and builders into a headlong dash to build before tighter controls brought an end to the 'good times'. Demand for housing was so great in the city in these years that a cottage with minimal dimensions of 12 foot frontage and 13 foot 6 inches depth would cost about £100, of which between 35 and 50% represented the price of Land (Cairncross and Weber, 1956-57). The inspectors of England's Victorian prisons considered nothing less than 1,000 cubic feet of space for every prisoner to be essential for health, yet in Liverpool's slums many inhabitants made do with 70 cubic feet. This state of affairs prompted the city to experiment. Its council housing development of St Martin's Cottages in 1869 charged two shillings and six pence (2s 6d) a week for one room flats; four-room flats cost 5s 3d (Burnett, 1986, pp 153-4). These were attempts to escape the grip of the 'jerry builder', a term first applied to the cheap builder in Liverpool about 1830 (derived from the nautical term 'jerry' or 'jury', as in 'jerry rig', meaning a temporary erection to cover an emergency). Small firms would build without laying proper foundations, placing basement boards within inches of damp ground and using badly burnt bricks to build flimsy walls, soon riddled with damp. London also passed a Building Act in 1844 in an attempt to improve the housing of the poor, but bribery of the inspectors was believed to be commonplace (Burnett, 1986, p 157).

The diseases of over-crowding

An investigation in Leeds in 1851 disclosed 222 lodging houses within a quarter of a mile of the parish church, in which 2,500 people slept at over two to a bed, often in filthy conditions (Harrison, 1971, p 61). Similar reports came from around the country. These dirty, insanitary and over-crowded properties were the focus of typhus fever, a cause of many hundreds of deaths each year in those days. The other 'spotted fever', not easily distinguishable from typhus, was 'typhoid' (like typhus). Though Coytharus had first suggested that the two were different diseases in 1578, it took 19th century science to separate them. The pathological distinctions had been described in 1832, but clinically the differential diagnosis remained difficult. Until 1869 the Registrar General of England and Wales did not differentiate the two conditions on the death certificate.

As long ago as 1685 Cober suggested that the human body louse was somehow implicated in typhus. Not until 1906, however, was it firmly established that insects could spread human disease when Howard Taylor Ricketts showed that a related disease found in America, Rocky Mountain spotted fever, was spread by a tick. Ricketts, who gave his name to these forms of bacteria (Rickettsia), died of flea-borne typhus acquired in the research laboratory in 1910. About this time Charles Nicolle in Algeria demonstrated that the transmission of epidemic typhus was definitely by human body lice. Epidemics of typhus are known to recur because some patients who recover have a recrudescence many years later. For example, some survivors of the concentration camps of the Second World War have had the disease return as long as 30 years afterwards. If lice are about at this time, there is a serious risk of a new epidemic.

Typhus, though a disease of the slums, could be spread to more affluent districts by lice-ridden children and adults. The disease was no respecter of social class. The Reverend Patrick Bronte lost his daughters Maria and Elizabeth when the disease got into their boarding school in Lancashire in 1826. Neither was typhoid a respecter of class. Queen Victoria lost her beloved Prince Albert to the disease on the 14 December 1861, and in 1872 she almost lost her eldest son Bertie in the same way. The organism that causes typhoid was identified by D. E. Salmon, a veterinary pathologist, together with Theobald Smith in 1885. The salmonella typhi bacterium spreads from one human being to the next, though sometimes by way of the housefly. Asymptomatic carriers of salmonella contaminate food and drinking water, and drinking water can also be contaminated with infected sewage.

Typhus and typhoid were responsible for almost 2,000 deaths a year in England and Wales throughout the 1850s and 1860s. To tackle this problem, Lord Shaftesbury created the Labourers Friendly Society, later to become the Society for Improving the Conditions of the Working Classes, with Prince Albert as its first President. In 1845 the Society erected a model lodging house in London's Clerkenwell, soon to be followed by another in the infamous St Giles. The Lodging Houses Act of 1851, introduced by Lord Shaftesbury, gave local authorities powers to register and inspect these places, as well as set standards by providing model lodging houses.

Cholera, another scourge, had raged in 1831-32 at the time of the first Reform Bill. Another outbreak in 1848-49, during the last upsurge of Chartism, added impetus to the movement for housing reforms. The outbreak of 1854 swept away 20,000 as it spread through England and Wales that summer. On Sunday 17 September, Charles Dickens' daughter

Mamie was struck down by the disease. With a house full of children, Dickens was terrified, but to his immense relief Mamie recovered and the others escaped.

Places like St Giles in London, Oxford Road in Manchester, Nottingham's 'Shambles' and Liverpool's Scotland Road posed major threats to health, and local medical officers of health were by now well aware of the direct relation between death rates and over-crowding. Not until 1891, however, was over-crowding first officially defined as more than two adults per room, a child under 10 years counting as half an adult, and an infant's presence being ignored. Building of those dark, badly ventilated, crowded back to back terrace houses was banned in Manchester in 1844 and in Liverpool in 1861, but many years elapsed before their demolition. In 1866 the London member of parliament W.M. Torrens proposed a bill which would have permitted wholesale slum clearance and municipal housing. In the event, however, the Torrens Act of 1868 was watered down to empower local councils to demand improvements to individual properties only, or their demolition (Fraser, 1984, p 76).

Power to cover whole districts of slum housing awaited the Cross Act of 1875, otherwise known as the Artisans and Labourers Dwellings Improvement Act. Yet this Act was thwarted by private land monopoly. As soon as local authorities wished to buy insanitary areas at a price to be settled by arbitration, slum owners forced profits from rent to a peak by yet more over-crowding. Property values were calculated from commercial rents, so slum dwellings became a source of excessive profit when bought out. Amendments were introduced, but compensation crippled the Act and discouraged local authorities from demolishing houses which blighted their citizens' life and health.

Central government and the 'slum problem', 1890-1920

Up to 1980 local authorities had powers only to enforce demolition of insanitary housing, but in that year under Part III of the Housing of the Working Classes Act they were given the right to build houses. In London, local authorities were ordered to re-house at least 50% of those displaced by demolitions (which up until then had contributed to shortages and driven up rents of the remaining stock). The Act of 1900 of the same name established similar powers and obligations for provincial boroughs, together with powers to acquire building land. The response was weak, however, and between 1890 and 1914 only 5% of houses built were for local councils. In many respects, Liverpool again led the way. The filthy Gildarts Gardens area was pulled down and rebuilt. The prize-winning block of tenements in Victoria Square had already been opened by Lord Cross in 1885. Between 1901 and 1907 Dryden Street, Adlington Street, Kew Street, Kempston Street and Hornby Street came down and went up again. The City Engineer, J.A. Brodie, built experimental tenements of prefabricated panels of concrete in 1905. All this cost Liverpool's ratepayers £56 per person. Other cities modelled their approach on Birmingham which chose to force repairs of existing properties on the private owner, thereby keeping costs to ratepayers at less than £1 per head for administrative charges only (Burnett, 1986, p 184). The government struggled on. John Burn's Housing and Town Planning Act of 1909 at long last put a national ban on building back to back houses, and allowed local authorities to go in and repair insanitary houses at the owner's expense. But the rent of new or improved property always tended to drive poor families back into the cheaper slums, thereby raising the return to the slum landlords and the costs of buying them out.

The nation's 'slum problem' was very much in existence in 1914, leading Lloyd George to declare that a primary objective of the wartime coalition government was to plan a post-war housing programme to provide 'homes fit for heroes'. The Victorian experience had finally driven home two messages: that it was not simply a matter of building houses, but of building to a proper standard; and that private builders and landlords could rarely provide houses at affordable rents for British working people in general. Then something strange happened soon after the start of the First World War. In areas where the industry of war was booming, increased local prosperity was soon followed by sharply rising rents. In Glasgow there was a little revolution – a rent strike. Government quickly responded with the Rent and Mortgage Restriction Act of 1915, pegging rents at levels charged at the outbreak of war. Nevertheless, after the Armistice and demobilisation men returned to a nation short of 600,000 houses. This influx created a great danger of rising rents and house prices, and the government found it impossible to repeal the Act of 1915. Faced with the high costs of labour and materials at that time, private builders did not build for the poor.

The government had foreseen some of these problems, and in 1917 had asked the member of parliament Sir John Tudor Walters, a major contributor to the Garden City movement (see below), to "consider questions of building construction ... of dwellings of the working classes" (Burnett, 1986, p 223). His Report of 1918 was revolutionary, laying down standards for local authority housing which remained as such even beyond the Second World War. In quick response, the Local Government Board had by 1919 issued a *Housing manual* giving advice and instructions for local authorities. Its call for planning to develop beauty of vista, with good exteriors in harmony with the surroundings, was reinforced by Dr Christopher Addison's Housing and Town Planning Act of 1919, soon to become the responsibility of the new Ministry of Health. Local authorities were required to survey their housing needs and report within three months. Thereafter they were to plan and carry out their re-housing programmes with the approval of the Ministry. Costs to local ratepayers were to be limited to an extra penny in the pound, the Treasury picking up the rest of the bill. The whole crisis was expected to be resolved by 1927, and up to then the rents of new council houses were to be fixed in line with the Act of 1915, irrespective of building costs. The nation was going to war again, but this time on a home front against slum housing.

Housing subsidies are taken into Rent

Government consistently under-estimated the power of the landholder and his ownership of Rent. As soon as central government funds became available for land purchase, up went the price, to thwart government's intentions. Although in 1920 the nation was plunging into yet another economic recession, the cost of house building boomed. While general prices had doubled since pre-war days, homes were costing four times as much. What cost £250 to build in 1914 cost £1,250 in 1920, barely 12 months after Addison's Act. As Sir J. Walker Smith, Director of Housing at the Ministry of Health wrote in these years: "... money alone will not permanently cure slums ... subsidies of any kind are apt to produce unexpected results.... The experience of the 1919 Act under which approximately 178,000 houses were built at an estimated capital cost of £178 million – £1,000 a house ... is a warning to us not to disregard economic laws" (Townroe, 1928, p vi). Understanding these economic laws, especially the law of Rent, is the first prerequisite. The Archbishop of Canterbury was moved to declare in 1928 that the "continuance (of bad housing) in a Christian country is contrary to the Will of God". Yet the Addison approach to the housing problem left government the legacy of a debt of more than £7 million a year, estimated not to be cleared until 1980 (Townroe, 1928, p 2). Far from everything being put right by 1927, Leeds, Birmingham, Bradford and Sheffield had between them in that year 165,000 back to back houses still occupied, even though the death rate in such badly ventilated houses was at least 15% higher than in houses with good ventilation.

Using the definition for over-crowding of more than two adults per room, the Chief Medical Officer of Health, Sir George Newman, pointed out that although between 1911 and 1921 the situation had improved in London, in many other regions it had deteriorated. Local councils were neglecting to condemn insanitary properties, the defence being that they had nowhere to accommodate the displaced families. In some districts, known cases of people with open tuberculosis were sharing their bedroom with other persons. Nearly every house in which tuberculosis had been notified was over-crowded, badly ventilated or damp. The bitter fact was that most manual workers and agricultural workers were unable to afford the commercial rent of a cottage suitable for healthy living. Even local authorities, forced to keep in step with the private rented sector, could not offer cottages at a rent that many poor families could afford. As Sir George put it: "Over-crowding, with its attendant evils, will continue until some scheme can be devised to provide wholesome housing accommodation at a rental within the reach of an agricultural labourer with a family" (Townroe, 1928, p 28). This had been known for many years. Liverpool's model tenements in Victoria Square were not occupied by those who had formerly dwelt in the demolished slums, as intended, but by a wealthier class of working man's family.

In the 10 years after 1918 the London County Council built more than 37,000 dwellings for rent, accommodating nearly 160,000 people. Families in slums whose circumstances demanded immediate attention were seen by a medical officer of health and given preferential consideration. Nevertheless, this amounted to only a small bite at the slum problem created over the previous century. It took Addison's grant of powers to local authorities for the compulsory purchase of land and insanitary houses, to the loss of the owners, in order to move forward in the capital. Land cost 12s to 18s per square foot north of the River Thames, as compared with 5s to 8s on the south side. A nine storey block could accommodate 3,000 people in a small area, so the Council began experimenting with high rise housing to the north. The highest apartments were the most popular, being above the smoke and pollution at street level, and therefore commanded the highest rents. The Council planned to include children's playgrounds on roofs, centralised laundries and electric lighting, but in 1925 these were all in the future. The problem for the Council was the private landlord, as illustrated by the following example.

There is a block of small cottages that is certainly ... an unhealthy area. In the old days the cottages were built around a central garden, but as land became more valuable, buildings were erected on this inner ground. Consequently, the rooms that formerly looked out on the open ground have no direct access to light or air. They ... have been rightly condemned ... by the health authorities.... But every attempt so far to deal with this block of property has completely failed.... The houses are owned by three different landlords who would be only too glad to dispose of the property at a price. Various attempts have been made to obtain a reasonable figure, but the site is one of the most attractive in London, and an adjacent house that had been empty for some time as it was collapsing and dangerously insecure, sold easily for a high price. ... Site value might run a very high figure. It is consequently an almost insuperable task to know how to deal with this ... property without asking the local ratepayers to pay an extravagant sum.... (Townroe, 1928, pp 49-50)

Under the 1890 Act the London County Council paid the market value for 40 acres of insanitary areas up to 1914, placing on the local ratepayer a charge of over £750,000 (roughly £23 million at 1993 prices) *after* deduction had been made for land resold and for the housing value of the land retained (Townroe, 1928, p 52). Many other cities faced similar problems. Nottingham, for example, had tackled its slums with vigour since 1880, but in 1925 there were still 5,000 back to back houses to clear. This was nowhere near the 72,000 back to backs in Leeds and 33,000 in Bradford.

Of the many problems facing those bent on improvement of the nation's housing stock, that of compensation to the landholder proved one of the most difficult. The desire of slum landlords to profit excessively at the State's expense forced the State on to the attack. Under an Act of 1925, the local authority became obliged to compensate the owner of slum property for the site value only, which the owners saw as confiscation. The site value fixed was not that governed by free market forces but one commensurate with the local authority's determination to use it for working-class housing. The law laid down that the value for purposes of compensation was that as a cleared site available for development in accordance with local by laws. Consequently a property in good repair could be caught up in slum clearance and the owner lose much capital, including the goodwill of a small business. There were numerous examples of injustice, with destruction of a family's capital, in misguided attempts to overcome the problems posed by the private landholder.

Complacency and concern: slum clearance in the 1920s

Many asked how the economy could be re-ordered so that those struggling to eke out a mere existence could be re-housed. Could their incomes be raised through wages or did the money need to come from local and central taxes? Others, enthusiasts of eugenic arguments of the day, saw little future for the dwellers of slums. Here is one Dr Hanschell in a letter to *The Spectator*:

> As a medical practitioner I have had to tend professionally ... the slum denizens and their broods in the slum and in the hospital.... I suggest that the true slum-making slum denizen is a valid sub-species of *Homo sapiens* ... I have observed this sub-species in the tropics – where minus 'housing difficulties' ... it appears as 'poor white trash'.... There exists evidence ... that some ... of this sub-species' young are like the parent, hopeless and helpless by reason of stamped-in mental defect.... It is important to find out ... how much of these unfortunates' misfortune be environmental only; how much, if any, actually inherent in the stock. ... They belong to no herd but their peculiar own ... they are entirely unblameworthy. Only savage ignorance blames and punishes a mule for its mulishness. (Townroe, 1928, pp 19-21)

Fortunately local authorities did not see eye to eye with the eugenicists.

The economic nonsense of slum housing had been acknowledged for many years. In Glasgow, council housing came in 1922, and over the next three years the annual number of admissions for pulmonary tuberculosis in the city fell by 742 cases. Each case admitted cost the community on average more than £43, so the housing scheme had saved £32,000 a year. If this figure were to represent commercial rent at an interest on the capital of 5%, the capitalised total would add up to more than £600,000, enough to build 1,200 houses in 1925. King George V was under no illusion about the housing problem. In 1919 he declared: "It is not too much to say that an adequate solution to the housing question is the foundation of all social progress. Health and housing are indissolubly connected" (Townroe, 1928, p 31). But the solution to the chronic housing problem has not been correctly identified by governments in the 80 years since then.

Public concern for housing of the poor led to a large number of voluntary bodies and private initiatives, some in collaboration with the local authorities. All aimed to provide new dwellings for the poor at an affordable rent. Slum properties were taken over and renovated by voluntary housing associations, often with capital donated at a very low rate of interest. Many associations had prominent citizens as figureheads. Lord Balfour of Burleigh was chairman of the Kensington Housing Trust Ltd, registered as a public utility society in 1927. The St Pancras House Improvement Trust had the patronage of the Magdalen College Mission, behind which were some very wealthy men of Oxford. Plymouth's housing trust was financed with capital provided by Lord and Lady Astor. Oswestry's trust had Lord Harlech for its President. In addition, the building societies would lend to any man who had saved a deposit and could show that he could repay the principal with interest over about 15 years, but this was a feat beyond most of the working class.

The inability of poor families to afford rents for housing determined in the market is well illustrated by the plight of the agricultural worker of the 1920s. By 1928, Addison's Housing Act of 1919 had stimulated the construction of 177,000 houses by rural councils and more than 100,000 rural houses by private builders. But government subsidies had driven up land prices and rents, and builders needed to borrow capital at interest in order to commence construction. The agricultural worker's wage would not cover the rent determined by these land prices and interest charges. Consequently what was meant for the rural poor went to others who could afford a weekend home in the country.

The Housing Act of Wheatley (1924) tried to stimulate building at rents affordable for the low paid worker. A subsidy was offered to builders of rural housing of £12 10s for 40 years. Added to a subsidy already offered by the local authority, this was equivalent to a capital of £250 on a 5% basis. At once the subsidy was captured in Rent, driving up commercial rents of which Rent is a part. The effect was fully exposed when government subsequently reduced the subsidy in 1926. Costs to the builder and consequently rents fell back appreciably (Townroe, 1928, pp 131-2). The Act, which remained in force until 1937, largely failed to provide working-class homes, even though generally regarded as the most successful of inter-war housing measures. Local authorities built almost 500,000 houses, while private builders put up about two million in the same period up to 1934. This meant that the number of middle-class houses increased by at least 50%, while that of working class houses for rent rose by less than 20%. Furthermore, council houses went largely to the better off among the working class such as semi-skilled workers with secure jobs. In Liverpool, for example, the income of successful applicants for council housing was on average 20% above that of the working class in general. Not until the 1930s were housing schemes aimed specifically at the poor.

The Inland Revenue's stimulation of privatised Rent

In the 1920s the Inland Revenue began to permit refunds in respect of tax on the amount of mortgage interest paid. This 'perk' at the taxpayers' expense immediately raised the level of demand, only to be translated to a rise in the selling price and commercial rent of properties. In the final analysis, this subsidy to house-ownership settled into the sink for all such subsidies – Rent. Once introduced, the 'perk' proved extremely difficult to withdraw; by 1974 it was costing the Treasury over £1 billion a year. This figure was only £250 million less than the total central government subsidy to local authorities (Timmins, 1996, p 329). Because the perquisite went mostly to the better off, it more or less cancelled any redistribution of income and wealth to the poorer sector through Welfare housing policies.

In 1985, Michael Meacher got a cool response to his suggestion that mortgage interest tax relief should be phased out (Timmins, 1996, p 488). Instead, the encouragement of private house-ownership by the Conservatives in the 1980s, and efforts to reduce the costs of local authority housing, caused mortgage interest tax relief to counter even further the redistribution of income under the Welfare State. Not until the 1990s did governments bite the bullet and begin to phase out the subsidy, after almost 70 years of existence. Throughout, however, the building societies pleaded that withdrawal of mortgage interest tax relief would damage the housing market (ie prices would fall). It is not that house prices would fall, but rather that for too long land prices had been boosted by a tax subsidy which raised Rent. The scheme made housing even less affordable for poor families, who lacked the resources to get in on the racket. Most house purchasers remained blissfully unaware that they were unintentionally thwarting a primary purpose of the Welfare State, regretting the fact that by 1998 mortgage interest tax relief had been reduced to 10% of the interest on the first £30,000 of the loan, and in 2000 disappeared altogether.

The rise and fall of the Garden City movement

Another major development in the early 20th century was the Garden City movement. The official definition of a Garden City was "a town planned for industry and healthy living; of a size that makes possible the full measure of social life, but not larger; surrounded by a permanent belt of rural land; the whole of the land being in public ownership or held in trust for the community" (Townroe, 1928, p 155). The founder of the movement, Ebenezer Howard, saw the Garden City as one answer to Britain's transformation from a largely rural to largely urban society during Queen Victoria's reign. The new towns would combine urban advantages with rural pleasures and benefits, all secured by public ownership of the land. The movement chimed well with the enthusiasm for national planning and social engineering which abounded after the First World War.

The ideas stemming from Ebenezer Howard's book of 1898, *Tomorrow*, were discussed at the Garden City conference in Bournville in 1901. Work on Britain's first such private green field development at Letchworth in Hertfordshire was undertaken between 1903 and 1906. The plans laid out a town for about 35,000 inhabitants on almost 4,000 acres of what had been farmland. The concept was largely destroyed, however, by the construction there of a large munitions factory during the First World War. Welwyn Garden City Ltd was founded on the 26 April 1920, as part of the 'homes fit for heroes' campaign. Almost four square miles of land near Hatfield, Hertfordshire, were bought for around £90,000 (£1.3 million at 1993 prices) from Lords Salisbury and Desborough. Manchester built its satellite city of Wythenshawe between 1927 and 1941, motivated by the same movement, but Wythenshawe is now simply another suburb of the city.

Overall, the Garden City movement made little impact on the nation's housing problem (Burnett, 1986, p 293). Even in these new developments the most serious difficulty faced by planners seeking to move families out of the slums into new accommodation was the high probability of an increased rent. The transferred tenants were frequently unable to raise such a figure, as well as local taxes, out of their family income. This mismatch between land prices and income continues to thwart the best efforts even today. It has meant the continuation of a survivor of Poor Law relief in the form of housing subsidies and rent rebates.

The slum problem in the 1930s

The problem of low income combined with high land prices dragged many newly housed families down into debt. In the early 1930s, the 90,000 residents of the Becontree estate outside London grew accustomed to crowds of passengers taking their bundles of belongings for pawn every Monday morning on the bus to Barking. A much publicised study in Stockton-on-Tees showed that in a sample of families moved from a slum area to a new council estate, there remained only 2s 11d per week per man for food after increased rent and travel expenses had been taken into account, as compared with 4s formerly. The standardised mortality rate actually increased from 23 per 1,000 per year before the move to more than 33 per 1,000 afterwards. By contrast, another sample from the same slum area, which remained there, showed a small reduction in mortality over the same period (M'Gonigle and Kirby, 1936, pp 108-29).

The housing problem persisted throughout the 1920s and 1930s because, by and large, private builders could afford to build only for the private middle class buyer, local authorities could not acquire land commensurate with an affordable rent for the majority of the working classes, and among working people unemployment grew to three million by 1931. As one writer emphasised, "The fundamental problem was the level of rents in relation to earnings" (Burnett, 1986, p 239). Even the heavy Wheatley subsidies, specifically designed to reduce rents, simply raised the price of land and were self-defeating. Surveys showed repeatedly that the lower the family income, the higher the proportion taken as rent. Just before the Second World War, families with incomes of less than £2 per week were spending one third on rent.

Faced with these difficulties, some local authorities introduced sliding scales of rent for the poor of the 1930s. Leeds found that even with the Wheatley subsidies its rents of 10s or more per week, plus the local rates, excluded much of the working class. In 1934 the Council therefore introduced a system of differential rents based on a means-tested scale, itself based on the British Medical Association's requirements for an adequate diet. The result – by 1935 as many as 11% of Council tenants were living rent-free. The political complexion of the Leeds City Council changed from Labour to Conservative within a year and the scheme was abandoned, leaving the problem unresolved.

The 1930s saw a swing in housing Welfare policy back to the Victorian aim of helping those in most need first and foremost. An interesting forerunner of the 1980s 'trickle down' notion of the Conservatives, whereby Wealth going to the rich was supposed to gravitate in part to the poor, emerged within housing policy in those days. It was called 'filtering up' rather than 'trickling down' (Burnett, 1986, p 242). The idea was that as the better off moved into new houses provided by private builders and local authorities, the poorest would occupy the accommodation vacated, thereby finding themselves better housed. This did not happen. Many could not afford the rents of these properties demanded in advance by the landlords, especially the one million or more new families added between 1923 and 1934. The housing stock was growing more rapidly than the population, but family size was falling in all sectors of society. The additional young working class families tended to be stuck in a room in the parents' home.

So intransigent was the housing problem, given the unwillingness to consider Rent reform, that one commentator could write in 1935: "No other civilised country has such vast tracts of slumdom.... For size and density, foul air and wretchedness, the slums of Britain are a class apart" (Burnett, 1986, p 243). To this problem the Greenwood Act of 1930 and the Housing Act of 1933 were specifically addressed, providing subsidies from the Treasury for slum clearance. The problem for the local authorities was how to define a slum for purposes of mandatory demolition and rehousing. The Acts were unclear. Nevertheless, work got underway, especially on multiple storey flats for the poor, for which the Greenwood Act offered a special subsidy. Thousands of flats were going up by 1939, mostly in blocks of up to five storeys, but one third of the population still lived in slum or near-slum conditions at the outbreak of the Second World War.

Public housing policy and national reconstruction, 1945-65

Six years of war between 1939 and 1945 set Britain's housing situation back considerably. Building had been curtailed, properties had aged, and almost half a million houses had been made unusable by German bombing. Labour set itself a target of "a separate dwelling for every family desiring to have one" (Ministry of Construction, 1945), but there was a serious shortage of building materials. The task was made all the more difficult when the marriage rate increased dramatically in the late 1940s, bringing in its wake the 'baby boom'. As part of national planning for reconstruction, private firms needed a licence to build, building materials were controlled, and every encouragement was given to local authorities to construct council houses and flats. The money came, like the Addison Acts of 1919, from Treasury subsidies for general housing needs in the Housing Act of 1946. Large subsidies of £16 10s annually per house for 60 years, on condition that the local authority add another £5 10s, plus extra grants for highly priced land, certainly stimulated council house building in the early post-war years.

Aneurin Bevan, born in 1897, was old enough to be strongly influenced by Tudor Walters and Ebenezer Howard, insisting on high standards for post-war council housing. Just as in the 1920s, however, high costs forced reductions in standards by 1951, and the Conservatives were to cut them further. The New Towns Act of 1946, designating as such 10 towns from Stevenage (1946) to Corby (1950), and another 10 from Skelmersdale (1961) to Central Lancashire (1970), eventually led to 25 new towns accommodating two million people. William Beveridge, his famous report completed and his skirmish into politics ended in defeat in an election at Berwick, found himself free to accept the chairmanship of two new town developments at Newton Aycliffe (Prime Minister Tony Blair's constituency in 1997) and Peterlee in County Durham, about 15 miles from each other as the crow flies. He had advocated development along Ebenezer Howard's lines ever since his days as a writer for *The Morning Post*, and town and country planning suited his philosophy. A mismatch between available funds and the cost of land and materials meant that, to his disappointment, his new towns lacked schools, libraries and playgrounds. They became vast housing estates, occupied almost exclusively, yet again, by the skilled working class (hit by closure of the Fujitsu high technology plant in 1998). Much to Beveridge's open annoyance, under Harold Macmillan and the Conservatives social amenities were given even less attention. In consequence, the Conservatives asked for and received Beveridge's resignation in 1952. He died in Oxford 11 years later, on 16 March 1963, with a final utterance, "I have a thousand things to do" (Harris, 1977, p 470).

Had land been more affordable, as it would have been had not landholders kept the Rent to play with, Labour's record on housing would not have been branded a failure for falling short of declared building targets. A million good quality homes went up between 1945 and 1951, but there could have been many more if the private land market had not been pitted against, and taken advantage of, public needs. Private developers such as Max Rayne began to buy up London's bombed sites, and other developers 'in the know' bought up sites alongside roads designated for widening by London County Council. Herein were the seeds of the spectacular flowering of the publicly listed property company in the 1950s.

In 1952, more than four million families were sharing dwellings (Timmins, 1996, p 182). The number of new families was rising rapidly, as was the number of pensioners, raising demand and, inevitably, land prices for housing. Macmillan recognised overcrowding to be mainly a problem for the poorest, often crammed into slum property. Rents had been controlled since 1939, some at levels that had not changed since the 1920s, and landlords frequently refused to maintain properties in a decent and uncrowded condition on the resultant income. Macmillan knew that, fast though he was building, old houses were becoming uninhabitable at least as rapidly. In response, he proposed a 1920s type of remedy in 1953, that local authorities could acquire slum property for the site value alone and rebuild at a new rent using increased subsidies from the Treasury.

Still the problem would not go away, and so in 1956 Duncan Sandys attempted to overcome the cost issue by providing preferential subsidies for high-rise flats. By 1966 high-rise blocks accounted for a quarter of all new 'starts'. Savings were few if any, however, because the methods of construction cost more than traditional building and the blocks themselves soon started to crumble and run up costs for repairs. Dismayed politicians realised they had thrown up new slums into which had been 'decanted' close to two million people. Subsidies for high rise buildings were abandoned in 1967. Meanwhile there were still too many of the poorest families living in slum private dwellings at controlled rents. The Rent Act of 1957 had triggered 'creeping decontrol' in the hope that higher rents would mean better landlords. By 1960, rents were soaring, but decidedly not the rate of repair. Indeed, the private rented sector was actually diminishing (Timmins, 1996, p 189). To sell was more profitable than to rent.

In the early 1960s came the non-profit housing association, an import from Scandinavia. A few two-bedroom flats in Birmingham, opened in July 1963, were the first fruits. This was publicly funded housing, but unlike council housing, an early manifestation of a renewed tendency to place central government Welfare revenue in the hands of an agency whose mentor is private enterprise. Sir Keith Joseph loaned the recently formed Housing Corporation £100 million to promote the scheme. When Richard Crossman took over for Labour in 1964 he complained that there was "no housing programme ... no information and no plan ... just a lot of meaningless figures" (Timmins, 1996, p 233). The 1965 White Paper sounded pathetically like a voice from the early 1920s: "Once the country has overcome its huge social problem of slumdom and obsolescence and met the need of the great cities for more houses at moderate rents, the programme of subsidised council housing should decrease. The expansion of the public programme now proposed is to meet exceptional needs ... the expansion of building for owner-occupation on the other hand is normal; it reflects a long term social advance which should gradually pervade every region" (Timmins, 1996, p 234).

Private housing and the mortgage: a question of ownership of Rent

To encourage private owner-occupation, the Labour administration of 1964-70 introduced a low interest loan scheme for house purchase on 100% mortgages by those with incomes too low to benefit from tax relief on mortgage interest. Such measures were bound to raise the price of land for housing, but by 1990 half of households in England and Wales were officially classified as 'owner-occupied' for the first time. What 'owner-occupation' means for families with a mortgage is highly debatable. The law as set down in the Law of Property Act of 1925 is highly convoluted on this point, and some very peculiar phraseology is employed for reasons not a little suspect when the Act is set in historical context.

Mortgage of land goes back to the 12th century, but modern systems using land as security for loans can be traced from the late 15th century (Simpson, 1986, pp 242-3). Essentially there were two forms of arrangement. Under the first alternative, the mortgagor (the borrower in possession of the land) transferred his ownership of the estate outright by conveyance to the mortgagee (lender) as security, who then had possession of the title deeds and the estate until the debt was repaid in full. The mortgagor was reduced to a tenant. The alternative, known as the mortgage by demise, allowed the mortgagor to hold on to ownership but to grant the mortgagee a long lease (500 years to 3,000 years), rent-free. The mortgagee would then grant a sub-lease to the mortgagor who then became a subtenant of the mortgagee at a fixed rent. This arrangement remained in force until either the debt was cleared, in which case the mortgagor was re-instated as outright owner-occupier, or the rent fell into arrears and the land was forfeited to the mortgagee.

The mortgage of freehold land by demise became obsolete in the early 19th century when the court took the view that the title deed was indissoluble from the estate to which it pertained. This meant that under the mortgage by demise the mortgagee would have no right to the title deeds. For this reason, right up to the Law of Property Act of 1925, the standard mortgage was one in which the mortgagee took ownership of the estate and the deeds, leaving the mortgagor as tenant until he cleared the debt and the freehold was redeemed by re-conveyance. But the Act of 1925 ruled that from 1 January 1926 the right to possession of the title deeds to the freehold was independent of the estate itself.

By the Act the legal mortgage consists of three tiers:

a) The mortgagor holds the land with an estate in fee simple.
b) The mortgagor obtains a loan of money from the mortgagee by granting as security a rent-free lease of 3,000 years to the mortgagee.
c) The mortgagee grants a sub-tenancy to the mortgagor who thereby falls back into possession.

Under the Act, transfer of the fee simple to the mortgagee is illegal as a form of security. The mortgagee remains entitled to hold the deeds to prevent the mortgagor from dealing in the land, but here is where the Act becomes less than transparent. The Act states that: "A mortgage of an estate in fee simple shall only be capable of being effected at law ... by a demise for a term of years absolute.... Provided that a first mortgagee shall have the same right to the possession of documents *as if* his security included the fee simple" (author's emphasis) (*Halsbury's Statutes of England and Wales*, 1987, vol 37, p 194). Why does the Act portray the mortgagee as one with a peculiar species of right, *as if* he had the ownership of the fee simple, rather than permit the mortgagee the right *to be* owner of the fee simple?

The Law of Property Act also invented a new form of mortgage called the Legal Charge. Under this arrangement (charge by deed by way of legal mortgage), the chargor (borrower) keeps both a form of ownership and possession of the land, but gives the chargee (bank or building society) the right to take the property if the loan is not repaid in the agreed manner. Most people buying houses in the UK are now so doing by Legal Charge. Again, the wording of the Act is peculiar: "Where a legal mortgage of land is created by a charge by deed ... the mortgagee shall have the same protection, powers and remedies ... *as if* – where the mortgage is a mortgage of an estate in fee simple, a mortgage term for 3,000 years ... had been thereby created in favour of the mortgagee" (*Halsbury's Statutes of England and Wales*, 1987, vol 37, p 198). Because the mortgagee by demise has already been given the same right to the deeds as if he or she had the fee simple, in reality mortgagors and chargors are both left with a form of ownership which is very far from complete. Certainly the borrower does not have a property right which is anywhere near being 'good against the world': a right to exclusive use, profit and disposal by sale or gift, which is what is meant by ownership of real property such as land. The mortgagor is obliged to keep the property in good repair, to insure it, and not make structural alterations without the mortgagee's approval. The mortgagor is unable to repay early without penalty, and is denied the right to grant tenancies without the mortgagee's consent.

Why does the Act speak of the lender *as if* he or she is the legal mortgagee and the owner of the fee simple? Why not state with clarity that the lender *is* the owner of the fee simple, as the law had done hitherto? What in reality is the essential difference between a law which states that one man is master of another, and a law which states that one man has the right to act *as if* he is the master of another? For the servant there can be none at all, and for the man with the powers of master also none at all. The answer to the riddle becomes transparent when the Act is set against the background of the Land clauses in the Finance Act of 1909-10, introduced by the Liberal administration of the day.

As explained in more detail in Chapter Fourteen, the Finance Act introduced a small 'land tax' (collection of a very small proportion of the Rent) for central government revenue, much to the horror of landholders. The Act empowered the Inland Revenue to assess the Rent (value of the site excluding capital improvements) of all land in the United Kingdom as a preliminary to its part-collection. Payment was to be made by the owner (rather than the occupier) of the land, defined in the Act as: "... the person entitled in possession to the rents and profits of the land in virtue of an estate of freehold, except that where land is let on lease for a term of which more than 50 years are unexpired, the lessee under the lease ... shall be deemed the owner instead of the person entitled to the rents and profits ..." (Short, 1989, pp 25-6). It is immediately obvious that as the law stood before 1926, the mortgagee as owner of the freehold would be eligible for payment of rent to government and not the mortgagor. Something similar had happened briefly in 1431, when persons receiving rent because they had a charge on land by deed were made liable for a land tax. The land clauses of the Finance Act were repealed well before 1925, but under the contorted arrangements of the Law of Property Act the mortgagor and not the mortgagee would be liable for payment of Rent in any future similar 'land tax'. The mortgagee was safeguarded against any Rent collection, and therefore made more secure than hitherto.

The whole exercise looked like yet another case of the conveyancer's 'sleight of hand', giving priority of consideration to the wealthier client with money to lend before the client needing to borrow. This device of the conveyancer, the '*as if*', had a long precedent, however (see Chapter Nine).

The fact is that under the Law of Property Act the mortgagee or chargee is given substantial ownership of the Rent to the extent of debt outstanding. For the duration of the loan, in practical terms virtually all of the characteristics of ownership reside with the 'lender' and not the borrower. The money transferred is called a loan, but a more realistic interpretation would be that the bank or building society has purchased an ownership of Rent on the land site (and interest on the capital in the buildings) in the same proportion as is the loan to the purchase price of the property. The borrower as occupying tenant enjoys exclusive use of the opportunities afforded by the site, but pays for that part of them covered by the loan as the principal is gradually cleared.

Banks and building societies finance mortgages in two ways in indeterminate proportion, one of which employs the deposits of savers. A key to their enormous wealth, however, is their ability to create money 'out of nothing' for this purpose (Rowbotham, 1998, pp 10-11). A line of credit is opened for the prospective purchaser, which when drawn upon creates an overdraft. This overdraft need have no backing in real wealth, being simply a statement that the tenant in possession as mortgagor owes the bank as mortgagee and deed-holding owner, in return for undisturbed enjoyment of the property under agreed terms. For this enjoyment the tenant turns over the Rent on the site and the interest on the capital in the buildings, usually as a monthly payment. The bank conflates the land and buildings as 'the property or hereditament', and the amalgam of Rent and true interest is thought of as 'interest' in the property. As the principal is reduced the numbers in the overdraft are altered accordingly. But what the bank is counting is its acquisition of real wealth generated by the productive sector represented by the tenant family's wages and interest on private capital. Therefore the mortgage payments do not go into the mortgagor's overdrawn account as might be thought, for real wealth is not required to eliminate an empty piece of financial wizardry. Instead, they are accounted to the bank itself as an asset which is quickly loaned out to secure more Rent. The productive sector, to whom Rent rightfully belongs for the benefit of the public, pays a 'fine' to the non-productive sector for access to this wealth (the mortgage rate). It follows that if governments were to collect the Rent for the nation, 'house prices' would fall, mortgages would not need to cover any element of Rent, and the nation would not be so much in debt.

Of Great Britain's total land area of 240,000 square kilometres, only 7% is classified as urban or suburban (Central Statistical Office, 1995, Table 11.18). Hence in reality, the modern day system of purchase of home-ownership hardly alters *land* monopoly. (Land monopoly is possible because each site is unique, fixed and non-reproducible.) The land occupied by housing development accounts for a high proportion of the total national Rent, however, illustrating how *land* monopoly and *Rent* monopoly are not necessarily one and the same. In 1991, according to the national census 24% of British households owned their houses outright; 43% were called 'owners' but were in reality forms of sub-tenants to their lenders under a mortgage or legal charge; and 33% were either renting or without permanent accommodation. In 2000, outstanding mortgages on houses totalled £505 billion, making banks and building societies together a most formidable Rentholding institution.

To sum up: the Law of Property Act states that the lender is entitled to virtually all of the privileges of ownership, but avoids any liability to taxation of the freeholder in law. The borrower has drawn the short straw, having few of the privileges of the freehold owner in fact, but the responsibility for any taxation of the freehold in law.

Retrenchment of state housing after 1979: the 'Right-to-Buy'

Edward Heath's Conservative administration of 1970-74 introduced another shift in policy. Old properties were to be renovated once again, with subsidies for the same to boot, a policy re-inforced by Peter Walker while at the Department of the Environment. In the wake of the realisation that demolition of slum areas also demolished viable communities, this new policy was in part designed to preserve what had only recently been threatened with destruction. Under the home improvement grant scheme, almost 500,000 such improvements were approved in 1973, 60% being to owner-occupied properties and 40% to council housing. Labour continued this policy between 1974 and 1979, but did not stop a steady sell-off of council houses (Timmins, 1996, p 330). The development to watch, however, was the Housing Association. With the private sector and local government having failed so many poor families, this young hybrid accounted for 20% of housing starts in the 'public sector' in 1978.

Change in direction of the nation's policy on social housing was emphasised by the Conservative administration after 1979. Mrs Thatcher's government sought to re-establish the ascendancy of the private sector, both owner-occupied and rented, and to reduce the public sector as far as was politically feasible. The sale of council houses for owner-occupation under the Conservative housing programme in the 1950s had continued under Labour. This approach was subsequently turned into the centrepiece of housing policy after 1979 under the title of 'Right-to-Buy'. In 1970, 6,000 council tenants in England and Wales bought their houses, and in 1979 42,500, but by 1982 the number had risen to 207,000 (Timmins, 1996, p 330). The reason was the Housing Act of 1980, giving the right of purchase to all tenants of more than three years occupation and granting discounts of up to 50% on the assessed value of the property. Council tenants had up to then looked on while owner-occupiers profited from speculation in the land market and capture of Rent. With the shift from one-earner to two-earner families between the 1950s and the 1980s, the combined incomes had been taken largely in increased rents and purchase prices. In 1953 an average of 9% of household income was devoted to housing, but by 1983 this had risen to close to 17% (Department of Employment, 1983, p 22, table 8). Unearned Rent was soaring ahead of earned income. Wealthier council tenants, like most house owners not understanding what was really going on, now wished to 'take the money' and get in on what seemed a good way to enrich the family.

The combination of certain rises in Rent and land prices, the hundreds of millions of pounds to be claimed in income tax relief on mortgage interest, and now the hand-out of similar amounts (on average 41% of the value of the property in 1983) was too good to miss. No wonder the policy was so popular – privately owning taxpayers thought they were getting council tenants off their backs, while the new owners of ex-council houses were convinced that they could not lose. Most bought on the promised 24 years mortgage (ie Rent capitalised over 15 years could be repaid with interest over a 24-year term). However, the vulnerability of those on low incomes and in insecure employment under this form of ownership was soon apparent, insurance or no insurance.

Amazingly, discounts on sale prices were raised soon after to as high as 70% for apartment residents. The result was the 'sale' of 20% of all council housing, yielding almost £18 billion in the decade after 1979. Over this period, largely as a result of this policy, 'owner-occupation' rose from 55 to 65%, while council housing tenancy fell from 32 to 25%. Yet, strange to say, the government failed to cut the cost of Welfare housing under this scheme. The gift in discounting at least equalled the savings on subsidies to local rates and council rents. Of course, the better stock was bought by better-off tenants. Families left in council housing were the poorer, unable to afford the purchase of their sub-standard housing even at a discount under other government 'low cost' home-ownership programmes.

To add the 'stick' to the 'carrot' of price discounting, government changed the system of subsidies for council housing, reverting (because it resembled means-tested outdoor relief of old) to a system of subsidies to tenants rather than the properties they occupied. In other words subsidies went no longer to local authorities so they could reduce the rents, but as means-tested benefits to enable the poorest to pay unsubsidised rents. The rules of means-testing effectively made council housing less affordable for all but the poorest, leaving the option of purchase increasingly appealing on balance for the not-so-poor. Between 1979 and 1984 council house rents increased about 40% in real terms (Esam, 1987, p 113), and more and more families resorted to 'housing benefit'. By 1993 rents had increased more like 80% in real terms, rises ranging from 65% higher for the poorest to 155% for the wealthiest among council tenants. Many of the better-off tenants avoided those rents by opting for Right-to-Buy.

Central government policy caused local authorities to revert increasingly to their original source of funding for housing the poor – the local property rate. Conservatives saw this development threatening victory in their battle to place private housing in ascendancy. Thus in 1984 the Thatcher administration introduced its Rate Bill to acquire powers to 'rate cap' what it termed 'high spending' councils (Pierson, 1994, p 81). This desire to disarm local government led Mrs Thatcher's administration to introduce its 'community charge' or poll tax in place of the traditional local taxes: a move which proved 'one step too far' in her political career. Still the Conservative administration was not satisfied. Further dominance over local government was sought in the Housing Act of 1988 and the Local Government and Housing Act of 1989. Under the 1988 Act, bids from outside agencies were encouraged to acquire local authority housing, with tenants as arbiter. Staggeringly, as bold as brass, government stipulated that voting abstentions were to count in favour of the bid! Even more brazenly, the 1989 legislation prohibited the use of local taxes for housing purposes. This astounding step went as far as to deny local authorities what even the Poor Law of 1601 had deemed the very least to offset destitution, transferring the function to central government.

Local authorities had no choice but to raise their rents towards the market rate, the unthinkable alternative being to let properties decay until they became uninhabitable. Then, as unemployment increased in the 1980s and 1990s, the bill for housing benefit and the numbers of beneficiaries climbed alarmingly. The response of central government was to withdraw the entitlement to housing benefit at increasingly lower threshold levels of income. In the face of this onslaught, better to buy one's way out of the system on borrowed money, which is precisely what many did. In the private market the age-old mismatch was as strong as ever, however, frustrating the government's desire to see private housing fill the gap opened by the enforced decline in the public sector. As one observer of these years put it: "Landlords do not get the rents they want. If they did, most tenants could not afford the rent" (Crook, 1986, p 643).

Many who were persuaded to plump for owner-occupation in the 1980s soon discovered that they could not afford that option. House (and Rent) repossessions, triggered by failure to repay the mortgage in a timely manner, climbed alarmingly in 1990 to reach a peak of more than 70,000 in 1991. Even in 1996 repossessions were running at 1,000 per week. In the same year almost 900,000 houses stood empty, beyond the affordability of thousands of families in need of a home. Rent controls, which the Conservatives attempted to relax through the Housing Acts of 1980 and 1988, could never conjure an equitable balance, given the private monopoly on land. This was the administration which, more than any other this century, committed itself to expansion of the private sector of housing. Despite the determination of Margaret Thatcher, it failed. Lenders were still pursuing re-possessed borrowers in 1999, the average debt outstanding being £27,000; the total debt from this fiasco being £6.5 billion (*The Guardian*, 8 December 1999).

One wonders when those in power will finally admit that the responsibility for the mess that is housing policy rests with the entrenchment of land monopoly and private appropriation of Rent. Paul Pierson has written: "It is difficult to predict how this impasse will be resolved" (Pierson, 1994, p 87). The fact is that the impasse is a manifestation of an archaic and obsolescent land policy which cannot be overcome until the privatisation of Rent is overcome. Treated wisely by society, Rent could be its faithful servant; as matters stand, Rent is the servant of over-privilege, the taskmaster of under-privilege. Despairing, local authorities were by 1994 selling their stock to the 'new hope', the Housing Association. In 1999, even Glasgow and Birmingham were negotiating to transfer their entire stock to the associations, and the banks were only too keen to fund the deals! Private and public sectors having

Table 6.1: State expenditure on housing (in '1993 pounds')

Years	Total (million)	Per head of population	% of national income
1919	104.6	2.4	0.13
1920	804.3	18.4	1.02
1923	566.6	12.8	0.84
1927	1,962.2	43.4	2.67
1931	1,842.2	40.0	2.47
1938	2,358.1	49.6	2.49
1945	1,385.8	28.3	1.07
1948	5,468.0	110.2	3.89
1953	6,103.7	120.3	4.01
1958	3,875.3	74.6	2.22
1963	5,523.8	103.7	2.64
1968	8,142.1	148.9	3.32
1973	13,545.4	244.4	4.39
1974	20,832.0	376.1	6.59
1979	15,800.8	286.4	4.38
1984	11,239.0	202.5	2.94
1989	10,599.4	188.6	2.15
1993	15,705.0	276.8	3.24

failed to master the ungoverned force, what hope had this hybrid of solving Britain's housing problem, even if this were its purpose? Is it any wonder that Jim Coulter, chief executive of the Housing Federation, ushered in 2000 with the words:"The housing market is creating winners but also losers.... The winners are the ones lucky enough to own a home soaring in value, while the unlucky ones cannot afford a home ..." (*The Guardian*, 17 January 2000).

Taxation for public housing, 1919-93

The Board of Trade published the yearly expenditure of local authorities on housing across the inter-war years (Board of Trade, 1939). Data for 1938 onwards have been published by the Central Statistical Office (Central Statistical Office, 1949-96). Table 6.1 summarises the figures for selected years across this period. As a percentage of national income, spending by the State on housing increased about eight fold in the aftermath of the First World War, reaching 1% in 1920. By 1938 the figure had climbed to 2.5%. Cut-backs during the Second World War were followed by the expansion of spending on council housing under the Labour government, accounting for about 4% of national income around 1950. Under the Conservative administrations of Macmillan and Douglas Home the percentage fell back once more. The peak figure of about 6.5% appears to have been reached under Sir Keith Joseph's home improvement grant scheme of the early 1970s, when owners upgraded their houses through the generosity of the State. In the Thatcher years the proportion of national income devoted to housing fell back to the levels not seen since the 1930s. Expenditure per head of population looks much more generous, being in 1993 about two and a half times what it had been in 1948 (expressed in '1993 pounds'). Even so, Britain's housing stock remains deplorable in many areas.

Health and the 20th century home

A house is expected to provide adequate space for family living, a sheltered and protective environment in which parents and children can relax together, dine together and sleep together. The house contains the home in which children are nurtured and educated, offering both communal living and privacy. Here the family and its belongings are secure in a healthy environment, with the British winter kept outside. All modern reports acknowledge these needs. The Parker Morris Report of 1961, *Homes for today and tomorrow* (Department of the Environment, 1961), recommended that all houses should have kitchens and passageways heated to at least 13 °C and living areas, including occupied bedrooms, to 18 °C. The British Geriatric Society, recognising the peculiar vulnerability of the elderly to cold, has recommended room temperatures of 21°C. In Britain the house is of special importance for health in winter, always the season with the highest death rates. For every 1°C by which the winter temperature is colder than average, deaths rise about 8,000 above the seasonal norm (Curwen and Devis, 1988).

The gap between what ought to be and what is in modern British housing remains appalling. Millions of houses approach nowhere near Parker Morris standards. In 1994 the National Housing Forum reported that every thirteenth house in the nation was unfit for human habitation (although frequently occupied) and every sixth house needed urgent repairs (Leather, 1994). About a quarter of the housing stock had been built before the First World War, the era of the gas light, the penny-in-the-slot gas meter and the open coal fire. Government spending on housing fell by 57% between 1978 and 1987. Public housing was blighted by neglect, and much of private housing was decayed.

When houses lack insulation, doors and windows are drafty, and heating inefficient, the cost of a warm home reaches beyond the pocket of poor families. Surveys showing that even in slum areas the great majority now have access to a private bath, a refrigerator, washing machine and television should not be taken to mean that living conditions inside are better than outward appearances might suggest. Elderly couples have been found suffering from hypothermia in front of the television. Poor facilities for food storage, washing, drying and personal hygiene create hazards for health. Beds, cookers and the like could therefore be obtained as one-off payments under supplementary benefit, the State recognising that certain basic appliances and furnishings were essential for modern living and no longer luxuries. Up to one third of patients who visit their doctor are suffering some form of emotional distress, and the management of psychological and mental disturbance has been estimated to account for 20% of expenditure in the National Health Services (Department of Health, 1991). Much of this ill health is concentrated in areas with poor housing and few amenities, generated by 'living on top of one another', worries about the health of the family and a sense of hopelessness.

On one estate in Glasgow, almost 60% of dwellings were found to be damp in 1983. Residents receiving social security payments were entitled to an additional heating allowance because of structural defects. Over 500 households were contacted by trained interviewers, who found those living in cold and damp conditions were much more likely to report psychological or mental problems than the better housed (Hopton and Hunt, 1996). In parts of London, Glasgow and Edinburgh, mould growth was present in 45% of dwellings. Children living in such conditions had an increased prevalence of upper respiratory problems such as cough, nasal discharge and wheezing, and more frequently ran a fever. These effects were shown not to be the result of coincidental over-crowding, cigarette smoking by the adults, or low income (Platt et al, 1989). The widely held belief that children need to be kept warm and dry for their own health and happiness causes many mothers in poverty prolonged anxiety when they are unable to fulfil this basic role of parenthood. More than four million homes lack central heating, and unsafe alternatives made a large contribution to the more than 550 deaths in house fires during 1991.

Of course, ill health can be concentrated in poor estates when local authority or central government policies provide preferential assistance for the healthy to leave or for the sick to move in. Local authorities were granted powers to provide those in poor health with public housing at a subsidised Rent in 1949. In 1969 the Cullingworth committee advised housing authorities to give priority to groups with a range of social needs, including medical disability. This policy was re-inforced in 1970 in the Chronically Sick and Disabled Persons Act. One result of this legislation could have been to raise the numbers of persons in poor health in public housing, but this does not appear to have happened. Although at times as many as one third of applicants for local authority housing claim a medical need, the great majority of applications on such grounds appear to fail. Council housing is a scarce resource and its managers deal with claims based on a wide range of needs, disability being only one. In Liverpool, for example, only 6.4% of white applicants and 3.8% of non-white applicants were housed for medical reasons (Commission for Racial Equality, 1984). In Bolton, one in every three claims on medical grounds were rejected (Cole and Farries, 1986). Local decision making means that the success rate of medical claimants will vary considerably from one authority to the next, but the overall effect of this policy on the frequency of ill health found in run-down council dwellings has probably been small.

On the other side of the coin, Conservative policy in the 1980s and 1990s (Right-to-Buy) encouraged many of the better paid in public housing to buy their properties. The healthier took council houses of better quality into the private sector under these schemes, leaving poorer tenants and their poorer quality housing with the local authorities. Combined with neglected upkeep of this residual housing, such a policy would certainly have made a significant contribution to the intensification of ill health, crime and poverty in these pockets. However, we must not forget the sad story of those who, though at the margin, just about managed to buy their council house under a mortgage. In some cases even a temporary illness threw them into debt. The forced sale of the property to clear debt left them 'intentionally' homeless and therefore ineligible for public housing as a statutory right. Families in this predicament found themselves in emergency 'bed and breakfast' accommodation while their applications were considered. Though homeless in the real sense of the word, these hostel dwellers are not officially recognised as such. An unknown but very large number of families losing their homes through re-possession have been taken in by friends or family, and they too do not appear in the official statistics, which therefore mean little.

The nation has evolved for itself vast areas of social degradation which the present Labour administration is pleased to call today's 'Action Zones'. 'Hit squads for sink estates' declares the headline (*The Guardian*, 24 January

1998) as Cabinet ministers devise yet another scheme to fight the pockets of ill health, poor education, unemployment, low pay, crime, Welfare dependency and environmental decay in which millions of the future generation are being raised. The blotchy, unattractive rash which these areas of socio-economic pathology form across the British landscape is a disfiguring surface manifestation of a deep systemic disorder for which calamines are no remedy. The disease is self-inflicted, chronic, and no amount of money spent on it will buy a cure. There is an unwillingness to get at the roots of the disorder, because these roots are the source of the Rent which nourishes much that goes into the better life of privileged areas. To disturb these roots is to disturb what feeds social class.

These, then, have been the policies and strategies adopted by Conservative, Labour, Coalition and National administrations since the First World War in the name of social Welfare, at the end of which Tony Blair's Labour administration was left to announce: "Inequality and social exclusion are worsening, especially among children and pensioners, despite rising spending on social security" (Department of Social Security, 1998, p 1). Important though tailoring of subsidies to needs clearly is, inefficient delivery is not the main cause of the Welfare State's difficulties. Rather, it is the lack of consideration given to the proper source of public revenue which in large measure perpetuates the social problems that Welfare fails to solve. Most fundamentally, the Welfare State is struggling to succeed, because the system adheres to a textbook of economics written for other purposes.

SEVEN

Rent for reconstruction

Unruly blasts wait on the tender spring;
Unwholesome weeds take root with precious flowers;
The adder hisses where the sweet birds sing;
What virtue breeds, iniquity devours. (Shakespeare, *Lucrece*)

In a leading article entitled 'Slicing the cake', *The Economist* of 1994 commented: "One of the saddest features of the real world is that goods do not spontaneously present themselves for distribution. They have to be made. As a result, they arrive with property rights attached.... In this sense, the market-determined distribution of income is already just" (*The Economist*, 5 November, 1994, p 13). In the real world, however, the market in goods is not the only market. The market-determined distribution of income as Rent is most iniquitous.

Contrast the statement of *The Economist* with that of an earlier writer:

> What constitutes the rightful basis of property? What is it that enables a man justly to say of a thing, 'It is mine!'? From what springs the sentiment that acknowledges his exclusive right as against all the world? Is it not, primarily, the right of a man to himself, to the use of his own powers, to the enjoyment of the fruits of his own exertions?... As a man belongs to himself, so his labour when put in concrete form belongs to him.... That which a man makes or produces is his own ... to enjoy or to destroy, to use, to exchange, or to give ... the exertion of labour in production is the only title to exclusive possession. (George, 1979, pp 334-6)

Thus far there is a strong measure of similarity, but the earlier writer perceived a logical consequence of this reasoning upon which the later writer failed to comment:

> If production gives to the producer the right to exclusive possession and enjoyment, there can rightfully be no exclusive possession and enjoyment of anything not the production of labour.... When non-

producers can claim as Rent a portion of the wealth created by producers, the right of the producers to the fruits of their labour is to that extent denied. There is no escape from this position. (George, 1979, p 336)

As emphasised in Chapter Three, when there is one producer there is private and exclusive ownership of what has been produced. When there is Labour of two or more producers in the production of a single and indivisible entity there is joint ownership. On a community level of enterprise, joint ownership becomes communal property. Rent is created, the expression of an indivisible productive capacity inherent to the community. Rent represents the general economic surplus after all Wages have been returned to Labour and all Interest paid to Capital. The private market-determined distribution of Rent is therefore manifestly unjust. All discussions of the origins, meanings and consequences of impoverishment are fundamentally flawed if they fail to recognise and take account of the separateness and uniqueness of Rent.

Prospects in 2000

Count Leo Tolstoy, author of *War and peace* and *Anna Karenina*, wrote a letter to Ernest Crosby on 24 November 1894 in which he said: "If the new Tsar were to ask me what I would advise him to do, I would say to him: use your autocratic power to abolish the land property in Russia and to introduce the single tax system (collection of Rent with repeal of taxes on other forms of income) ..." (Redfearn, 1992, p 91). Despite many such calls, vigorous efforts to introduce the principle of Rent for public revenue in the early years of the 20th century were unsuccessful, as explained in Chapters Thirteen and Fourteen.

The world of today is very different from that of 1900, but for all that the message regarding Rent is as relevant now as then. Professor Frank Graham of Princeton University wrote:

> ... unearned income is that which accrues to an individual without his having done anything which contributes to production ... of such income; the most important is that which issues from the site value of land. The recipient of such an income does nothing to earn it; he merely sits tight while the growth of the community about the land to which he holds title brings him an unmerited gain. This gain is at the expense of all true producers, whether they be labourers ... or investors.... The (collection) of this gain can do nothing to deprive the community of any service

since the donee is rendering none.... Society creates the value and should secure it by (collection).

Professor Milton Friedman, the guru of monetarism, was reported to have said: "In my opinion the least bad tax is the property tax on the unimproved value of land" (ie the value of the land without buildings or other capital investments made within, say, the past 20 years) (*Human events*, 18 November 1978, p 14). Professor Joseph Stiglitz of Stanford University, who in late 1999 resigned as the World Bank's Chief Economist, disgusted with the International Monetary Fund, has written: "in an equalitarian society ... the tax on land raises just enough revenue to finance the (optimally chosen) level of government expenditures" (Stiglitz, 1977, p 282). President Reagan's chief economic adviser, Professor Martin Feldstein of Harvard University, wrote: "One of the reasons that economists have long been interested in the tax on pure Rental income is that it is a tax without excess burden. Because the owners of land cannot alter the supply of land, the tax induces no distortions and therefore no welfare loss" (Feldstein, 1977).

In her thorough review of Rent for public finance, Kris Feder has written: "It is my belief that (Henry) George's central economic principle (Rent for social purposes in exchange for taxes on the productive sector) is valid and profound – and that the reasons to pay attention to it are gathering power and urgency" (Feder, 1994). Mark Blaug has written: "The administrative difficulties of putting a Georgian tax scheme into action are no greater than those involved in distinguishing income and capital under the progressive income tax. Provided there is no deception that such a tax would raise much revenue except in rapidly growing cities, there would seem to be nothing wrong with the principle of site value taxation, that is, the taxation of land values with full or partial exemption of the improvements made on the land. Ultimately, of course, the issue rests on the violability of property rights" (Blaug, 1997, p 83). Blaug's final remark explains why this book has delved into the legal, political and social aspects of Rent in addition to its economic dimension. Later he stated: "the idea of confiscating the income of a leading social class was deeply shocking to a generation bred on Victorian pieties. In consequence the concept of site value taxation was never seriously discussed" (Blaug, 1997, p 83). In 1910, Davenport could write: "The economists have never seriously attacked the theoretical validity of the single tax program. In the main, in fact, they have come nearer to ignoring than to condemning" (Davenport, 1910). At the other end of that century

Kris Feder was forced to conclude: "economists have neither understood nor challenged the Georgist view of the abundant revenue potential of Rent taxation" (Feder, 1994). The reasons behind this lack of proper consideration have far more to do with class, over-privilege and property rights than economics – theoretical or applied.

There is one flaw in the way this idea is expressed. Since Rent belongs properly in the public domain, governments by collecting it are not *taxing* Rent, any more than the commercial landlord 'taxes' the tenant when collecting a fair rent. Rather, when *not* collecting the Rent due to it, the community is *subsidising* the private landholder, and only to the extent that Rent is collected is this subsidy withdrawn. There is nothing akin to taxation of Wages or Interest in collection of Rent.

Attitudes and opinions have changed dramatically over the 20th century in many positive ways. For example, during the extreme distress of the working class in the winter of 1904-5, which led to disorder on the streets, the Local Government Board proposed a scheme for the provision of relief of the unemployed and the establishment of Labour exchanges subsidised by local taxation. The Bill was denounced by back bench Conservatives as a "dangerous concession to the right to work" (Harris, 1977, p 114). Such sentiments are a far cry from New Labour's declaration: "Work for those who can; security for those who cannot" (Department of Social Security, 1998, p iii). Work is seen today not only as a right but a duty – a duty which the State assists the worker to fulfil when needed through the taxation and benefit system.

Even more amazing has been the change in official attitude to the scientific evidence for material deprivation as a major cause of illness and premature death. As recently as 1987 Ray Whitney, Conservative Under-secretary of State for Health, could confidently declare to the House of Commons that the excessive rates of sickness and death in the poorest paid occupational classes, "do not mean that those diseases are a function of poverty. Other reasons and issues are neglected by those who write these reports and those who pounce on them and seek to benefit politically from them" (Whitney, 1987, col 54). Only 11 years later New Labour was to set down in black and white: "it is clear that people's chances of a long and healthy life are basically influenced by how well off they are, where they live and by their ethnic background" (Department of Health, 1998, p 10). These developments offer realistic hope for the future.

In 1931, hardly more than yesterday in the lifetime of the nation, a leader of the Conservative opposition in the House of Commons stood to declare that, if and when he was returned to power, any measures designed to collect Rent for public revenue would 'never see daylight' (Baldwin, in *The Times*, 15 July 1931). The landed interest and its agents have not changed their spots in a mere few-score years, but the non-landed interest is, relatively speaking, a far more powerful political force than it was back then. An enlightened use of the vote and full participation in the democratic process, while still faced by the vested interests of 'those who have got', present more of a match today. Surely, the nation now more than ever is willing to root out those inequitable ways of the past which determine the distribution of income and wealth, and which damage health in ways over which the afflicted have little control.

The abolition of Rentery

The economy of the future should be framed upon the following:

First and foremost: the abolition of Rentery, by which is meant an end to Rent as private property and its resultant injustices.

Second: the reduction of taxation on Wages and Interest, and hence the socio-economic harm that flows therefrom, to the absolute minimum.

Third: the common understanding that these reforms subserve justice, equity, fairness and efficiency by removing iniquitous differentials in income and health while raising the standard of living of all and protecting the environment and ecology for future generations.

These prizes are too precious and long-sought for the nation to duck hard choices in the transition from the out-dated to up-dated.

Economic theory has much to say on efficiency, but relatively little on fairness and equity, which is why the ordinary citizen finds little attraction in this discipline. Surveys of national opinion never fail to confirm that the great majority of British people believe in public expenditure for medical research, help for the elderly and the disabled, and the protection of the family. Yet the paradox seems to be that this sense of fair play and fellow feeling is not matched by a willingness to pay for such causes through increased taxation on the earnings of their labour or their savings. Few relish the thought of income tax rates of 80% or more for a massive expansion of spending on Welfare. In reality, however, there is little contradiction or disingenuousness; only a canny intuition that high taxation is not the solution for social evils and inequities. There has to be a more satisfying remedy that roots out causes and re-distributes wealth and income in accordance with an easy to appreciate political morality. People are unwilling or uneasy to act until they are certain of the rightness of what is proposed. Faced with the undeniable evidence that under-privilege and material impoverishment are major causes of sub-health, illness and premature death, minds can no longer be closed to the wrong in the privatisation of Rent.

The foundations for a programme of reform need to be set down in a Declaratory Act of Parliament stating in unequivocal terms the State's insistence on its inalienable right to the full value of Rent for public revenue, current arrangements and laws notwithstanding. It is the wish of the people that Rent be disbursed on social expenditure according to their will as expressed through their democratically elected representation in parliament. Such a declaration would provide the moral authority for what follows as the political economy moves through the transition of Rent from private to public revenue.

Rent of the Realm Act

With this statement of rightness and purpose in place, the preparatory groundwork for collection of Rent needs to be authorised through a Rent of the Realm Act that establishes the mechanism for the valuation of all land sites in their unimproved state and the identification of all freeholders. In the case of agricultural land, or when there is no such thing as unimproved land, then the proper valuation is of the land in the least improved condition in which it is customarily found (Tideman and Plassmann, 1998, p 150). Is such an approach feasible? Can land be valued in its unimproved state, even when the site is highly developed? The answer is that this is what was done in response to the Finance (1909-10) Act under Chief Valuers Sir Robert Thompson and Sir Edgar Harper, as described in Chapter Fourteen. London County Council had not forgotten this lesson when in 1939 it sought to bring a private Bill permitting local 'taxation' based on site value rather than on the combined annual value of the existing use of land as developed with its buildings or other improvements (the 'rates'). The House of Commons determined that the proposal was not a matter for a private Bill, but then defeated the measure as a public Bill on its first reading.

The national Rent

Of all national secrets guarded by laws of privacy, the total value of the national Rent is the best kept secret of all. Not even government seems to know. Despite the enormous difficulties, however, attempts were made to value Britain's land in the 1980s (Banks, 1989; Richards, 1989). The

Department of the Environment had monitored land usage in these years and the Inland Revenue Valuation Office published estimated values for bulk residential building land and 'typical' industrial and warehouse land. These figures, together with data allowing estimates of the value of land used for public services, agriculture, forestry and mines, produced a total Rent of £120 billion in 1990. Residential land accounted for more than half of this figure and land devoted to commerce and industry about one quarter. Compare this estimate of national Rent with the cost to general government of all social services including health and education in 1990, about £125 billion: education, £27 billion; health, £28 billion; social security, £62 billion; housing, £8 billion. What we want to know, however, is not the value of the national Rent in the economy as presently constructed, but its value in an efficient, modernised economy unburdened of taxation on its productive powers.

Just how much better off would be the people of Britain and their Welfare State if the transition was made from taxation to Rent for public purposes? This question was addressed in 1998 by economists at the Virginia Polytechnic Institute and State University (Tideman and Plassmann, 1998). So little interest has been shown in this question that the authors stressed that their trail-blazing study needed independent confirmation. Yet so staggering were the findings that little doubt can remain about the extent of damage inflicted on the nation by outdated fiscal practices developed by governments of yesteryear for the landed constituency.

The approach was to use data for the G7 economies (Canada, France, Germany, Italy, Japan, the UK and US), including their economic output, the proportion of total income going to wages, taxation rates and revenues, and to apply a set of parameters modelling the functional characteristics of these economies. The results showed that economic performance had ranged from 52% (France) to 77% (the US) of full potential in 1993. The UK had performed at 55% of full capacity, nett domestic product running at $14,972 per capita that year. A switch to Rent for social revenue would have raised this figure by 81% to $27,105 per capita. In other words the burden of taxation has caused the national economy to run at half speed on full throttle.

Let us now use our imagination. In our simple model of the operation of Rent and taxation in a market economy described in Table 3.9, Land of six differential levels of economic performance yielded a nett productivity, after Wages had been paid, of 45 units. Of this total, taxation took 6 units, Interest after taxation 24 units, and Rent 15 units. Now let us release this economy from taxation, and accepting the limited confidence we can have in predictions of subsequent economic growth, say that output increases by 88%. Nett productivity therefore rises to 85 units. With marginal Interest in this economic model being 4 units, and nett productivity increasing by 1 unit for each standard input of Labour and Capital as the quality of Land rises by one level, this increase in nett productivity will have been accomplished by raising the differential levels of Land from 6 to 10 (13 + 12 + 11 + 10... + 4 = 85). Interest will claim 40 units (10 x 4) leaving the total Rent standing at 45 units as compared to 15 units under taxation. Although only an illustrative model, the exercise serves to demonstrate the suppressed potential for unrivalled improvements in health, education, housing and social security suffered by a 21st century economy shackled to taxation. The possibilities for Welfare Capitalism when social spending is funded by Rent in an unburdened economy are immense and exciting.

Conventional economics is apparently blind to the foregoing – it stares but cannot see. This is why when asked, economists of the popular school say that what they see of Rent could not possibly provide the revenue for public finance in a modern economy. Physicists know that white light is produced by mixing three primary colours, green, blue and red, in the correct intensities. They also know that mixing green and blue produces the secondary colour cyan, and that mixing cyan with red also gives white light. So it is in the world of economics. The primary incomes were long ago recognised to be Rent (green), Interest (blue) and Wages (red). Rent + Interest + Wages equals Wealth (white). But Rent (green) + Interest (blue) equals profit (cyan), and profit (cyan) + Wages (red) also equals Wealth (white). A physicist who is fully satisfied that white light consists of two complementary colours only, cyan and red, is utterly unable to explain the nature of two other secondary colours, magenta (red + blue) and yellow (red + green). An economist who is content to accept that profit and wages are all we need to know about wealth is left equally bereft of explanations for certain secondary phenomena in economics, namely cyclic recession and the persistence of maldistribution of Wealth produced. How can this economist, unable to discern Rent from ·Interest in profit, enlighten the rest of us as to the amount of Rent there is in the Wealth we create as a society?

Mervyn King, Deputy Governor of the Bank of England, looked at the national income blue books and pronounced: "... the total of economic rents, of all kinds, is not now a sufficiently large proportion of national income for this to be a practicable means of obtaining the resources needed to finance a modern state" (Kay and King, 1990, p 179). In the US similar conclusions have been reached (Solow, 1997, p 8). All that appears in official accounts of the US national income is the superficial rental value of homes belonging to owner-occupiers, estimated at less than 2% of this total (Harrison, 1998, p 67). Once the accounts are re-worked with a true concept of what constitutes Rent, this estimate rises to approach 10% of national income. A partial explanation for this staggering discrepancy is to be found in the horrific way Rent is ignored as a component of the profit made in the real estate market (Hudson and Feder, 1997).

Comparison of Tables 3.1 and 3.9 showed that government's income collected in ordinary taxation of Wages and Interest is drawn indirectly but ultimately from Rent. This effect of taxation cuts deeply into what landholders retain as unearned income to appear as the annual rental value of land in official accounts. Add collected and uncollected Rent together, and then add the growth in Rent that will follow when the dead-weight of ordinary taxation is lifted from the economy, and the final figure will be much more than enough to finance Britain's Welfare State.

Rent collection: an outline proposal

Having mapped the distribution of the national Rent site by site with modern aids such as the computer and satellite, the task is to initiate the transition from taxation to Rent. In considering the proportion of Rent that is to be collected at the start of this process, and the length of the transition to collection of Rent in full, several points have to be borne in mind. Two major purposes of reform are an end to damaging speculation in Rent at times of economic advance, and effective unburdening of the productive sector of the economy. Neither of these objectives can be realised if the rate of collection commences at a proportion as low as 5 or 10%. On the contrary, instead of denying the speculator the power to distort economic performance, such low rates are likely to intensify speculation with what remains in private hands in an attempt to make good what has been lost. The danger is that this is exactly what the land monopoly will do. Those who are eager to undermine the reform, driven by private interest, will then claim prematurely that the benefits of reform have been wildly exaggerated. For this reason the initial rate of Rent collection should be set at least at 30%, with *commensurate relief of the economy* from taxation of Wages and Interest. Increments in subsequent years should achieve virtually complete collection within 15 years (say a rise of 4% annually). This rate, however, need only be the average. Freeholders of Rent could be classified and the rate tailored to suit each class in order to smooth the transition as much as possible. As a general rule, Rent collection should be in full by 15 years, except for specified reductions and exemptions in the public interest. Rent rebates would be one mechanism of social security for rentholders unable to work.

The collection of Rent for public revenue will in general raise the value of properties as the economy flourishes, relieved of the weight of taxation and the distorting stresses of land speculation. What will happen is that this value and its associated rights and privileges will be split into two bundles. One bundle containing Rent goes to the State. The other bundle continues to hold everything except Rent and remains the property of the freeholder. The landholder retains title to all improvements on the site and the right to exclusive and beneficial use.

At present, Rent is bought and sold as a valuable asset in its market. When a property is sold the purchase price includes a figure to cover the sale of the right to enjoy Rent for the next 15 years (sometimes 20 years or even more). Tenants pay over an element of Rent in the commercial rent going to landlords. Landholders who occupy their own site enjoy an imputed Rent which forms part of their income, though an income in kind rather than cash (this was taxed under Schedule A until 1963). Those occupiers who have purchased under a mortgage or legal charge are in the final analysis sub-tenants of the bank or other lender (Perrins, 1995, pp 140-1), and as such they too turn over to the lender an element of Rent in the repayment of the principal. These concepts may be unfamiliar but they are the realities of the obscure market in Rent, discussed in Chapter Six.

The multiplier of 15 to 20 years for Rent when sold appears again and again. Where does it come from? Once again the answer is rooted in times past. Over the centuries until as recently as about 1870, average life expectancy in England was never more than 35 to 40 years (Wrigley and Schofield, 1989). Hence a young adult who purchased land could not expect to enjoy its advantages for much more than 15 to 20 years. Thus the purchaser literally bought a life interest in Rent. Never was Rent knowingly given away. Without a doubt, the steady increase in length of life after 1870, set against an unchanged multiplier, has been the principal motivating force behind fundamental changes in attitude to ownership of land – even a little land, from 1900 onwards. Buy land, clear the mortgage over 15 years, then sit back and enjoy Rent as unearned income, as did the traditional landocracy by inheritance.

Before the First World War the position was much more simple. In those days most of the population, including many of the rich, would rent their homes rather than buy. The income going to landlords was declared to the Inland Revenue and appeared as part of the national income. From the 1920s more and more families bought under a mortgage or legal charge and Rent itself was split into two smaller bundles in a rather complicated manner. Part of the Rent went to the borrower, mortgagor or chargor and part went to the lender, mortgagee or chargee. The portion of Rent inherent in the purchase price that is covered by the lender is in the same proportion as is the loan to the cost of the property. Suppose, for example, a house was bought for £100,000 with a 10% downpayment and £90,000 mortgage. Suppose also that the Rent or value of the unimproved site accounted for 30% of the purchase price or £30,000. Then while the full mortgage was outstanding the occupier would owe the equivalent of £27,000 of the Rent in the principal.

While paying Rent to the lender at its value at purchase under the mortgage, the occupier has the right to any 'unearned increment' in the Rent as time goes by. Supposing after five years the property is worth £105,000 on the market. Most of this rise in value probably represents an increase in the capitalised value of Rent over 15 years from £30,000 to £35,000. This increment goes to the occupier, increasing the value of Rent in the mortgagor's bundle from the original £3,000 to £8,000. Capture of the unearned increment is what makes land and house purchase so attractive. It is truly something for nothing.

In collecting Rent, the Inland Revenue needs three facts: the value of Rent at the time of purchase, its current value, and the size of the loan outstanding under mortgage or legal charge. With respect to our example, if the full Rent is collected then in the first year the occupier pays to the Inland Revenue one fifteenth of £3,000 (£200) and the lender one fifteenth of £27,000 (£1,800). Remember that the occupier is paying £1,800 per year as Rent to the lender in the principal of the mortgage. In year five the occupier will pay one fifteenth of £8,000 (£533) and the lender £1,800 if none of the principal has been repaid. If Rent collection were introduced at a rate of 30%, rising to 50% by five years, the occupier would pay £60 in the first year and £267 in the fifth, while the lender would pay £540 in the first year and £900 in the fifth. As discussed in Chapter Six, lenders cannot escape the fact that, under the legal terms of the agreement, they have a very substantial property right to the Rent, secure in the event of default on the part of the sub-tenant-occupier who aspires to but is not yet owner-occupier in the true sense.

Supposing a mortgage is taken on land (usually as part of house purchase) for repayment of the principal over 15 years. Supposing also that the purchase price of the property included the annual value of Rent capitalised over 15 years. Finally, suppose the borrower secured a 100% mortgage from the bank. Then in repayment of the principal over 15 years, the borrower hands over to the bank each year the full Rent as it stood at the time of purchase. If the mortgage amounts to 80% of the purchase price, then 80% of Rent at purchase is transferred to the mortgagee over 15 years. Thereafter the owner-occupier can enjoy the full Rent. Before that time the mortgagor effectively pays the mortgagee for the right to private enjoyment of the amenities of the site, at Interest (the mortgage rate). This Rent is turned over from the productive sector, as explained in Chapter Three, that is out of the tenant family's Wages and Interest on their Capital. Of course, once the period of transition of Rent from private to public income is complete, and Rent no longer forms part of the sale value of real property, entanglement of Rent in the standard mortgage would be a thing of the past.

The banks as rentholders

In the US, about 70% of business loans made by banks go to real estate credit. The banking and loans industry and real estate investment trusts are today the largest monopoly holders of Rent (Hudson, 1997), collected on the land they essentially own until the mortgage is cleared. Failure to make repayment will immediately result in repossession of the whole property, including the Rent attached to the site.

Purchasers on mortgage in the real estate business make money in two ways. First, they capture any rise in Rent of the land they hold. Second, the interest paid to the mortgagee is sometimes legally deducted from the mortgagor's income before taxes are calculated. Mortgage interest is a pre-tax deductible expense in the US. This horrific state of affairs exists because society allows it to exist. A political morality that cries out for an end to this abuse of public revenue is drowned out by the clamour for private profit out of unearned income.

The dereliction of Rent

The cardinal rule of Rent is that it is communal income, the surplus created by the indivisible productive energy of society as a whole. There will be times when a superficial impression is gained that rental values in a particular district are determined largely by the activities of a specific agent or agency, perhaps a supermarket or large employer. But as Chapter Three showed, Rent on any site is the indirect product of economic activity on sites of inferior quality, not on the site itself. Further reflection will confirm that this agent is merely taking economic advantage of the opportunities created by the local, regional and even national economy. No single agent can expect private reward for influence on Rent. Those who might object to this position should remember that by the same token, no single agent or agency can be held solely responsible for any deterioration in the value of Rent. Landholders have a trinity of rights in law wrapped up in the bundle called land; *ius utendi, fruendi, abutendi*: to use, profit from and 'abuse or use up'. In profit-seeking and 'using up', the Rent of the land is likely to deteriorate (the site sinks in quality to a lower stratum), but the forces of decay never arise solely from a single agent. The web of causation ramifies throughout the local, regional and national economy. Nobody wants dereliction of land, and because Rent is a communal product the control of dereliction is a public responsibility.

The industrial use of land is 'as old as the hills'. Cicero's tutor Posidonius watched tin being mined, melted, shaped and exported during his visit to Cornwall around 100 BC. Lead mined in the Mendips ended in the plumbing of Roman villas and public baths. Copper was mined in Shropshire and Anglesey and its alloy with tin had long before ushered in the Bronze Age. Coal was mined in Northumberland in Roman times. Siderite was mined for iron 1,000 years before the arrival of the Romans, and iron founding became so central to the economy that wood burning for the process threatened deforestation by the 16th century. 'Where there's muck there's brass' (money) runs the old Northern saying, but the problem is that where there is brass there is muck. Britain's landscape and ecology have been completely transformed by centuries of economic activity, leaving widespread damage and dereliction. There is an appalling legacy of spoil heaps, disused mine workings, worked-out quarries and pits, rubbish dumps, abandoned industrial sites, contaminated sub-soil, polluted waterways and shorelines, oceans of flotsam and jetsam, and atmospheric pollution. Capitalism or Communism, Monarchy or Republic, Democracy or Dictatorship: it makes no difference where exploitation of land is concerned. Yet here too there have been some remarkable changes in public attitude in recent years in the face of ever-mounting scientific evidence.

In 1977 the Department of the Environment claimed to have no reliable information on the extent of idle land in Britain, arguing that such data could be collected only at 'disproportionate cost' (Norton-Taylor, 1982, p 200). This statement did not reflect complete disinterest, however. In 1974 local authorities had attempted a survey of derelict land with the assistance of the Department, and the less than sanguine attitude may have stemmed from that experience. Twenty years later at least three major reports on the extent and characteristics of derelict and dormant land were available, including Groundwork's report on *The post-industrial landscape* (Groundwork Foundation, 1996). Damaged and idle land is placed into several categories. Vacant land is that for which the previous productive use has ceased for a significant period of time (Shepherd and Abakaks, 1992). It lies idle and awaiting re-development. Some vacant land is derelict, meaning that it has been so damaged by industrial or other exploitation as to be incapable of beneficial use without treatment (Wickens et al, 1995). Some derelict land is contaminated, meaning that it poses an actual or potential hazard to health or to the environment. Land in productive use can also be derelict and contaminated. Such sites are 'operational' but continually add to vacant dereliction when abandoned. Working waste disposal tips and obsolescent industrial plant are in the queue for dereliction. In some districts the records show little land as derelict, although much is obviously damaged and despoiled. In the area of St Austell in Cornwall there are extensive workings of china clay extending over 60 square kilometres, yet only 283 hectares were reported as derelict in 1993 (Coppin, 1993).

There has been much imaginative reclamation of vacant and derelict land in recent years, with landscape restoration and provision of public amenities. The Environmental Protection Act of 1995 has raised awareness by requiring local authorities to identify contaminated land. However, there is a very long way to go. A recent survey estimated that there were close to 60,000 hectares of urban vacant land in England in 1990 (Shepherd and Abakaks, 1992). In northern England as much as 11% of urban land was waste but suitable for redevelopment. Altogether, England's waste land probably covered about 80,000 hectares. The extent of dereliction in the UK as a whole approached 60,000 hectares (Groundwork Foundation, 1996), of which there were about 40,000 hectares in England on 10,400 sites (Wickens et al, 1995). General industrial dereliction accounted for 25% of total dereliction in England, with spoil heaps making up a further 23%, railway dereliction 14%, and excavation 15%. Despite the valiant efforts of development agencies, the area of derelict land has changed little in 25 years because ex-operational land enters as fast as reclamation proceeds. Overall, derelict vacant land in England has been reclaimed over recent years at a rate only 180 hectares per annum in excess of that created. "If these rates remained constant it would take 200 years to clear the backlog!" (Groundwork Foundation, 1996).

People detest dereliction and contamination, especially in their own vicinity. They dislike the eyesores, they worry about risks to the health of their children, and they object to the adverse effect on Rent which lowers the price of property. Rats and vermin thrive on such sites unless contamination has poisoned them. Yet strange to tell, when in an opinion poll more than 2,000 adults were asked who had responsibility for cleaning up the mess, most named the local authority or the local community *per se*. Apparently very few considered reclamation to be the responsibility of the landholder or of local businesses (Groundwork Foundation, 1996). Perhaps this reflects an underlying understanding that the value of land is determined by the actions of the local, regional and national communities in the final analysis, rather than a particular agent.

If deep-seated practices continue to generate dereliction, can 'Rent as public revenue' contribute to the solution of the problem? The answer is 'yes'. Rent can be used to further the declared aim of government in a White Paper of 1991: "... making the best use of our finite supply of land. An important part of this is to bring previously developed land back into constructive use" (cited in Groundwork Foundation, 1996). For more than 30 years governments have made available derelict land grants amounting to full cover of the reclamation costs for local authorities and 80% of approved costs for private enterprises. Rent rather than taxation would be a better way of covering this public expense.

There are several aspects to the problem of idle land. Vacant land suitable for productive or recreational use but held out of the economy by the private speculator is easily solved by charging full Rent. This would immediately encourage the holder to put the land to good use or to sell it to someone who could. To discourage dereliction and pollution of the operational site and spillage on to other sites, imaginative schemes of Rent subsidy could be introduced which give an economic advantage to those enterprises that are ecologically considerate. Such subsidies would be meant to encourage investment of resources into pollution control and site protection. Rent turned over to the Treasury could be used in part to finance derelict land restoration grants, on the understanding that, unless exempted for the public good, Rent would become payable on the restored site. To that extent reclamation schemes would be self-financing in the longer-term. Land restored and turned over for 'soft' end uses such as nature reserves and open spaces, being for public enjoyment, could be designated Rent-free or Rent-subsidised. With no taxation on their income, such public places should thrive whenever they fulfil a public need. The restoration of Rent to the mainstream of politics and economics would help to keep the care and protection of the environment in the forefront of public consciousness.

Rent collection and housing

In 1885 the Royal Commission on the Housing of the Working Classes focused public attention on the horrors of housing suffered by the Victorian poor. The outcome was the Housing of the Working Classes Act of 1890 (Royal Commission on the Housing of the Working Classes, 1885). Exactly one century later and another Inquiry into British Housing, organised by the National Federation of Housing Associations and chaired by HRH The Duke of Edinburgh, again stressed the seriousness of the housing problems faced by poorer families (National Federation of Housing Associations, 1985). The National Federation urged that more energy and more money be devoted to the improvement of the housing stock, but apparently the words of Sir J Walker Smith, Director of Housing at the Ministry of Health just after the First World War, had been forgotten: "... money alone will not permanently cure slums ... The experience of the 1919 (Housing and Town Planning) Act ... is a warning to us not to disregard economic laws" (Townroe, 1928, p vi). Chapter Six has described the miserable consequences of failing to work within economic laws, especially the law of Rent as it operates in the housing market.

The fundamental problem with housing for low-income families is the yawning gap between the Rent (or purchase price) and what they can afford. Rent-for-public-revenue will go a long way to restoring the balance. Once a sufficient proportion of Rent is collected the activities of a speculating Rent monopoly will be curtailed, thereby increasing the security of low-income families in the housing market. Unlike the situation today, families with little financial reserves who buy in boom years, only to end in dire straits when the market collapses, will become a very unusual phenomenon. The removal of the burden of taxation will create new job opportunities for many families who hitherto have known little but low pay, financial insecurity and bouts of unemployment. Purchasing power will be raised across the board. Of course, Rent diverted from private pockets to the public purse is Rent that still has to be paid unless exempted. Nevertheless, housing will become more affordable for the poor as the economic margin of a thriving economy brings into productive activity land previously idle, stimulating the building of new dwellings free of market speculation. Families on improved incomes free of taxation at the point of receipt and point of expenditure will not find Rent the barrier to a better life that it had once been. For those excluded from the Labour market because of old age, sickness or disability, social security can include some form of Rent rebate.

Rent and the health of the nation

Taxation of wages and interest in lieu of Rent for public revenue creates haves and have nots in two ways, as already described. Rent monopolised by one sector of the population creates economic and social distance, re-inforcing over-privilege by providing this sector with unearned income to the exclusion of the less affluent sector. The resort by governments to taxation in recompense for Rent lost creates economic distortions which inflict most damage on the sector already the victim of Rent monopoly. The end result is the inequity in the distribution of income and judgements of social worth that, through diverse pathways, are a major cause of inequalities in health and life span.

Despite her venerable maturity, Britannia displays a lack of parenting skills unbecoming for her years, showing favour to some of her offspring to the relative neglect of others. In 1980, Britain's infant mortality rate was more than 12 deaths for 1,000 births, second only to the US which led the field of countries in the Organisation for Economic Co-operation and Development (OECD) with a rate of almost 13 per 1,000 births. Sweden and Norway had achieved respective rates of 7 per 1,000 and 8 per 1,000 by this time (Wennemo, 1993). What was striking, however, was that whereas fewer than 5% of families were in relative poverty in Sweden and Norway, more than 11% were in this position in the UK and a horrific 16% in the US, the most affluent nation in the world and leader of global Capitalism. This pattern, so clear in infancy, was similarly apparent throughout life. When allowance had been made for family size, life expectancy at birth was highest in Sweden, Norway and the Netherlands (about 74 years), with the least inequality of post-tax income, while it was least in nations such as France, Spain, West Germany and the US (72 years or less), where income inequality was greatest among the OECD countries. In sharp contrast, life expectancy in these wealthy nations is not influenced significantly by economic growth (Wilkinson, 1994, pp 17-24). What matters most for average life expectancy in affluent populations is the way the wealth is distributed. As the ratio of over-privilege to under-privilege increases, as the gap between richest and poorest enlarges, so average life expectancy falls away. The sudden increase in income inequality experienced in Britain during the 1980s was enough to put a temporary hold on improvements in infant mortality, which up to that time had shown dependable gains over very many years (Wilkinson, 1994, p 5). The proportion of children living in relative poverty tripled during this period.

If the distribution of wealth and income could be shown convincingly to be equitable, based entirely on merit, then society might be forgiven for believing that the alleviation of ill health in families at the bottom of the scale was simply a case for charity, fellow feeling, and a benevolent Welfare State. Indeed, there are many who self-assuredly regard this as the end of the matter. Those at the bottom find themselves there for a variety of genetic and environmental reasons amounting to collective hard luck, but that is the way of the world, so the comforting argument goes. This abbreviation of thought will not do, however. The inequity in the distribution of wealth and income, rooted in Rent monopoly, permeates through society with an inseparable inequity in the distribution of health and life expectancy, a form of social 'poison' that injures even the infant and the child in the womb. For those who retort that what matters most is efficiency and growth of the economy, raising absolute income levels for rich and poor alike, Rent-for-public-revenue should be applauded for the relief from taxation it permits and the rapid economic growth that will follow. For those who say that in economically advanced nations what matters most for health is the distribution of the national income, Rent-for-public revenue should receive equal acclaim for the removal of material and social over-privilege on one side of the average, and material and social under-privilege on the other. Together, these two basic characteristics of Rent-for-public revenue ensure that as the poor catch up, the wealthy do not fall back in absolute terms.

It is all too easy to be impressed by what strikes the senses. Want sits begging on the pavement and stands in the queue for dole. Disease fills the waiting rooms of the doctors' surgeries and the hospital wards. Ignorance displays itself on the streets, in remedial classrooms and in unemployability. Squalor blights town and country alike. Idleness frequents the job centres and between times hangs around in boredom seeking petty amusement. Certainly the statistics of modern Britain, not to mention the sights on its streets, are enough to send the minds of all concerned citizens into a frenzy. Take the list recently assembled in a report for Barnardo's: reports of crime rose by 80% between 1981 and 1991; the number of young drug offenders doubled between 1979 and 1989; deaths from solvent abuse more than quadrupled between 1980 and 1990; the number of children under five years coming on to child protection registers following serious injury increased by 50% between 1979 and 1989; the suicide rate among men aged 15 to 24 years increased by 75% between 1983 and 1990 (Wilkinson, 1994, p 1).

By 2000 the New Labour administration was tackling these problems with new vigour. To reduce crime £1.2 billion was being invested in the police force and £400 million in other preventive strategies. An extra £217 million was being invested in measures against drug abuse. There was a new statutory minimum wage for those aged 18 or more. A £5.2 billion windfall tax on the privatised utilities was invested in several 'New Deal' programmes to assist the unemployed back into work, and 'action teams' were backed by £40 million to tackle long term unemployment. A Working Family Tax Credit had been introduced in 1999 to ease the transition from Welfare to work. Government's claims of rapid success (Social Exclusion Unit, 2000, p 6) were soon to be disputed, however, by others who claimed that, given the strength of the economy in these years, most placements under the New Deal would have occurred anyway. The real test of the government's initiatives would come when the economy was creating unemployment rather than employment (*Sunday Times*, 16 April 2000, pp 5-6).

Surely nobody doubts that, better reporting notwithstanding, these signs and symptoms of social exclusion and material deprivation hang as a syndrome on a common thread of social pathology. The underlying disease, not one of flesh and blood but of the body politic and its political economy, calls out for diagnosis. Yet all too often the response has been to look away, to take the Rent and to say a prayer for one's less fortunate brethren. This complex, whatever we like to call it, is the Evil Giant behind Beveridge's giant evils. It is not Want, Disease, Squalor, Ignorance and Idleness that block the road to reconstruction, as Beveridge phrased it (Harris, 1977, p 431), but something altogether more sinister in its omnipresence and omnipotence. This insensible force, cloaked in social respectability, decency and virtue, walks abroad not even pretending but believing itself to be something it is not. It pervades the most august of institutions, the most hallowed of places, as well as dens of vice and the middens of the throwaway economy. This all-pervasiveness denies a foothold for 'Rent for reconstruction'.

William Blake, poet, painter and engraver, was largely ignored in his day and regarded as close to madness for his revulsion at deism, atheism and materialism. He died in 1827 of neglect, in poverty, yet few hearts do not swell and voices rise to his words:

> I will not cease from Mental Fight,
> Nor shall my Sword sleep in my hand,
> Til we have built Jerusalem,
> In England's green and pleasant land.

Blake's Jerusalem, the soul of the nation regained by acceptance of universal brotherhood, cannot be built while the natural wealth of this green and pleasant land and the fruits of communal economy remain the province of a private monopoly. *La perfide Albion* referred to England's treachery in foreign affairs as perceived by other nations, yet a certain perfidy prospered at home. Rent coursed with blue blood through the veins of Old England. How Rent came to be privatised, and how it has remained a species of private property to this day, forms a fascinating thread running through the tapestry that is the nation's history. To follow this thread, as we do in Part II, is to see that it leads nowhere but to anachronistic privilege which has no place in the political economy of the 21st century. We cannot unthread what ran through the past, but we can sever it now rather than weave it into our future.

Part II:
The lethal legacy

EIGHT

An aristocracy of service: Rent before its privatisation

Wrongs do not leave off there where they begin,
But still beget new mischiefs in their course.
(Samuel Daniel [born 1562] *Civil War*)

In 1797, Thomas Paine advised: "It is only by tracing things to their origin that we can gain rightful ideas of them, and by gaining such ideas that we discover the boundary that divides right from wrong ..." (Paine, 1987, p 476). In similar vein, Arnold Toynbee told his audience in London 90 years later: "If you want to propose a scheme of practical reform ... patiently look into the history of the country" (Toynbee, 1884, p 50). The kingdom of England is very old, and to trace its history of Rent is in large measure to recount the domestic history of the nation itself over the past millennium. Rent is a common thread linking the feuding, civil wars, party politics and law-making of the land, from ancient times to what we have today. But the Englishman's disposition towards Rent is far more than a domestic matter; his lawmakers propagated it as the foundation of land law in Britain's former dominions and colonies overseas.

The mind-set of the English landholder

To the English landholder of yesteryear, who handed down the law, land was much more than the ground on which stood our houses, factories and farms. Rather, land was everything he succeeded in holding for himself, a mind-set encapsulated by the legal draftsmen responsible for the Law of Property Act of 1925:

> (ix) 'Land' includes land of any tenure, and mines and minerals ...
> buildings or parts of buildings ... and other corporeal hereditaments ...
> and a rent and other incorporeal hereditaments, and an easement, right,

privilege, or benefit in, over, under, or derived from land.... (*Halsbury's Statutes of England and Wales*, 1987, vol 37, p 330)

Land as defined for economics encompasses all opportunities, forces and materials provided by nature for productive purposes. The land of the lawyers is much more, enriching the Land of economics with many opportunities, forces and materials created by human ingenuity for private gain. Now a man who can claim this complex species of property for himself is rich indeed, for the definition is unbounded. What is more, ever leaving the door ajar, the definition was left deliberately incomplete, as if there was not enough. The wording states not that 'Land *is*', but that 'Land *includes* ...'! The landholder wants to call this bundle of wealth and privileges his own, to claim 'ownership'; to be able to show, in court if need be, that of all the people in the nation, the land he possesses is his alone – all of it; every penny of profit, every smidgen of privilege.

Landholders have not always had such astounding power and possessiveness. The complex of land and the right to do more or less what they want with it were gradually acquired by the landed over centuries that shaped the nation's character. Even sinecures of public office were once regarded as freehold property, as Pitt reminded parliament in 1797 (Roseveare, 1969, p 126). The end product is a bundle of assorted assets and privileges tied together in the red tape of the lawyers. Entangled in this bundle, somewhere among the incorporeal hereditaments, the rent, the privileges and the benefits, is Rent. In its process of assembly many citizens were denied fundamental rights.

The usurpation of Rent is still exposed by modern legal teaching, nowadays no more than perpetuation of a myth, that no one *owns* land. In law, on paper everyone who possesses land merely holds that land for some superior lord (the whole bundle including Rent), and nowadays for most landholders, large, small, and very small, the Crown is sole temporal lord paramount. The lawyers who safeguard land ownership recognise the myth and the immensity of power given to the landholder, who has the legal right to exclusive use and the right to exclusive profit. The landholder can 'alienate' these rights by selling them, giving them away or destroying them, as desired. What we have to ask ourselves is whether the entrapment of Rent in this bundle held by the private landholder serves the best interests of Welfare Capitalism, or is merely another source of private profit for what we call nowadays the capitalist?

In days long since passed, the contents of this bundle were originally distributed between the community and the private individual in a more meaningful way, of which the reminder of today is simply a drop of ink in the legal archives. The original arrangement meant that the State held not merely the surface of the earth within the nation's boundaries, but also had first claim to the surplus wealth created within these boundaries once citizens had received a fair return for their own labour. The waste, the impenetrable forest, the moorland and the bogs offered little opportunity for wealth creation. The fertile lowlands, the riverbanks, the shoreline, afforded far greater returns for labour. Hence there was Rent, and to a greater or lesser extent Rent was collected in cash or in kind as revenue for the protection and development of the State. But as Rent was gradually transferred from the Crown to the private landholder the State was obliged to depend increasingly on the taxation of labour and interest for its revenue, a system originally devised to meet only the extraordinary exigencies of natural disaster or war. We take up the record in fifth century Britain.

The early English – lords and vassals

Events on the European mainland in AD 406 forced Constantine to pull back his legions from Britain into Gaul. In 410 the Emperor Honorius wrote to the cities of Britain instructing them to look after their own defence, and by 450 all links were irrevocably broken between Britain and Rome. The indigenous Britons were once again free to re-establish their kingdoms. However, they were left exposed to the threat of invasion. The Roman system of forts on both sides of the English Channel, the Saxon shore system centred on Boulogne, was no longer operational. Their vulnerability was emphasised by the sparse numbers of families in the numerous small kingdoms that arose, and their lack of unity.

The early Germanic communities who gained a foothold in Britain from the middle of the fifth century, Jutes, Angles and Saxons, were probably also small in scale. The dominant male of each invading group was acknowledged as '*cyning*', Old English for member of the (ruling) family or cynn (kin), from which came such royal names as Cynewald and the eventual derivative 'king'. Citizens of these forming nations expressed their commonality by turning their eyes to their ruler and giving allegiance. A good monarch was one who could raise 'the king's peace', that is secure the safety and prosperity of his people through good law and civil order, strong defence, and a general advance in the civilisation of the nation. But he needed resources to achieve these goals, resources locked up in the Rent of land.

When lands were sparsely populated, communication unreliable, and gathering of intelligence fraught with difficulty, the only way to secure the king's peace was to divide the land into units and place each in the care of a statesman, usually a relative or trusted friend of established competence. These men of high office, the king's *thegns*, administered their lands in turn by parcelling out settled areas to lesser thegns. Landholding by thegns was never a gift from the king for their own pleasure, but a grant with a greater purpose of service to the nation. The word 'thegn' meant a servant, disciple or follower (Toller, 1898, p 1043). But such a system of government was inherently weak, for it depended utterly on the bond of fidelity between lord and vassal, and this weakness was often exploited for personal advantage. Even kings are only mortal. "Remember that absolute monarchs are but men", wrote John Locke much later, "and if government is to be the remedy of those evils which necessarily follow from men's being judges in their own cases, and the state of nature is therefore not to be endured, I desire to know what kind of government that is, and how much better than the state of nature, when one man commanding a multitude has the liberty to be the judge in his own case, and may do to all his subjects whatever he pleases" (Locke, 1948, p 9). This vexed question as to the bounds of the king's prerogative, and the prerogative of his great lords, which is to ask to what extent they retain the right to behave according to the laws of (their) nature and escape the common law, was a perpetual source of trouble and conflict. Thus the most elaborate arrangements were made to re-inforce the bonds between lord and vassal; the ceremony of homage was the foundation of a system that was to evolve into high Feudalism, a system ultimately found wanting.

A code of national administration and justice based upon homage, so vulnerable to human fallibility, could not and did not endure. Slowly there evolved an alternative infrastructure for national justice, administration and defence, operating through king and counsel, parliament and the royal courts, funded increasingly through national taxation of wealth and income other than land. In the process, the burdens of feudal tenure were gradually off-loaded, yet at the same time the aristocratic class endured and strengthened its hold on Rent bound up in landed estates through legal inventions of their own devising, aided by their servants, the land lawyers. The historical process by which the shepherds were transformed into shearers was a long one and not easily summarised, but can be illustrated up to the Norman conquest by following the fortunes of the little Anglo-Saxon kingdom of the Hwicce and its powerful southern neighbour, Wessex.

The forging of an English aristocracy

The kingdom of the Hwicce came to be centred around what is modern Winchcombe in Gloucestershire, stretching north into the high Cotswolds around Cutsdean, and immortalised in place names such as Wychbold and the forest of Wychwood. (In 2000 the forest's owner, the third Baron Rotherwick, lost his claim to £1.6 million in compensation for loss of privacy when the County Council created a public footpath across this land.) Not until the latter part of the sixth century were the lands which became the kingdom of the Hwicce affected by incursions of English settlers, probably from the Thames Valley, who began to colonise the south west Midlands. Later tradition remembered the battle of Dyrham (577) as the turning point between British and English control in the region, but though after 600 the ruling family of the Hwicce was English (to judge from the names of the kings), the bulk of the local population was probably of older British stock.

In the seventh century, little kingdoms like that of the Hwicce co-existed with the greater kingdoms of the West Saxons, Mercians, East Anglians and (in the North) the Northumbrians. By the beginning of the eighth century the smaller units had largely been absorbed into the larger and, south of the River Humber, Mercia and Wessex were emerging as 'super kingdoms', dominating all others. In the eighth century Mercia predominated, but by the end of the ninth century the West Saxons were the dominant political force south of the Humber. By this process less successful realms came to be subordinate to stronger neighbours and eventually melded into larger and administratively more complex units.

The history of the Hwicce came to be bound to that of the Mercians, an Anglian people who emerged from the shadows of history under Penda, their warrior king from 626 to 655. Penda's aggressive wars created a greatly enlarged kingdom covering most of England between the Humber and the Thames. He may have developed the Hwiccian kingdom as a buffer zone to secure his south western borders against the Welsh and the equally aggressive West Saxon kingdom south of the Thames. Consequently the Hwicce fell increasingly under Mercian domination. In the closing years of the seventh century King Oshere of the Hwicce is recorded as donating lands, but with the consent of Aethelred his Mercian over-king.

Charters and bookland

About 680, the see of Worcester was created to serve the Christian kingdom of the Hwicce. Indeed, the old boundaries of the kingdom are probably contiguous with those of this medieval diocese (Bassett, 1989, p 6). Osric, who was king at that time, founded monasteries at Bath and Gloucester and endowed them with lands. His brother and successor Oshere gave lands to the noblewoman Dunne and her daughter Bucge for the establishment of the minster in what is now Withington in Gloucestershire. The records of this grant illustrate the sophistication of administration in many Anglo-Saxon parts of Britain by the late seventh century.

Oshere's grant to Dunne and Bucge was recorded in a charter or landbook, now lost. The charter was introduced into England by the Church to provide ecclesiastical institutions with land to be held in perpetuity, free from the claims of the heirs of the original donors. Charters, which were issued only by kings, freed the land concerned not only from hereditary claims, but also from the majority of renders and dues normally owed to the Crown by all landholders. With the issue of a charter, a particular kind of tenure was created called 'bookland'. From the eighth century onward such grants by charter were also made to lay nobles. In effect, the charter allowed the recipient to intercept the renders and dues formerly owed to the king, as his local representative, for the king's peace. But the recipient remained liable for those dues which were not exempted, usually military service in its various forms and the fines for more serious judicial offences. These services still had to be rendered to the king.

Bookland was thus a privileged tenure whereby the lord rendered service to the king, while himself enjoying customary services from the people who dwelt on the lands covered by the landbook or charter. In this way the Crown diverted revenue to regional institutions, providing them with the means and authority to meet their delegated temporal and spiritual responsibilities to that region of the State. Of course, some of what was diverted went to the private uses of the ecclesiastics and lay lords, for them to maintain the standards expected of men of high status. All too often this went too far.

The lands of individual manors, lay and ecclesiastical, were not contiguous but scattered to provide the best mix (some land in the valleys, higher land for grazing, woodland areas etc). Dunne and Bucge were given a well-defined endowment of twenty *hides*, one hide being an area of land at least notionally sufficient to support a peasant family, allowing for local conditions. Their land lay in the district centred on the nearby *vill* of Wycomb. Oshere as grantor would clearly have known how many hides of cultivated land were in his province, and what he could expect in revenue from each manor. The *tribal hidage*, which may have been a tribute list produced for Penda's son and successor, Wulfhere (658–675), recorded that the lands of the Hwicce held 7,000 hides. By the eighth century about a quarter of land had been granted to the Church, leaving three quarters to support the lay institutions of the province.

By the end of the reign of Offa, king of Mercia between 757 and 796, with the exception of Wessex all the kingdoms of the Midlands and south eastern regions of England had been conquered by his powerful and prosperous nation. The Hwicce was now absorbed into Mercia. A charter of 855 freed the manor of the minster at Blockley, north east of Cutsdean, from 'feeding and maintenance of all hawks and falcons in Mercia, of all huntsmen of the king or ealdorman' except those in the 'province' of the Hwicce (Sawyer, 1968).

Large and powerful though it had become, Mercia was not without its share of conspiracies, plots, civil wars and invasions. Its hegemony over the other English nations finally collapsed when King Ecgberht of Wessex, King Alfred's grandfather, emerged victorious against the Mercian forces at the Battle of Ellendune (south of modern day Swindon) in 825. In addition, throughout the late eighth and early ninth centuries the Vikings repeatedly raided Britain's eastern and southern shores. By 875 King Burgred of Mercia had capitulated to the invaders, leaving the south west kingdom of Wessex as the only territory unconquered. The original lands of the Hwicce now had a Viking over-lord.

A pivotal development occurred in May 878. Alfred, King of Wessex, had been forced to flee to Athelney in the Somerset marshes in the wake of a surprise attack by the Dane, Guthrum. However, Alfred emerged to lead a victorious counter-attack at Edington, midway between Bridgwater and Glastonbury. Over the following 14 years of relative peace Alfred the Great went about strengthening the defences of his kingdom, such that he was able to contain the next Danish invasion of 892. These fortifications or *burhs* were listed in the *Burghal hidage*, showing the extent of land attached to provide for military and civil requirements.

When Alfred died in 899 the task of conquest was taken up by his son, Edward the Elder, and his daughter Aethelflaed. By 924, the southern settlements of the Danes had been over-run by Wessex. Leicester and Derby were taken by Aethelflaed, Nottingham and Stamford by Edward, leaving only the regions of Lincoln and York in Danish hands. Brother and sister also took the Danish southern settlements in East Anglia, south east Mercia and the north east Midlands, bringing administration of their conquered lands into line with the shire system they were familiar with in their homeland.

The massive and sustained period of territorial conquest and fortification by the Wessex dynasty demanded major reforms to the systems of government, taxation and landholding to sustain the successes. The garrisons required to defend the burhs probably comprised about 30,000 men, and many of the population must have moved in for protection and to meet the needs of the army in quartering and rations. Add to this the mobile army of thegns and the labour working on their lands to support it, and the enormity of a Wessex geared for war becomes apparent.

The task of subduing the Danes of York fell to Alfred's grandsons, Athelstan, Edmund and Eadred. Between 927 and 954, a series of bitterly fought campaigns brought final victory and the incorporation of the last Danish settlements in York and Lincoln into the West Saxon kingdom: a vindication of the claim, first made by Athelstan, to be 'King of the English'. As for the kingdom of the Hwicce, it was by this time reduced to no more than a district of the united kingdom of England, its lands apportioned between neighbouring parts of Gloucestershire, Worcestershire and Warwickshire.

In the closing decades of the 10th century a fresh phase of Viking raids began, coinciding with the opening years of the reign of Æthelred II (978-1016). In the 11th century the scale of Viking attacks escalated. Swein, King of Denmark, and the Danish warlord, Thorkell the Tall, led devastating attacks from Scandinavia between 1003 and 1006, and 1009 and 1012, respectively. In 1013, Swein was actually acknowledged as King of the English and Æthelred fled to Normandy, returning only when Swein died in February 1014. One of Æthelred's last actions before his exile had been to grant four hides of land in the manor of Mathon near Great Malvern to Leofwine, *ealdorman* of the Hwicce.

The struggle was continued by Swein's son, Cnut, who in 1016 concluded a peace treaty with Æthelred's son and successor Edmund when they met in Hwiccian country, at Alney near Deerhurst in Gloucestershire. Between 1019 and 1035, Cnut ruled a North Sea empire embracing much of Scandinavia as well as England. The old West Saxon line enjoyed a brief return after the death of Cnut and his sons, Edward the Confessor ruling between 1042 and 1066. His death revived rivalries between three claimants: for Norway, Harold Hardrada; for Wessex, Harold

Godwinson; and for Normandy, Duke William (whose claim arose because Edward's mother was his aunt, Emma).

By this process of treaty and conquest a host of ruling families were forged into an aristocracy of thegnships owing allegiance to the ruling house of Wessex, which after a long campaign finally provided the early monarchs of England. King's thegns, bishop's thegns and lesser thegns were bound by homage, lesser lord and greater lord together, preliminary to the lords temporal, lords spiritual and knights of later centuries. Not until 1660 was homage abolished, and even today remnants remain as various oaths of fealty. It was an institution used for more than 1,000 years, reaching its highest expression in the 12th century (see below).

Some idea of Anglo-Saxon society as it evolved during this 10th century of territorial aggression can be gauged from a unique manuscript that was probably produced in the scriptorium of Worcester Cathedral, the *Rectitudines Singularum Personarum*. The king himself held vast tracts of land, having seized many royal estates in Mercia and East Anglia. Then there were the great thegnly families holding land charters from the king: ecclesiastics and lay lords. Land grants indicate that in the early 930s there were about 120 families of such status, many connected with the royal families of Wessex and Mercia. The men heading these families were responsible for overseeing great wealth through their offices, managing lands running into tens of thousands of acres. Wulfgar of Inkpen (west of Newbury), for example, held several thousand acres of rich farmland in Cambridgeshire's Kennet Valley (Wood, 1990, pp 107-9). With territorial expansion the thegnly class expanded. Men found trustworthy and capable when tested in battle were granted the increased status and responsibility of thegnhood and the resources of landholding in order that they could fulfil their responsibilities. But thegnly status appeared to depend not only on the qualities of the man himself but also the track record of his family. According to the Promotion Law, thegnhood apparently required satisfactory tenure of at least five hides of land for three generations by charter from the king, in return for services.

The common people of early England

On the lands of the thegnly class, both ecclesiastic and lay, lived and worked ordinary families farming hides held on the customary terms of their lord. Some of these commoners, called *geneats* (origin of gentlefolk?) in the *Rectitudines* (which probably described west Midland practice), were free men: free in the sense that they had entered into an understanding with the lord on more or less equal terms and of their own free will. Some such free men would have negotiated a fixed term in return for services, the term covering either one life or three lives, with reversion to the lord or his descendants at the end of the 'contract'. Such land was called loanland (*laenland*). There were other still more privileged free commoners who held land without any fixed term demanding eventual reversion to the lord, but nevertheless on condition of payment of customary rents and services. This form of tenure appears to have been modelled on the king's grant of bookland, whereby services due to the king had been diverted to the lord and his heirs in perpetuity for use according to the terms of the royal charter. In the *Domesday Book* such land tenure was called '*sokeland*'. The remaining commoners, the *geburs*, were unfree in the sense that their agreement with the lord was distinctly one-sided; they were bound to provide rents and services to the manor on terms which could change with the lord's mind. Wulfgar's estates seem to have been worked by between 700 and 1,000 unfree families, some of whom were virtually slaves (Wood, 1990, pp 107-9). The terms under which they remained on the land were often spelt out to the last penny, cartload of firewood, and measure of wheat to be handed over.

Early English administration

Local administration in early England was based on the shire and its court. Beneath the shire was the hundred with its own court, notionally containing 100 hides, though the actual size and assessment of individual hundreds varied considerably. Beneath the hundred was the tithing, a unit notionally of 10 hides and the vill (which might include one or several actual settlements). The vill also possessed a court, though it rarely surfaces in the surviving evidence. This structure provided the king with a most efficient system for raising additional revenue in times of emergency, at a variable rate to the hide. Collection of revenue based on landholding was facilitated by the circulation of coinage coming from the royal mints (which used 30 tonnes of silver in 1018, for example). Only the king could impose rounds of taxes upon his subjects, or grant exemption. Heaviest of all were the Dane-gelds used to buy off the Danish enemy. According to the *Anglo-Saxon Chronicle*, King Aethelred was hard put to it between 991 and 1017, the Dane-geld of £48,000 in 1011 being dwarfed by another of £72,000 raised to pacify Cnut a few years later (Dowell, 1965, vol 1, p 9). Note, however, that taxation was not routine. The day-to-day material and spiritual needs of the State were met through services of the thegnly class. Of course, conquerors and over-lords frequently turned taxation into a system of tribute, an acknowledgement of dependence of the weaker nation upon the stronger. Supported by their charters and manorial lands, the great minsters (the word is derived from monastery) provided for the spiritual and intellectual needs of the lay manors in their jurisdiction. In later years the boundaries of many lay manors came to define the smaller parish boundaries of churches erected on estate lands. Estate churches serving the manor were a popular innovation in the 10th century, adding to the minsters, abbeys and hermitages yet another ecclesiastical feature to the landscape. The new 'offspring' churches intruded on the 'mother churches' or minsters, and many disputes arose over tithes and burial fees, but the new parish system added a third administrative unit to the shire and the borough as the minster parishes broke up. By 1066 as much as one third of the cultivated land of large stretches of England in the south and south west had been endowed for the support of Christian institutions, a growing practice which led to increasing conflict between the lords spiritual and the lords temporal.

Norman Feudalism

The framework of landholding developed by the Saxons as they forged England was thrown into upheaval with the arrival of Duke William of Normandy and his army at Pevensey on England's south coast on 28 September 1066. William defeated King Harold at Hastings on 14 October, opening a new era. The heads of the great Norman families who formed his military entourage, among them Aubigny, Beaumont, Grandmesnil, Mandeville, Tosny and Warenne, were landholders in their own homeland. There they had their own system of Feudalism, and English concepts such as bookland puzzled them. As victors, they suppressed this English system beneath their own to suit themselves, but leaving its remnants supporting Feudalism. The Normans handled landholding by inheritance, whereby land passed automatically (first by custom and later by law) to the person recognised as the landholder's heir – usually the eldest son. So forcefully was this applied that inheritance of land in this strict sense became deeply ingrained in the national psyche and was not abolished (with minor qualifications) until the Law of Property Act of 1925. Even then, the Act was forced to frame its definition of land in terms of 'hereditament', the very system it was essentially abolishing in law. So from then on 'land' meant that complex of the tangible and intangible that was *in the past* inheritable.

What the Normans inherited was a tenure called *feodum*, the rules governing which formed the feudal system of landholding (not landowning). The 50 years after 1066 were a period of high Feudalism in England, which is to say high colonialism under William and his successors William II and Henry I. The lands of much of the Anglo-Saxon aristocracy were confiscated and vested directly in the colonising monarchy. From then on all entitlements to hold land (titles) were granted only by the king either directly or indirectly. As early as 1067 William was granting land to the military generals, his barons, as well as English collaborators. This was the start of an appropriation that was to take 20 years. Many former English freemen found themselves landless and in bondage, part of a labour force used, for example, to construct fortifications around the countryside.

Feudalism and inheritance as systems were anything but trouble-free, and the king's court was repeatedly called upon to settle situations which threw up conflict. Not even the king escaped the contradictions and confusion. Until William's death in 1087 Normandy and England were one lordship which just happened to be split by an inconvenient stretch of water. But William and his magnates held inherited lands in the Norman part and acquisitions by conquest in the English area. The law of descent applied to inherited feudal lands but not to land acquired by purchase (in law the term purchase merely refers to land acquired by personal action such as conquest, gift or bargain and sale, rather than by inheritance). Lands of purchase were useful as a means of provision for the cadet branches of the family headed by younger sons. This arrangement left the inherited estate intact under the eldest son. A proclamation of Henry I, set down in 1100, stated: "The ancestral fee (the heritable land held in return for service to the State) of the father is to go to the first born son; but he may give his purchases or later acquisitions to whomsoever he prefers" (Holt, 1972).

Bequests of land by will do not appear to have been a feature of the early Anglo-Norman period; land held by tenants on their deathbed was simply not in their gift to will away. Gifts to children had therefore to be made during the father's lifetime. If it happened that the eldest son and heir received both the inherited and acquired lands, the whole became a parcel of inherited estate from then on. Furthermore, what the younger son received through his father's purchase became the inheritance of the cadet branch. So, for example, in the Grandmesnil family the Norman inheritance went to the senior branch and the English acquisition launched the inheritance of the junior branch.

When, as in the Giffard family, lands in Normandy and England went to the same person, the seeds of confusion were sown because of what followed. With William's death in 1087, his eldest son Robert succeeded to the inheritance of the Duchy of Normandy while the younger son William II took the purchase of England. This meant that men holding land on both sides of the English Channel now had two lords – but how could one man serve two military over-lords at the same time? The whole edifice of Feudalism was structured on homage and fealty. Under Feudalism every man had his lord (the king's lord was God, whose spiritual representative was the Pope; hence the Church always had its degree of independence from the Crown). Military tenures of barons and under-tenancies of knights were buttressed by the ceremony of homage, in Norman culture more sacred than blood relationship. The tenant put his hands between those of the lord, signifying subjection and fealty on the part of the former and warranty of protection and confirmation of the tenant's *seisin* (possession of the land on a justifiable basis) on the part of the latter. A strict feudal rule was that no grantor may derogate from his original grant. Clearly, problems arose when a vassal paid homage to two lords, as sometimes happened. In a culture not averse to settling problems violently, the division of England and Normandy became a recipe for war. Robert, William Rufus and Henry (William's other surviving son) engaged in wars of succession as for 26 years between 1087 and 1154 England and Normandy were ruled separately.

Tenure, service and estate

In English Feudalism the king's immediate vassals, perhaps 2,000 of them, held land directly from the monarch as his tenants-in-chief. No other person was interposed between the king and these great men. They tenanted land of the king under a bundle of terms and conditions, the first and foremost condition being an understanding that in England no one *owned* land as their property; all tenants merely *held* land directly or indirectly of the king, whose powers of forfeiture of the land of traitors gave him a unique status among the lords. Tenure set down the continuous services expected of the tenant and the incidental obligations which might become due at certain times, essentially as forms of death duty. Medieval lawyers classified lay tenures as knight service and castlegard (both military), sergeanty (king's civil offices, several of which still survive in connection with coronations), and socage (a residual category, but still owing services of one kind or another). Spiritual tenures were classified as frankalmoign (services uncertain) and divine service (services fixed) (Simpson, 1986, pp 7-15).

In theory at least, the military tenants-in-chief were bound into service for 40 days in the year but never compelled to serve outside of the kingdom. They accompanied the king on his armed expeditions and were required to provide the number of knights stated in the tenure. The size of the knightly complement was not apparently related directly to the estate, by which is meant the land held under tenure and the duration of the interest granted, be it for a term, life, several lives (to the descendants), or in perpetuity by inheritance (the fee simple). The tenant-in-chief was left to establish the means by which his complement was assured. In general, however, he would settle each knight on his fee, a piece of land considered adequate to support his own needs and those of his servants and family. A knight owed his lord 40 days of service in a year, and the military tenancies were estimated to be capable of supporting 6,500 such fighting men. However, the king did not have need of 260,000 days of knight service each and every year. Furthermore, the knight might be a fine warrior at 25 years of age, but not at 45. Hence from 1100 we begin to read of scutage or shield money. In lieu of presentation of the knight in person, the king would accept a sum of money from the tenant-in-chief, who was allowed to recover the same amount from the absent knight. The cost of scutage was at least £1, and it was levied at least seven times in the 12th century. Civil and religious services could be commuted in a similar fashion, and even the magnates were sometimes able to buy a licence from the Crown to commute their services.

Inheritance of Land and feudal death duties

The important point to appreciate is that under Feudalism, as in pre-Conquest days, land was held by lords in return for service and incidents to the over-lord, and hence ultimately to the State. The landed estate furnished Rent. The lord in possession set aside a part to fulfil his local and national duties, and submitted another part as incidents for central revenue. Notions of land ownership simply did not exist (Palmer, 1985, pp 4-8). Fees were rather like squares on a chess board on which interpersonal feudal relationships were played out. The 'pieces' needed no proprietary claim to the spaces they occupied in order to comply with the rules of Feudalism. The tie of homage and fealty which secured the State's interest naturally was severed, however, at the death of either party, and something had to be done to strengthen this weak link in the feudal chain. So when the tenant died, whether this be knight or tenant-in-chief, the land held in fee reverted to the lord. This was a time when, during re-organisation, the lord would collect certain 'death duties' or incidents due from military tenancies. What the lord had granted the lord temporarily re-possessed. Under Norman custom those in line for the heirship knew the relative strength of their claims to inherit, but all too often an undisputed eldest son was not there when needed. What happened, for example, when there were twin firstborn sons, both surviving their father's death and both on the land? What happened when the deceased had eldest sons in two marriages? These were among the many problems for the lord and his court to sort out as best as possible; cases that eventually came before the courts of the common law which matured between 1066 and 1200.

Assuming the heir was generally acknowledged, then to obtain a grant of the land the heir was required to pay homage to the lord and pay a 'relief' that could amount to one year's profit of the land. When the heir was male and under age, which was 21 for military tenure and 14 for other tenure, the lord obtained custody or wardship of the tenant's land and retained the profits until he was of age. The lord also had wardship of the young tenant, protecting his interest and grooming him for his future responsibilities. When the ward came of age, release from guardianship was obtained by payment of ousterlemain (taking off of hands), often amounting to six month's revenue of the land. Wardship was indisputably a major source of revenue for the Crown.

The rules of inheritance of the fee were based on four principles, the first being that the 'issue of the deceased's body' took precedence. The second was that inheritance never ascended a generation on the deceased's death. The third was that males took before females of the same degree (brothers before sisters), and the fourth was that sons took in order of seniority, while daughters took equal shares. When the heiress was a minor, her lord had a right to choose her husband and to dispose of the lands. Whoever was favoured would often pay good money for acquisition in this way, and by the late 12th century the king was selling the marriages of both male and female heirs. If the minor married without consent, the heir forfeited '*duplicem valorem maritigii*', or double the value of the marriage.

When a feudal tenant died without heirs, the lord took back the lands by 'escheat'. In his own good time the lord was then free to grant the estate to whomsoever he favoured. A new tenant stepping into a knight's fee generally had to find a relief of about £5, but those taking up larger estates would have to find much greater sums. Another most important incident was 'forfeiture', under which lands were returned to the king in cases of treason. Not only the convicted tenant, but his lord also would lose the lands for assumed complicity or negligence. Lands were likewise forfeited for felonies other than treason.

The tensions in Feudalism were obvious, and homage was frequently not enough to paper over the cracks. The king was primarily interested in revenue for the State and the competence of his tenants-in-chief to deliver this revenue through services, death duties of various kinds, and rents as servants of the State. Their lands were split into the 'demesne' to provide an income for their own support, and that held in fee by under-tenants. Vassals of the lord were husbands and parents with ambitions of their own, however, and they were motivated to secure a balance in which the family came out of the arrangement as well as possible. Herein lay a battle over the possession of Rent.

Ownership and title to Land

The endless series of feudal conflicts meant that lawyers never even bothered to attempt to define 'ownership', even as land was evolving into a species of private property (see below). The word implies a right to assert that something is one's own. Rights are therefore assertions against others, which lawyers break down into rights in property (*in rem*) and personal rights (*in personam*). The latter category is enforcable only against a specified person, while the former has become enforcable against the world. English law has come to be focused on competing claims to property such as land, and seeks only to determine who has the better claim – better entitlement or 'title'. Thus it turns out that the law is concerned only with the strength of competing claims to Rent (as an integral part of the land complex). As the lord's powers under Feudalism receded, so Rent went increasingly in the vassal's favour, as he (or she) became less and less a vassal and more and more a tenant with an estate in fee *simple* (meaning an estate granted to the tenant *and the tenant's heirs in general*).

The legal brains that shaped the law of landholding between 1066 and 1300 generally came neither from the royal household nor the families of the great magnates, but from the talented sons of the under-tenants. The under-tenant wished to escape 'death duties', secure the inheritance of the eldest son and provide lands for the future of the younger children, while maintaining the value and integrity of the estate against 'stranger' families with similar motives. The first sign of escape from the dominion of the over-lord, so as to achieve these aims, came with a revision of homage. This we can take as the start on the road to an aristocracy of private landholding.

NINE

An aristocracy of privatised Rent

Wealth, however got, in England makes
Lords of mechanics, gentlemen of rakes:
Antiquity and birth are needless here;
'Tis impudence and money makes a peer.'
(Daniel Defoe, *The True-born Englishman*, 1701)

If the nature of Rent is obscure to the modern citizen, the legal processes through which it was privatised are doubly so. Descriptions of the history of land law are laced with comments such as 'peculiar', 'intricate and specialised', 'obscure', 'confused', 'tangled', 'mysterious', 'full of riddles and conundrums'. Cromwell concluded that the law of real property was an ungodly jungle. Law tends to follow custom, not make it, and as the nature of landholding underwent its long and tortuous evolution, so legal opinion and statute law shifted in like manner.

> To the layman the system became wholly unintelligible.... To the lawyers ... the law of property ... became a great mystery, an elaborate network of rules so inter-related that any radical legislative interference might destroy the assumed coherence of the whole, and throw men's security in their property into confusion. What enabled them to adopt this position was the extraordinary mastery of the law exhibited by the leading conveyancers of the late 17th and 18th centuries, whose model conveyances were imitated by the lesser members of the profession, and whose practice was treated with reverence by the courts. Their conveyances so manipulated the rusty machinery of the land law as to produce the social consequences desired by the more important and influential landowners. And, no doubt, the deeper the mysteries involved, the more money lawyers could extract from their clients for their arcane services. (Simpson, 1986, p 233)

This chapter traces two threads through the muddle: the struggle of landholders to wrest the right to Rent from the State, and the constant battle of the members of this dynastic class to keep their bundle of rights and privileges called land, which increasingly included Rent, within the family. In so doing, it cannot be stressed too highly that the rightness of Rent as public revenue stands on its own merits – needing no historical precedent for justification. Nevertheless the precedent is there, in the feudal services and death duties owed to the State by the tenants-in-chief holding land and its attached privileges of the king. Here is the root of the term 'real' property; *regalis*, Latin for 'of a king'. The argument that Rent should be returned to the State is not of course an argument in support of Monarchy or Feudalism of any sort. Rather, it demands from modern democratic government what the old undemocratic governments comprised of the landholding class refused to do, which is to fund government expense in peacetime by collection of Rent rather than taxation of wages and interest.

The Assize of Northampton: strengthening of the tenant freeholder's title

In the middle of the 12th century the ceremony of homage was still sacred. The lord's warrant of the vassal's title to the fee prevented the lord from asserting his superior title so long as the vassal was alive and keeping his side of the bargain. But homage traditionally lapsed on the death of either party, lord or vassal. On the lord's death all tenants had to swear fealty to their new lord; and when the tenant died the lord similarly accepted the homage of the new tenant. The rule of inheritance was powerful, but the lord had the prerogative of choice if he considered the tenant's own heir to be unsuitable. Many such disputes came to court.

A change in viewpoint evolved somewhere in the 12th century, when homage came to survive until both parties had died (Thorne, 1959). From then onwards, when the lord died his heir and new lord was barred by the homage of his ancestor from taking back the tenant's lands and demanding regrant only on condition of relief. Only when the tenant died did *his* heir owe homage and relief to the new lord. Similarly, when the tenant died before his lord, the tenant's heir stepped into the fee without payment of relief. Only on the lord's death did the tenant's heir need to pay homage and relief to the lord's heir.

This change in feudal practice clearly strengthened the rights of the tenant family, increasing their security of tenure and much reducing the occasions on which relief was due to the lord. Then by the Assize of Northampton in 1176, the heir acquired the automatic right to claim the land and the benefits that went with it before he had actually paid homage and relief. In the language of the day, the heir was 'seised' of the estate from the moment of his ancestor's death; not from the date of formal gift from the lord: "if any freeholder has died, let his heirs remain in such seisin as their father had of his fief on the day of his death.... And afterwards let them seek out the lord and pay him a relief and the other things they ought to pay him from the fief" (Hudson, 1996, p 132). To facilitate this arrangement a new procedure was introduced by the Assize of Northampton, the assize *mort d'ancestor*, to expedite the satisfaction of the tenant heir whose lord refused to acknowledge his right to automatic seisin.

The Assize of Northampton was an attempt by Henry II to ensure the fulfilment in good faith of feudal obligations between lord and tenant. When magnates prepared for armed conflict, they and their followers saw land tied up by minors, widows and men they distrusted as contrary to their best interest. Hence ways and means were frequently sought to remove such tenants and replace them with men of military prowess, even though in so doing feudal obligations would be trampled upon.

When Henry II came to the throne of England in 1154 his realm was racked by violence amongst his tenants-in-chief. He restored order but was determined to uphold feudal principles in future and prevent lords committing wrongs against militarily weak tenants who occupied knights' fees. One way to achieve this end was to grant the heir immediate enfeoffment. If the lord disagreed then he could take his dispute before the royal justices rather than settle the issue in his own court.

Enforcement of feudal obligations to tenants and their heirs threw a tremendous burden of oversight on the king's own court and justices. Full-time royal justices were therefore created by 1179, and bureaucratic procedures quickly evolved to standardise the administration of the common law. By 1205 the rule was that no freeholder need answer for his free tenement without service of a royal writ.

This shaping of the common law, designed to uphold feudal obligations, gave royal protection to the freeholder. Mort d'ancestor protected tenants' claims against their lords. Soon other novel procedures were created to protect the claims of lords against their tenants in the royal courts. The foundations were thereby laid whereby the common law became the instrument of the State, replacing feudal arrangements, and the forum within which land evolved into a species of private property (Milsom, 1976; Palmer, 1985). Rent, however, became private property through the operation of the Chancery court, one function of which was to ensure that those who held land in trust performed their duties in the manner for which they had been entrusted by the grantor, as described later.

The courts intruded further into the lord–tenant arrangement when another reform, probably introduced at the Council of Windsor in 1179, allowed land disputes to be settled not by combat but by the opinion of 12 knights of the district who, in the presence of the king's justices, testified as to which party had the better title (Hudson, 1996, pp 132-4).

The heir-at-law, and tenant's right of alienation

The strong principles of heritability in feudal landholding would suggest that the heir-by-expectation had an interest in the fee even while his predecessor still lived, and that on this account the father or whoever this predecessor might be could not alienate the land. This was not the position, however. By 1250 the tenant in fee had secured the right of alienation, selling or giving away land without the heir's consent. The rule which arose to explain this apparent contradiction was that a living person had no heir-at-law, for until his or her death the heir-at-law could not be identified with certainty. In early feudal times what the tenant could alienate was part or all of the fee in demesne. What he could not alienate, for they were not part of his fee, were the seigniorial rights to services and incidents for which the lord was seised. Hence Rent as feudal dues to the State was at first secure, only later to be lost as public revenue when, with the ending of feudal dues, it became a valuable part of the bundle which the tenant could sell or lease.

Alienation was illegal if it broke the feudal chain – no conveyance of land was valid if it created or opened the possibility of abeyance of seisin (for example, a grant to A for life, with the heir to inherit at the age of 21, threatened an abeyance of seisin if A died when the heir was still a minor). With this proviso, alienation was achieved in one of two ways. The method preferred by the lord (though he had no say in the choice) was for the tenant simply to substitute another in his place either by gift, sale or settlement of debt. The lord may or may not like the incoming tenant, but could influence the outcome only by way of the size of the fine of substitution he demanded of the outgoing tenant. Services and incidents would then be due from the new tenant in proportion to the value of the parcel alienated to him.

The method of alienation preferred by the tenant, and therefore the more common, was sub-infeudation of a parcel of his land, in which he created a new link on the end of the feudal chain, avoiding any fine of substitution in the process. He, the outgoing tenant, remained bound for services to his lord while the incoming tenant took the outgoing tenant for his lord, thereby creating a new feudal relationship. For the lord of the outgoing tenant this was potentially disastrous because he could effectively lose the value of the incidents. To illustrate:

> Let the lord be A and his tenant B ... A derives a regular income from the services and has the expectation of important profits at irregular intervals (the death duties). ... Now let us suppose that B sells his (interest in his) land (to C). He receives a large sum of money which, of course, is quite beyond the lord's reach. B then enfeoffs C (ie creates a new feudal association) ... by the nominal service of a rose at midsummer. ... We now have to consider how this arrangement will affect A. The regular services due from B to A are still secure, but the occasional profits of A's lordship are seriously impaired. Relief which is based on the value of the tenement will no longer be considerable, for B's tenement produces nothing but a rose at midsummer. ... Wardship and marriage of B's heir are ... worthless ... under the most favourable circumstances the guardian could only collect a few roses. (Plucknett, 1956, pp 539-40)

The forty shilling freehold and knighthood

With knights sub-infeudating their land and scutage becoming more difficult to collect, the concept of knight service became increasingly obsolescent. The end came in 1247 when by royal proclamation knighthood no longer signified military prowess but simply landed wealth. All freeholders of land worth in rent 40 shillings or more a year were from that date entitled to knighthood. It is important to remember, however, that the tenants-in-chief remained tenants by military service, and could still be charged the attached feudal dues by the Crown, a cause of much conflict in later centuries.

Quia Emptores: sub-infeudation outlawed

Should a tenant wish to secure his salvation by endowment of land to a religious institution, he would normally sub-infeudate, the new tenancy created being in alms for frankalmoign. The service he obtained from the new tenant would not even be a rose in midsummer, but prayers for his soul. Furthermore, no incidents such as relief or wardship could be expected from a corporate body that never dies. When the original tenant died there was now nothing for his lord to claim – the lord's seignory amounted to nothing with respect to the land granted to the religious institution. The outcome was the same when the land had been alienated by substitution. The lord found himself with a tenant who never dies, ruling out any prospect of escheat.

These problems were recognised in the statute *Quia Emptores* of 1290 (Digby, 1897, pp 236-9), which laid down several principles. First: "... henceforth it should be lawful to every freeman to sell at his own pleasure his lands and tenements or part of them, so that the feoffee (the person enfeoffed) shall hold the same lands or tenements of the chief lord of the same fee, by such service and customs as his feoffor held before". Secondly, the statute forbade sub-infeudation: "And if he sell any part of such lands or tenements to any, the feoffee shall immediately hold it *of the chief lord*...." But there remained the threat of alienation by substitution to a religious institution, and this was also dealt with in *Quia Emptores*: "And it is to be understood that by the said sales or purchases ... such lands or tenements shall in no wise come into mortmain" (ie into the possession of an ecclesiastical or other corporation). The final statement of the statute was equally important: "And it is to wit that this statute extendeth but only to lands holden in fee simple" (ie to the heirs general, an arrangement potentially of infinite duration). In other words, tenants were still free to sub-infeudate lands by a grant 'in fee tail', that is where the inheritance was restricted to certain classes of heir, such as male descendants of a particular wife, thereby allowing fathers to make gifts to the family.

From the point of view of Rent, *Quia Emptores* was highly significant. The statute forbade freehold lands held in seisin to be parcelled out by sub-infeudation in fee simple. This meant that when a mesne lord died without heirs and the land returned to the chief lord according to the doctrine of escheat, the chief lord took the deceased mesne lord's tenants and lands for his own. Hence with each escheat a link was removed from the feudal chain. The statute forbade the chief lord from replacing this link by a sub-infeudation. Thus *Quia Emptores*, coupled with the State's enquiries into the status of lands of deceased landholders through local officials called escheators, should have brought feudal dues under increasing control of the Crown and improved the flow of revenues to the State. What effectively opposed this trend, as discussed below, was the counter-development of the medieval use. As a result, Rent in the form of feudal dues was lost to the State as it found its way into the pockets of landholders. *Quia Emptores* remains the law today, a proposal for its repeal having failed as recently as 1967.

The threat of the heiress

For tenants wishing to secure what they were increasingly confident was theirs by right, the common law threatened when there was in the family an heiress-by-expectation. So long as he lived, a king's vassal wishing to marry off his heiress was expected to inform his lord. The king would neither interfere nor demand a fine in return for his acquiescence, provided the prospective groom was not his enemy. Thus, daughters who were heiresses-by-expectation were given in marriage by their fathers. The threat from the common law came with the death of the person from whom the heiress expected to inherit. She now became heiress-at-law, and by 1100 the king had established the right to sell her marriage to a man of his choosing on counsel of his barons (Plucknett, 1956, p 535). For the king this arrangement was quite satisfactory, for death duties were forthcoming whether there was an heir-at-law or an heiress-at-law. For the tenant with an heiress at his death, however, the king's powers threatened the family estate.

To recapitulate, males took before females of the same degree; sons took in order of seniority, while daughters took equal shares. If the father was lucky enough to have both sons and daughters who survived him, then the eldest son as heir-at-law took all land that had been in his father's legal possession. Unless, therefore, the father had taken care to provide for the younger branches of his immediate family during his life, they would be disinherited. When there had been no son of any marriage, the father's inheritance went to his daughters if any, the heiresses-at-law. There may be 'collateral' males, a brother or nephew of the deceased for example, but lineal descent was paramount. But 'heirs lineal' could be of either sex.

Under the common law, family fortunes meant that about one in four inheritances would go directly to heiresses-at-law. Furthermore, because co-heiresses took in equal shares, and in some cases of collateral descent the inheritor would be female, in all about 40% of women would inherit under common law (Spring, 1993, p 11). For the father there was therefore a significant probability that, without evasive action, part of his land would pass to other aristocratic families by marriage of his daughters to 'strangers'.

Even though the children of such marriages would still be 'the issue of his body', landholders preferred the land to go to a man within the family than to one without. The conveyancer specialised in solving such problems.

Initially, landholders provided for younger children by granting land at their marriage. The deed conveying the land to the new couple (*maritagium*) made the grant conditional on their having children, and sometimes more specifically a male child. The form was 'to my daughter and husband (or son and wife) and the heirs male of their bodies'. The couple were forbidden therefore from disposing of the land, in contrast to tenants in fee simple, because the inheritance was entailed (French: *taillé*, meaning curtailed to the lineal heirs of the original grantee). Should this junior branch fail to produce the specified heir then the land would revert to the senior branch on the death of the son or daughter. Only when the third generation of heirs of this junior branch was established were homage and services again due, and alienation of the land permitted. Absence of homage meant that the donor and his heirs had not warranted the title, and therefore could reclaim the land if the specified heir did not materialise. For three generations therefore the land could be 'entailed' to male heirs only, denying inheritance to any heiress–at–law in this junior branch.

De Donis Conditionalibus: the development of the inalienable entail

Lands granted in the maritagium were nevertheless disposed of in ways never intended by the original donor. Widows, for example, alienated land and the original grantor had no writ available to pursue recovery. The statute *De Donis Conditionalibus* of 1285 was directed solely at this problem: "... they to whom the land was given under such condition shall have no power to aliene the land so given, but it shall remain unto the issue of them to whom it was given after their death, or shall revert unto the giver or his heirs if issue fail ..." (Digby, 1897, pp 226-30). After decades of legal argument it came to be accepted that the entail would endure not merely for three generations but for as long as there were heirs of the prescribed class.

The underlying concept of *De Donis* was later extended to estates other than the maritagium. Landholders began to limit inheritance of alienated land to male heirs only, or to the descendants of a particular husband or wife. These entailed estates fell in their potential duration between the life estate and the fee simple. The tenant in fee tail was regarded as having merely a life tenancy and could not behave in any way that threatened the interests of the prescribed heir. He could not alienate family land, and could not grant a lease for longer than his own life. Even if he was a traitor the lands could not be forfeited beyond his lifetime – they then returned to the rightful heir. The fee tail created a sense of secure family property in which the prescribed heirs had a future interest. Insofar as Rent was part of the estate, the entail served to bind this within the family according to the original donor's wishes.

Barring the entail: landholders manipulate their own law

The donor who created a fee tail may have removed the threat of the heiress and the power of the heir to sell the land with its rights and privileges, but he had at the same time prevented future generations from providing security in land for all of their children. This difficulty of providing for family when land had been entailed to the male line eventually proved too much to tolerate as a means to secure the estate. By 1500, conveyancers had devised a way of destroying for the entailed tenant what his ancestors had invented. Barring the entail had a mysterious genesis, but by 1600 it was achieved by 'common recovery', a practice which illustrates just what a nonsensical tangle the conveyancers had woven to please their clients – so tangled that conveyance became a complicated, unfathomable and expensive business.

Many judges and lawyers were denied an inheritance because they were younger sons of families with lands entailed to eldest males. They therefore colluded in a fiction, using two actions in common law for their purpose. One was an action called 'levying a fine', the other 'suffering a recovery'. First, an action was brought against the tenant-in-tail by someone (say the younger son) claiming an imaginary title which he knew to be untrue. The tenant-in-tail then got the court usher to say that he (the tenant-in-tail) really had a fee simple (ie to the tenant and his (unspecified) heirs). This too was a lie known to the court. The tenant-in-tail then failed to appear in court to 'defend' himself, so the action went to the plaintiff by default, who ended up with a fee simple. Anybody disinherited could sue the poor court usher, but that would be financially a waste of time. (For details of variations on this method see Simpson, 1986, pp 126-37.)

The 'feoffee to use': the development of beneficial interest in Land

By 1250, almost two centuries on from the Conquest, lands originally acquired through warfare had found their way into the realm of inheritance. What happened to such lands on the death of the tenant was stipulated by the common law, and any attempt to determine the fate of inherited land by personal will was illegal. Wills could dispose of the deceased's moveable property, but not inherited land. To escape from this constraint, landholders and their conveyancers unravelled the bundle termed land and devised a way of redistributing its contents to defeat the law. They adapted an entity recognised in common law as the 'feoffee to use', the forerunner of the modern trustee.

The story goes that when knights went to war, being uncertain of their return, they would convey their lands to a friend who would act as a guardian in certain respects, perhaps collecting rents on behalf of the manor. The conditions under which such conveyances were made were termed 'uses'. Better still, if the conveyance was to a group of feoffees to uses, security was improved, especially when the feoffees had power to elect replacements. The feoffee to use had the legal title under common law, but had lost part of the bundle to another. He held the land not for his own benefit but for the benefit of the nominee of the original landholder who had requested the conveyancers to split up the bundle. The nominee would then possess the specified benefits (eg the wife gets the rents), but would not be possessed of the rest of the bundle, including the corporeal hereditaments, on his or her death. The beneficiary was known as the '*cestui que use*' (shorthand for 'the person to whose use the feoffment was made'). There was now separation of legal (the feoffee's) and beneficial (the cestui que use) aspects of landholding, the forerunner of the separate systems of law (legal 'ownership') and equity (equitable 'ownership').

Common law constraints circumvented by beneficial ownership: the will of land

Because the feoffee had only the legal title, and did not possess the profits (benefits) of the land, the arrangement denied the lord death duties due under common law. Furthermore, the beneficial owner – the cestui que use – free of common law constraints, could instruct the feoffee on the disposal of the beneficial ownership after his death. In other words he could make a will, not of legal ownership but beneficial ownership. At a stroke, two limitations of the common law were circumvented. The next step was for the landholder to make *himself* beneficial owner, which in time he did. Rent was thereby reserved for those who inherited through the will, and was lost to the State. All common law controls providing for the heiresses-at-law and a dower for the widow were also lost, such provisions being from then on entirely in the gift of the cestui que use. What proved particularly distasteful about this invention was the collusion of conveyancers and dishonest landholders in the enfeoffment of estates to avoid the distrainment of land. Fraudulent landholders gave away legal ownership to keep the land out of reach of creditors, while continuing to enjoy the benefits of the estate. Also, if a family in possession of land discovered that their title was weaker than that of another, then to avoid losing the land the head of the family would create an enfeoffment so that no common law action could be taken against him for recovery.

The feoffee to use and loss of Rent to the State

Estates were almost always held by feoffees to uses by 1400, and the will of the cestui que use took care of the needs of the family as the father saw them. When the cestui que use died, under the common law, the lands held to his use belonged not to him but his feoffees. The original donor had granted seisin to the feoffees to uses, trusting them to convey the benefits of the land to the cestui que use as directed. However, the cestui que use was not protected in common law against an untrustworthy feoffee to use, and it was Chancery he petitioned to defend his interest. Chancellors, trained in both the civil law and the law of the church, were motivated to act in good conscience, securing the original donor's wishes. However, the increasingly obvious abuse of the feoffee to use in order to avoid death duties caused the State increasing concern. When used in this way, the under-lord was defrauding the over-lord. The mesne over-lord who lost revenue in this way could recoup by applying the same strategy against his own lord, but when uses were manipulated by tenants-in-chief, the State was in jeopardy (Bean, 1968, p 180).

The State was not entirely powerless, because tenants-in-chief needed a royal licence to alienate their lands to feoffees to uses, and licences cost money. Licences to alienate were generally sold on condition that at least a fraction of an acre remained held directly of the king. This way the Crown retained the right to wardship of any heir of a tenant-in-chief when a minor and to the lands. Wardship remained the most valuable of feudal dues. However, the protection of the king's other interests on the death of a cestui que use created by a tenant-in-chief was more difficult and usually depended upon detection of technical flaws in the conveyancing or clear evidence of collusive enfeoffment to defraud the Crown (Bean, 1968, pp 197-220). All too often the use successfully evaded death duties due to the State, thereby diverting Rent from the public purse to the private pocket. Not for nothing was the cestui que use also known as the '*pernor*' or taker of the profits of land.

No Plantagenet king effectively tackled the problem of this diminishing source of revenue. Indeed, as tenants-in-chief themselves before accession to the throne, they were invariably either feoffee to use or cestui que use. One such was Richard, Duke of Gloucester. On his accession in 1483, Richard III, as feoffee to use, wished to transfer his seisin to the beneficiaries. The law obliged, enacting in 1484 a statute which allowed the cestui que use to act in certain respects *as if* he had legal ownership. The result was confusion, both feoffee and cestui que use having the same powers of conveyance! Here, however, was one of several important precedents for the '*as if*' in law, adopted by the draftsmen of the current Law of Property Act (1925) as discussed under private housing and the mortgage in Chapter Six.

With the disembarkation of Henry Tudor and his invading army in a secluded cove on St Anne's Head near Milford Haven on 7 August 1485, England was set to experience yet another turbulent era of land reform. On 22 August Richard III fell at Bosworth Field and Henry VII was, according to popular history, crowned there and then by his godfather Thomas Stanley. Good fortune went to those who had stayed with him. His uncle, Jasper Tudor, born a poor Welsh squire, found himself at age 54 the Duke of Bedford, one of the greatest magnates in the kingdom. Lord Stanley was made Earl of Derby. Henry's mother, Margaret, descendent of the Dukes of Somerset, regained the family's former estates and vast tracts of other lands including the town of Poole in Dorset, leaving her with an annual income of £3,000 in rents.

In 1489 Henry attempted to impose a new round of taxation to pay for a war in Brittany. There was riot in Yorkshire, a mob lynching the fourth Earl of Northumberland near Topcliffe. Lord Henry Percy, Earl of Northumberland (see below), the second most wealthy magnate of the realm, had enfeoffed much of his lands but had nevertheless died seised-in-chief. Yet in his will, knowing the rights of Henry VII to the wardship of his children, he nevertheless stated that the executors were to have governance until their 18th birthday. Henry couldn't afford such situations.

A statute of 1490 declared that whenever a cestui que use to landholding by knight service died intestate, then his heir when a minor should be placed in wardship, and when of full age pay a relief. But this Act hardly began to restore death duties. The minority of Henry, fifth Earl of Northumberland, lasted nine years, during which time his father's feoffees received revenue of about £14,000, all lost to the State (Bean, 1968, p 233). Only Henry VIII could do better, but even here there was compromise as the politics of Rent reached white heat.

Henry VIII and his proposals for land reform

Henry VIII looked closely at the laws that denied the Crown death duties. In 1529 two measures were drawn up for consideration by parliament. The first would have abolished the entail, leaving only the life estate and the ordinary title to land with the right of permanent alienation by sale or gift, the fee simple. Only the tenants-in-chief would be permitted to continue to entail their lands, and in return the king was to have the death duties of wardship and other feudal sources of income. The second measure would have required all uses to be recorded in the Court of Common Pleas. To avoid the possibility of fraudulent land-deals, quite frequent in those days, all deeds of conveyance were to be announced in church and registered in the shire town. The lesser nobility in the House of Commons were most displeased. Such enactments would deny them the right of secret conveyancing and the power of making secure family settlements protecting the estate from dispersal along the female line. Conveyancing in confidence helped in the perpetration of fraud and obstructed the State in the recovery of death duties, for it gave the legal tenant anonymity. Conveyancers were equally dismayed, seeing themselves deprived of a livelihood. Not surprisingly, therefore, neither measure survived the House of Commons (Holdsworth, 1924, pp 450-3).

The Statute of Uses: the Crown fights back

Henry began a war of propaganda against lawyers, listening to petitions complaining of their connivance in the abuse of the use for their own profit. The king had a stroke of good fortune when in 1535 a panel of judges declared that an enfeoffment made by Lord Dacre of the South had been intended to defraud the Crown. They had in fact been persuaded to do so by Henry's Secretary, Thomas Cromwell, and Chancellor Lord Thomas Audley. Something had to be done about the damage to the

State inflicted by the feoffee to use. Four draft Bills were before parliament at this time, out of which arose the Statute of Uses of 1536, much to the displeasure of the Court of Chancery lawyers. From 1 May 1536 this statute took legal ownership from the feoffees and vested it in the cestui que use (Holdsworth, 1924, pp 461-2). This meant that separation of the legal estate from the equitable estate was abolished and Henry VIII could recover his death duties. Common law lawyers were happy at the business coming their way, Chancery lawyers were annoyed at their financial loss, and the landholding class was furious at the disappearance of the power to make wills on lands of inheritance.

In the construction of their wills, landholders had been careful to ensure that the daughters of marriages without sons were not a threat to the integrity of the estate, by willing to collateral males whenever possible. The heiress-at-law would be cared for, but she would not receive what was due to her under the common law. Henry VIII with his Statute of Uses put a stop to this practice, restoring to the heiress-at-law her rightful inheritance. The fee in male tail was no protection since it was now barrable, and the old objections to entail still remained.

The gentry rebel: the Statute of Wills

There followed a rebellion for mixed motives known as the Pilgrimage of Grace, centred in Lincolnshire and Yorkshire. The nobility rose against the Statute of Uses and the clergy against dissolution of the smaller monasteries, while the labourers on the manors revolted against enclosure of common lands. The rebellion was crushed with many executions, but cooperation was restored only by returning to the landholder what he wanted, the power to make a will in land. The Statute of Wills of 1540 (the year after parliament had ratified the dissolution of the monasteries) allowed all those with lands held by ordinary (socage) tenure (see below) the freedom to "give, dispose, will and devise ... by ... will and testament ... or ... by any act or acts lawfully executed ... all hereditaments at free will and pleasure" (Holdsworth, 1924, p 465). But if the land in socage tenure was held directly of the Crown then the king held on to his rights of recovery on the death of the tenant-in-chief (primer seisin), reliefs and other payments. These were now to be paid by the beneficiary of land under the will (the devisee). Those who held land of the king by knight's service could will two thirds of their estate, the king reserving his right to feudal dues on the inherited remaining third. Here also the persons who took under the will were liable to feudal incidents.

The provisions of the Statute of Wills regarding liability to feudal dues were eventually evaded by more contortions of the law. The landholder would enfeoff his lands to a friend for his own use, the use in this instance being in the form of a legal fee simple which terminated on his death. On his death, therefore, the 'landholder' had nothing in the way of land to devise in his will, for his fee simple terminated. In the original conveyance, however, the 'landholder' had reserved the power to appoint further feoffees to uses by will. These new feoffees could dispose of the land in accordance with the deceased's wishes. This way of proceeding was not technically a will of land according to the letter of the law, and so protection of death duties for the State under the Statute of Wills was lost (Simpson, 1986, pp 191-2). Thus we can now perceive, if but dimly, the extent to which the evolution of land law represented a ceaseless battle between landholders who wanted to privatise Rent through the evasion of services and (especially) incidents, and the king who wished to secure as much Rent as possible as revenue for the Crown. The common law, through *Quia Emptores*, was gradually removing mesne lords from the feudal chain, bringing death duties closer to the king. Equity, through protection of the cestui que use and a lack of determination to protect the Crown's right to feudal dues, was allowing the State to lose the revenue from land.

Socage and the landed gentry

The Norman system of military fees, with its magnates and knights, had been superimposed by colonisers on the older system of English landholding. Medieval lawyers, struggling to organise the legalities of land, lumped together the terms and conditions of the great residue of landholding falling beneath military service and serjeanty as 'socage' tenure. The link here with the Anglo-Saxon freeholders, the *sokemen* with their *sokeland*, is obvious. Indeed, many holding 'in socage' were English by descent with non-Norman names. Here feudalism shaded imperceptibly into commoner status.

Looking back to Domesday, in 1086 the proportions of commoners in unfree status varied considerably across the country, the highest percentages in enslavement being towards the south west, especially around the lands formerly held by the Hwicce. Bonded villeins were widespread, unfree in status but sharing the common lands of the manor. Freemen at the bottom of the heap were very noticeable in the eastern shires, in some parts of which more than half the population were sokemen; as much as

70% in Bolingbroke, for example. Here the freemen paid homage and services to their lord but were free to sell their interest in the land should they wish. Many were conveying their interest as smallholders using charters and a personal seal in the manor court, either by sale or 'in alms' as a gift to the church. What they could not do was sell the interest of the lord in the services and rents. The successful were able to buy into the land market and increase their holdings in one or more manors; the exceptional few even acquired lands with rental values entitling them to knightly status.

It was among freeholders with non-military tenures, and the smallest tenants subjected to feudalism, that ideas of 'the Norman Yoke' were kept alive. Thomas Starkey's work, *Dialogue between Pole and Lupset,* alluded to the "tyrannical customs and unreasonable bonds" imposed by William I "when he subdued *our* country and nation" (Hill, 1954, p 18). The gentry were flexing their muscle against the feudal insistence on service (mostly commuted to rents by then) and incidents. They wanted freedom to dispose of their estates in ways that suited themselves, to escape the feudal powers of the monarch and the tenants in chief, while at the same time protecting the privileges and benefits they held from the desires of the more ambitious among the lower classes. Their representatives in parliament were mobilised to achieve these goals.

The land market after the dissolution of the monasteries

Buying and selling of land was relatively uncommon even in Tudor times. Land was highly valued for the powers it conveyed, so little was on the open market until Henry VIII dissolved the monasteries. By Act of Parliament and deeds of surrender vast tracts of monastic, chantry and bishops' estates were acquired by the Crown for disposal by grants of inheritance, leasehold and sale of freeholds. Much of this land was in fact sold, there being more than 300 purchases in 1589-90 alone (Youings, 1991, p 159). The commissions established to sell these lands were instructed to sell at a price equal to 20 times the nett current annual rental value. In the 1590s some estates were offered at 40 years purchase, and in 1599 with the Crown desperate for money to defeat Hugh O'Neill, Earl of Tyrone, and his comrade in arms, Hugh O'Connell, the commissions actually managed to sell some land at 60 years purchase (Youings, 1991, p 161).

So much land coming on to the market caused anxiety among the middling gentry, who feared that the social mobility created would destabilise society. A statute of 1445 had excluded from the House of Commons all men whose lands were insufficient to generate an annual rental income of at least £20, thereby re-inforcing monopoly of the bundle of rights called land, and closing the Commons to those below the lesser nobility. Now, a century later, it appeared possible that too many would be able to buy the privilege, using land as a tax shelter at the same time (see Chapter Ten). Cromwell entertained the idea of forbidding merchants to purchase land worth more than £40, to keep their wealth within the productive economy (Elton, 1973, p 127). In 1559 a proposal was put to parliament that husbandmen and yeomen should be forbidden to buy property worth a rental or more than £5 a year, and merchants restricted to purchases of property of £50 or less a year. However, the idea never reached the statute book.

By 1600 the trappings of a modern land market were in place, if still relatively primitive. Lawyers and others regularly undertook conveyancing, agents were introducing buyer to seller, and surveyors were valuing properties for sale or lease. In 1539, for example, Sir Christopher Hales bought the manor of Appletreewick in Yorkshire for £314 and sold it that same year for twice that amount (Youings, 1991, p 166). John Fry, a lawyer, bought three manors in Devon for £839 in 1545, and by 1558 had sold them to John Willoughby, a clothier, at a profit of £161 (Youings, 1991, p 166). Much of this purchasing was to create estates of inheritance, power and prestige. Younger sons of landed families, displaced by the eldest son and heir, found such acquisitions attractive.

The feoffee to use evolves into the trust to restore beneficial ownership

In the early 16th century a popular method of land conveyance was 'bargain and sale', but its technical performance, like the will, involved feoffees and the use. As stated earlier, the use became so common in the scheme of landholding that by the middle of the 15th century it was held to exist even when no express purpose could be identified. Originally, to escape from beneath the common law, the tenant would grant his land by deed to the feoffees (usually paid lawyers) for the beneficial use of himself, rather than share these benefits with the State. Now, it came to be regarded that when the tenant made a grant of his land to another, but received no payment in return, then the grantee must be the feoffee awaiting the tenant's instructions as to the uses with which he was to be entrusted.

Thus by the mere grant of the legal estate, the beneficial ownership automatically returned to the tenant. On the other hand, if the tenant sold his land to another, but purchaser and vendor had not completed the formalities of enfeoffment, then the relationship was assumed to be the other way around. In law the tenant was the feoffee holding the land for the beneficial use of the purchaser. One of the effects of the Statute of Uses was to give those with the beneficial use a legal estate in such circumstances, whether they be tenant or purchaser.

The two parts of that bundle of land, the legal ownership and the beneficial ownership, gave the landholder more scope and flexibility when kept separate. Faced with the Statute of Uses, landholders therefore put the conveyancers to work once more. It did not take too long to fabricate ways to circumvent the law. If the father (A) granted his land to the feoffee to use and his heirs (B), to the use of his son and his heirs (C), then under the Statute of Uses the son's beneficial ownership became a legal fee simple. The conveyancer would therefore draft the conveyance to uses to say 'to D and his heirs, to the use of B and his heirs, to the use of C and his heirs'. By the Statute of Uses B's beneficial use was converted to a legal ownership, making D as feoffee redundant. Now B was back in possession of the legal estate (as he had been originally as feoffee) and C, the son, once more had beneficial ownership rather than legal ownership. Eight additional words was all it took in the land of conveyancing to thwart statute law. The feoffee as a legal concept was now obsolete. The use to C became known as a trust; the feoffees the trustees (Simpson, 1986, pp 201-7).

Registration of titles to land: a proposal in 1535

One of four draft Bills before the parliament of Henry VIII in 1535-36 proposed a system for recording all uses and other dealings in land. This record would have been the responsibility of masters of enrolments appointed by the king, one for each shire. The permanent records were to be kept in the Chancery, and all-importantly they would have been open to public inspection. There would then be far less risk of dealings in land of which the general public and government were unaware, and the collection of revenue from those holding land would have been put on a much sounder footing. Land in the boroughs would continue to be registered before the mayor and his officials.

This (draft legislation was) a remarkably comprehensive scheme for the registration of conveyances; and, if it had been passed and efficiently carried out, we should have today in working order a series of county registers, which would have considerably simplified the land law. We should not have been faced with the difficulty of fitting a scheme of registration on to a system which the large powers of landowners and the ingenuity of conveyancers have made more complex than any other modern system ... the causes which render a scheme of registration so difficult today are largely the result of the failure to pass the Bill proposed in 1536. (Holdsworth, 1924, p 459)

So wrote William Holdsworth, Professor of English Law at Oxford University, barely a year before the introduction of the Law of Property Act and the Land Registration Act of 1925. He doubtless reflected on the self-interested opposition to registration displayed by conveyancers before and immediately after the First World War (about which, more later). The reasons for the failure of the Bill of 1536 are unknown because, as Holdsworth recorded: "We could only learn the truth if the missing records of the proceedings in parliament were to come to light" (Holdsworth, 1924, pp 459-60). This sounds like an early version of the phenomenon of 'missing files' during a public enquiry, but maybe the loss was innocent.

Instead of a comprehensive Act of registration, parliament passed a short Act of limited purpose. An advantage of enfeoffment during the process of bargain and sale had been that a record existed of the arrangement and the feoffees could ensure that the title for sale was good. This safeguard was unintentionally removed by the Statute of Uses. Therefore parliament introduced the Statute of Enrolments, whereby from 31 July 1536, the sale of *freehold* land had to be registered. Registration of land under the Statute of Enrolments was in time circumvented by another fabrication attributed to Sergeant Moore of the Court of Common Pleas, known as the 'lease and release'. Should the tenant wish to sell without record, he would first create a lease. To achieve this he 'bargained and sold' his land for a term of one year (estates of limited duration do not amount to freehold). Thus the purchaser acquired the beneficial use of the land for a year. The Statute of Uses automatically converted this beneficial use to a legal term without any need to register, because what the purchaser got was not a freehold estate. Secrecy was therefore assured in the privacy of the conveyancer's office. The next step was for the vendor to execute a deed of release to the purchaser, who then became tenant in fee simple. The Statute of Enrolments, in referring only to 'freeholds', had not foreseen this manoeuvre. Again, the conveyancer outwitted the legal draftsman (Simpson, 1986, pp 189-90).

Landholders seek to abolish feudal death duties

Elizabeth I and James I attempted to enforce the collection of incidents through the Court of Wards and Liveries that had been established by Henry VIII in 1540. The nett annual profit in Elizabeth's reign, averaging about £15,000 (Hurstfield, 1955-56), was not much, but perhaps 75% of what was paid had been siphoned off as unofficial salary for the Court and its middlemen. Parliament, the seat of the Rentholders, argued that the Court was behaving in an 'unparliamentary' way, for the concept was strengthening that there should be no taxation without approval of the representatives of those being taxed. Lord Salisbury had proposed the abolition of all feudal dues in 1610, but failed because knights and gentry of the Commons refused other taxes to substitute for the loss of revenue to the Crown. In fact the House of Commons was proving more and more unwilling to grant taxes of any kind. In 1580 a group of intellectuals had formed the Society of Antiquaries to popularise the notion of the Norman Yoke imposed upon free Anglo-Saxon institutions. Its members promoted parliamentary opposition against the powers of the Crown. They argued that William the Conqueror had reduced the English to a state of servitude little better than villeinage, supplanting the laws of holy Edward the Confessor with harsh Norman law. Much of their belief was myth of course, but nevertheless served to challenge monarchists. The Conqueror and later monarchs had consistently claimed to hold by conquest all land as chief lord in the national interest, and with it a right to raise revenue for the Crown off all estates according to their prerogative powers. The landholding interest in parliament indisputably had a good case against royal prerogative, but while seeking more control over revenue-raising they were intent upon establishing a superior claim to what previously went to the State, that is the Rent of their estates. The shepherds were increasingly putting the shears before the crook, and what was shorn they planned to bale for themselves.

When Charles I came to the throne in 1625 he tried to rule for 11 years without the assistance of parliament. With the Exchequer running dry Lord Cottington, Chancellor and Master of the Rolls, attempted to raise more revenue for the Crown through the Court of Wards and Liveries. The lords were outraged. Noblemen were claiming that laws devised for their protection and preservation were being turned into instruments of their destruction. The Court collapsed during the Civil War (1642-48), ceasing to sit after February 1645 (Dowell, 1965, vol 2, p 18). The following year, parliament abolished feudal tenures as stigmas of bondage.

Unfree landholding: villeinage, copyhold and leasehold

Parliament's victory in the Civil War knocked the monarchists' argument into a cocked hat. If kings could gain absolute power by conquest, they could lose it in the same way. Charles I was executed in 1649. The House of Lords voted against regicide, for which it was abolished by the Commons for 11 years as 'useless and dangerous'. But the landholders who believed themselves the representatives of earlier Anglo-Saxon heritage, which they claimed to defend by common law, found themselves challenged by another radicalism in the form of the Levellers and the Diggers. The Levellers were advanced thinkers, the democrats of the English Revolution. They too rejected the claims of monarchy through conquest, but they also questioned the origins and value of the common law. They were not 'sold' on claims to rights simply because they were supposed once to exist, but sought to establish which rights *ought* to exist (Hill, 1954, pp 28-37). They thought they saw a unique opportunity for parliament to re-think the common law and the powers of the lords. Then came the Diggers, the most radical of all, who wanted an end to private property in Land. They established communal colonies in Cobham, Surrey, and sought unsuccessfully the release of those tied to the manorial courts, a remnant of unfree tenure which they saw as another feudal imposition.

Little has been said about the mass of labouring families at the bottom of the heap, the unfree villeins tied to the manor. Villeins were subject to the lord's manor court, but that did not prevent some organising to fight what they considered to be excessive or uncustomary demands in the hundred or shire court. As early as 1276 the manorial tenants of Stoughton in Leicestershire took their lord to court, refusing to accept his demand for certain services (Wood, 1990, pp 192-3). Such cases came before the Court of Chancery, which by 1350 had existed for some years. The Court of Equity was tentatively venturing into the realm of protection of the unfree by this time, whereas not until the 16th century did the courts of common law show signs of moving into this area.

As the feudal system of lord and vassal weakened, so did villeinage. Originally, when a villein wished to leave the manor and another was ready to take his place, the transfer required the lord's permission. A copy of the transfer was kept in the manor's records, and the new tenant paid a 'fine' for the transaction to the lord. Gradually, however, labour services were commuted to a 'quit-rent', and by 1500 villeinage had become known as copyholding as its servile status diminished. Another popular arrangement was leaseholding, originally simply a contract in which the lessee acquired permission to use the land for a fixed term on certain conditions. If the lessee was evicted before the lease expired he could sue for compensation, but not for repossession. Only in the middle of the 15th century did the court use the writ *de ejectione firmae* to recover possession. From then on the lessee had a claim of sorts to the land, and so leasehold came to be regarded as a weak form of land tenure.

The practice evolved of conversion of tenure from one sort to another. Copyhold could be converted to freehold by sale, and both yeoman farmers and minor gentry would make such purchases. Other copyholds were converted to leaseholds, for which the fine payable to the lord could be as much as 200 times the annual quit-rent. Tenants could at times acquire by these means sizeable portions of the manor or even neighbouring manors, holding many parcels of land under different tenures. For example, by Tudor times the former monastic manor of Chippenham in Cambridgeshire had passed into lay hands, Thomas Bowles acquiring leases for the former farm of the manor and 20% of the open fields. Another farmer, Thomas Rawlings, held 101 acres by copyhold, and there were six freeholders of small parcels (Youings, 1991, p 51).

The Tenures Abolition Act of 1660

The new Convention parliament met in April 1660, inviting Charles, son of Charles I, to take the throne. An early action was the Tenures Abolition Act, seemingly in line with the rule of the Long Parliament of 1640 that all extra-parliamentary taxation was illegal. This Act converted tenures in knight service to 'free and common socage', thereby enabling all landholding to be willed and removing services and incidents such as scutage, wardship, ousterlemain and licences. Also abolished were all tenures by homage and all fines of a feudal nature. The justification was: "Whereas it hath been found by former experience that the Court of Wards and Liveries, and tenures by knight-service ... and the consequents upon the same, have been much more burdensome, grievous and prejudicial to the kingdom than they have been beneficial to the king" (Digby, 1897, pp 396-7). The Act did not touch the spiritual tenures, but frankalmoign depended upon the land having been held continuously by the same ecclesiastical tenant since before 1290 (that is before *Quia Emptores*). The one important incident not removed was escheat, the right of the lord to recover land when the tenant had been convicted of felony or had died intestate without an heir.

Copyhold was untouched by the Act, and the country squirarchy, as lords of the manor, continued to receive their copyhold rents and incidents. The one compensation for the copyholder, his rights of common pasture, he was soon to lose. Looking forward, although much copyhold was turned over to freehold during the 19th century with the decay of many manors, large amounts of land remained copyhold until as late as 1925. In that year all copyhold was turned over to freehold (socage tenure) by the Law of Property Act.

The Tenures Abolition Act deprived the Crown of about £100,000 a year and this had somehow to be replaced. The first proposal was to impose an equivalent land tax on all shires, and a careful valuation of lands was made for this purpose by a prominent committee. Objections were raised, however. The Tenures Abolition Act benefited only those who held land directly of the Crown, while the proposed land tax would affect all landholders irrespective of their lord. So then the proposal was made simply to tax the tenants-in-chief, bringing revenues from land under parliamentary control in an equitable manner, it was claimed. Again there were objections. In the 15 years since the collapse of the Court of Wards, heirs of the tenants-in-chief had succeeded free of the incidents of relief and wardship. Others had mortgaged land, and most serious of all, much land formerly subject to incidents had been sold. Buyers objected that there were no grounds to claim compensation from them for the relief of financial burdens they had never carried (Dowell, 1965, vol 2, pp 19-21).

The Act of the Hereditary Excise: taxation in lieu of Rent collection

The House of Commons took the line of least resistance. The knights and gentry imposed a tax on the ordinary man and woman without the parliamentary franchise. The legislation through which this was accomplished was the Act for the Hereditary Excise, which settled upon his majesty, his heirs and successors, "in full and complete recompense and satisfaction, as well as for the profits of the Court of Wards and Liveries and the feudal tenures and incidents, as also for all manner of purveyance and pre-emption then taken away and abolished", a set of excise duties on home-made beer, ale, cider and perry, mead and other liquors. The brewers were to pay the duty weekly, while innkeepers and retailers were to pay monthly. King and Council immediately saw the advantages. The excise would bring in far more than what had been lost under the troublesome system of dues from land. They therefore urged the Commons to take this route, and the Act was soon law (Dowell, 1965, vol 2, pp 19-22).

Barring right of tenants to the commons, landholders now had the whole bundle of land as they wanted, wrapped up in red tape – Rent and all. So when in 1670 Charles II granted to his cousin Prince Rupert, in gratitude for Rupert's support for Charles I and his distinguished career in the Dutch wars, the right to all those lands 'in whatsoever latitude they shall bee that lye within the entrance of the Streightes commonly called Hudson's Streightes', he did so according to the law of landholding in England. Rupert and his colleagues were granted this vast and unexplored stretch of Canada, "in free and common socage, on the same terms as the manor of East Greenwich". Rent service was commuted to two elks and two black beavers whenever the king should visit Rupert's Land (Morris, 1979, pp 116-17), in return for an area which turned out to amount to nearly four million square kilometres. Today, more than three centuries on, 'free and common socage' is the only freehold tenure. 'Free' indicates that the extent of services due to the lord (ie the Crown) remains fixed and agreed – it is simply that the agreement is that no services are demanded. 'Common' indicates that there is immunity from any special customary incidents. Under such terms, Rent is well and truly privatised.

The law of Rentholding was now like a pyramid prised from its broad base in society and forced over so as to stand unnaturally with its apex in the lap of a handful of aristocratic families: topsy-turvy and certain to topple without the strong arm of the law as a prop. The conveyancers were creating for themselves a perfectly unfathomable but lucrative monopoly, shoring up Rentholding against the forces of logic and equity. The apex of this inverted ancient edifice has crumbled with the weathering of time, but the props are still there. Land could and would be taxed after a fashion during the 18th century and beyond (see Chapter Ten), but bundled in with all other sources of income, and on terms and conditions set by landholders themselves.

The settled estate

Landholders could once again keep their dealings in sales and purchases out of the gaze of the public. They could will their land. They could place their land in trust and had abolished the common law requirements of death duties. Now they sought yet more security for their estates, not against the State, but against their own kind, in the event that providence failed to give the father a responsible son as heir. The will and the use had enabled the landholder to subvert the common law, but the will had its own problems. Wills are personal deeds, vulnerable to personal feelings and eccentricity. What the landholder craved was the whole bundle of land, including Rent, wrapped in as much red tape as possible. The Tenures Abolition Act did away with a prime motive for the will of land and the use by abolishing feudal dues. For those so inclined, the Act also opened new scope for locking on to Rent, not merely for two lives but for at least three in succession.

A conveyancer of the late 17th century, Sir Orlando Bridgman, is believed to be the man who around 1655 (Habakkuk, 1950) took a number of pieces out of his box of tricks and put them together to provide the ultimate in estate planning. Under the old arrangement, at the time of the marriage of the eldest son, the father had a life interest and the son was due to inherit by entail on the male side (tail male). However, any son who came to inherit on these terms could bar the entail and create a fee simple, thus enabling himself to alienate part or all of the land. This the father did not want, but the son and wife were willing to cooperate in alternative arrangements meeting his wishes. They needed to finance a new family and could not wait until the father's death. So, particularly after 1660, father and son accepted an arrangement modelled on that proposed by Bridgman – the Strict Settlement. Settlements arise when several specified persons are entitled to the same property in succession. In this instance the succession is father to son, to the as yet unborn grandson. The settlement is 'strict' because it includes a limitation to trustees to preserve the interest of the grandson, protecting it from any damage that the son may otherwise cause. The principle is simple. A tenant in tail must never actually acquire the land. Rather, the estate must always be in possession of a tenant for life, because a tenant for life can lawfully alienate the land only for the duration of his life. In a sense the tenant for life holds the legal estate on trust – he is trustee of the land having powers of management with the interest of all parties to the settlement in mind. The trustees of the settlement, often more distant family or neighbouring landholders, are guardians of the settlement, watching over the behaviour of the tenant for life.

At the marriage or coming-of-age of the eldest son, father and son agreed to a re-conveyance, whereby the son took a life estate in remainder after his father, and there was an entail in remainder to the son's as yet unborn son. Provision was made for an income for the son charged on the lands, and for a rent charge to provide his wife with a personal allowance. Should there be a grandson who survived to maturity, then usually at his marriage he and his father repeated the process, and so on down the generations. Provisions were made to ensure that the estate went to a male heir if at all possible, in the eventuality that no grandson was born or survived to maturity, and to provide younger children with capital sums called portions.

So the Strict Settlement avoided the danger to landed estates threatened by the will. Fathers were now committed before they developed the emotional attachments of actual parenthood, and perhaps an overwhelming desire to give land to their beloved daughters rather than a remote brother or nephew in the absence of a son. The common law heiress-at-law would not take her legal estate but merely a portion set aside before she was born. This ruthlessly dynastic settlement, perpetuating the power of wealthy landed families and maximising their grip on Rent, had an immense effect upon the distribution of wealth, income and political influence in the nation. The ancient common law, although still there to ensnare the fortunes of the unwary landholder, was now even more effectively evaded.

Land registration: limited successes after 1700

Land law went through a relatively peaceful period in the 18th century. Local registries of land conveyances were secured for the West Riding of Yorkshire in 1703, the East Riding in 1707, Middlesex in 1708 and Yorkshire's North Riding in 1735. Ireland secured the registration of deeds in 1707. This trend culminated in a Bill for a general registry passing through the House of Commons in 1739. The Bill never became law, however, and thereafter life settled down again for landowners. Conveyancing was legally regulated for the first time in 1712, when the Company of Scriveners (drafters of documents) was granted monopoly for the City of London. In 1804 lawyers extracted the monopoly of conveyancing from William Pitt as a concession at a time when government wished to raise stamp duties on legal documents to help fund the war against France. By this means solicitors secured a lucrative source of income (Simpson, 1986, pp 272-3).

Looking further forward, the appointment of the Real Property Commissioners in 1829 led to four massive reports over the following four years, largely concerned, however, with the mechanics of conveyancing. As far as the substance of that bundle of rights and privileges called land was concerned, the Commissioners were most content to state: "the Law of England ... appears to come almost as near perfection as can be expected in any human institution" (Simpson, 1986, p 275). The obvious sense in a national register of land transactions led to many attempts to establish such a system, but all failed. Progress got as far as Lord Westbury's Act of 1862 and Lord Cairns' Act of 1875, allowing voluntary registration. Landholders did not respond, however, many fearing scrutiny of titles which might be found deficient. Attempts to introduce compulsory registration from 1873 onwards failed miserably (Simpson, 1986, pp 272-3), partly owing to resistance from the law societies which ran on beyond 1900. We shall pick up this theme later.

The surrogate heir

Landed dynasties extinguished in the direct male line were forced to take desperate measures for survival of the family name. An ancient remedy was to adopt the husband of an heiress or a more remote male on the distaff side as surrogate heir. The adoptee, often a younger son of another noble family, would assume the surname and take the arms of the family in distress, which thereby was rescued by a 're-creation'. The great Percy dynasty has undergone three creations in its thousand year history. The founder was William de Percy (1030-96), a follower of William I of Normandy. For his services, de Percy received from his king a huge fief in Yorkshire and Lincolnshire. William de Percy's grandson was the last of the direct male line, leaving heiresses Maud (childless) and Agnes de Percy on his death in 1175. Agnes had married Joceline, who assumed his wife's surname to establish the second creation. Agnes' descendent, Henry, purchased lands in Northumberland and Percy, Fourth Baron Alnwick (1341-1408) was elevated to First Earl of Northumberland. The direct male line of this family survived until 1670. With the death of Joceline, 11th earl, in that year, the Percy estate went to his heiress Elizabeth Seymour, who had married Sir John Smithson (1715-86). Sir John assumed the Percy name to establish the third creation, and was elevated to First Duke of Northumberland. Earl George Dominic Percy, heir to the 12th duke of Northumberland, was page of honour to the Queen in 1996. In 1998 the Duke (reputedly worth £250 million) created a stir by pronouncing his intention to reassert his right as lord of the manor of Alnwick to charge the town £2,000 annually for licence to hold its market.

The surrogate heir assumed increasing popularity after 1730. In the 1740s John, Duke of Montagu, went so far as to procure by private Act of Parliament a ruling that any husband of any heiress of the Montagu family was obliged to adopt his wife's surname and arms if he wished to secure his inheritance to the Montagu estate. Perhaps one of the most famous of serial re-creations is that of the Lytton family of Knebworth. A succession of deaths without heirs or only heiresses from 1705 forced four surrogacies on this family to secure the estate. Edward Robert Bulwer-Lytton, Viceroy of India from 1876 to 1880, could claim not a drop of true Lytton blood (Stone and Stone, 1984, pp 130-2).

The new Domesday of 1874

In 1880 landholders were in the minority in the House of Commons for the first time. Even so, the relative proportions of landholders and others in parliament still nowhere near reflected those in the country, where the landholders were in an extraordinary minority. The national census of 1861 had identified no more than 30,000 landholders in a population of 30 million. This hold on Rent and other privileges placed inordinate political and economic power within the ranks of the high Tories and the Conservative Party. To the left of this deep divide were assembled the land reformers, taking up the cause of those without any title to land whatsoever, especially the poor. Lord Derby was angered over the use of the census figures by his opponents to justify their cause. The Census 'quite obviously' had included only landowners who had declared landownership to be their principle occupation, Derby claimed, thereby missing a great number who owned land but not as a main occupation. In 1872 he therefore requested the Local Government Board to draw up a new census of all landowners, listing the size of their holdings. The 'new Doomsday Book', ready by 1874, did not please him. The concentration of landownership revealed 7,000 persons owning between them 80% of the land of England, a figure which astonished the nation and strengthened the determination of land reformers (Bateman, 1971). Numerically the largest group of landholders was the cottagers, 800,000 of them owning less than one acre each. Public and institutional landowners accounted for no more than 1.4 million acres, 5% of the total land area (Clemenson, 1982, p 20). The land of England and Wales, exclusive of London, of roads, Crown lands, wastes and commons, and houses and gardens of less than one acre, amounted to 32,862,343 acres, owned by 269,547 persons. As many landholders held estates in several counties, however, there was considerable double-counting. In addition, leaseholders with leases of over 99 years were wrongly treated as owners. Thus the count was a considerable over-estimate.

These revelations, public reaction to them, and the drastically altered composition of the electorate and their parliamentary representation in the Commons, gave land reformers hope that more could be achieved in future to loosen the red tape around that bundle of rights and privileges and bring more of them into the public domain, especially Rent. But to imagine for one moment that the electoral concessions granted by the landholding interest could be used to deprive them of their unearned income in Rent was to overlook the power of the greatest bastion of landholding privilege of all – the House of Lords. Nevertheless, the cause was taken up more vigorously than ever.

The Strict Settlement is no longer 'strict', 1882

The landholders' increasing dissatisfaction with Strict Settlement was assuaged with the passage of the Settled Land Act in 1882 under a Liberal administration. Many landed estates were in debt for reasons connected with Strict Settlement and entail, and properties were falling into decay. The owners of such estates, that is the tenants for life or the trustees of encumbered estates, needed an escape route. The president of the Incorporated Law Society, which represented solicitors, suggested that the tenant for life should be able to approach the Court of Chancery for powers of sale. But a Bill introduced in parliament in early 1880 went much further in proposing that the tenant for life be granted full powers of sale, irrespective of the views of trustees or other interested parties, save for the principal mansion house and its park where permission would still be needed. What was left as capital after clearance of debt would remain an estate subject to the Strict Settlement. This amazing acceptance of legislation to over-ride the former interests of the tenant-in-tail in the peripheral parts of the landed estate shows how laws relating to land are laws of convenience which can be dispensed with when their obsolescence or awkwardness become sufficiently widely accepted. The legislation of 1882 did not abolish settlement, life tenant or entail, but simply increased the powers of the holder of that bundle called 'land' to alienate if so desired (Spring, 1977). The reform was another of those '*as ifs*' in land law. The tenant for life was given powers of disposition over something which according to strict law he did not possess. From then on he could act '*as if*' he had powers of alienation.

The transformation of British society between 1880 and 1920 has given rise to a lasting but mistaken impression that concern for Rent bundled up in land is nowadays an anachronistic occupation. Roughly two thirds of members of the House of Commons in 1868 were landed, but less than half in 1886, and only one tenth in 1906 (Thompson, 1977, p 15). Whereas only seven businessmen had entered the peerage prior to 1885, more like 50 were so honoured between then and 1911 (Pumphrey, 1959). The Settled Land Act opened the way for wealthy industrialists to acquire parts of landed estates and for landholders to cross over into business on the floor of the board room and Stock Exchange. From 1892 the courts ruled that industrialists with the money could have the lot, main mansion and park included.

Reference will be made again to the heavily encumbered estate of the Marquis of Ailesbury. The fourth Marquis finally threw in the sponge and agreed to sell the Savernake estate to the Guinness family of Dublin, which in 1886 had converted its brewing business to a public company. Guinness was now in a position to buy Savernake in its entirety, but the family of the Marquis objected. The case went to the House of Lords, which upheld the ruling of the appeals court that the purpose of the Settled Land Act "was to prevent the ruin of agriculture and the distress of those who lived upon the land by making land alienable"; "the public interest ... ought to outweigh all the considerations of sentimental interest in the family" (Spring, 1977, p 55). Edward Cecil Guinness retired from the brewery business in 1889 to undertake philanthropic work through the Guinness Trust for construction of working class homes in Dublin and London. He was created first Earl of Iveagh in 1919.

The new land market: registration of landholding still resisted

So now the Land market was fluid and the bundle called 'land' could be bargained and sold more easily than ever before. *The Economist* was very pleased. Estates could be transferred in part or whole as often as desired. Thus the ancient landed aristocracy crumbled, but not the bundle of land – this was as secure as ever. Rent transferred hands at a quickening pace, as often as the bundle itself changed hands – but it remained firmly in private hands. Large bundles were broken down into smaller bundles, but each with its Rent. The increased conveyancing that this new land market called for re-opened the old question of registration of transfers to facilitate the process of sale or lease. A revived movement to establish a land register failed however, as in the days of Henry VIII.

Her Majesty's Land Registry was founded in 1862 under Lord Westbury's Act to allow voluntary registration of legal title. Self-financing and responsible to the Lord Chancellor, the objectives of the agency are to provide State guarantee of legal title, to simplify land transfer, and reduce risk of fraud. Registration of land is now compulsory on sale, but much land has not come to sale during the life of the agency, so that millions of properties remain unregistered and the index maps show large gaps. More than 16 million records are held, but none on unregistered sites, tenancy agreements, or land held under a lease for a term of 21 years or less. Since 3 December 1990 the register has been open to public inspection for a fee. The proprietorship register identifies the legal owner, while the charges register gives details of registered mortgages (but not value). The purchase price of properties was removed from the register in 1976 but is due to be restored in 2000. Publishing quarterly reports of average sale prices and sale volumes of houses, the Registry is today, as it was ever, the natural repository of updated site values of Rent for purposes of State.

One hundred years ago, conveyancing fees accounted for about half of the income of the ordinary solicitor. Their privileged knowledge of the land market placed them in a very favoured position to act as paid go-between for dealers in land, including auctioneers, builders and financiers. The opinion gradually gained support that an efficient system of land registration would cut out this inefficient and expensive method of conveyance by private treaty. In 1897 the Conservative government was finally forced to introduce the compulsory registration of title to land in the County of London. The Law Society had resisted this move and managed to secure what was called the 'county veto', which meant that any extension of compulsory registration to other parts of the country could only be initiated by the relevant local council. The lawyers, thinking of their fees, were relying on their heavy representation on these councils to suppress local attempts to replicate the London experience.

In the following years a bitter hostility ensued between Sir Charles Brickdale, Chief Registrar at the Land Registry, and a group in the Law Society representing many provincial solicitors. Their spokesman was JS Rubinstein who was connected with the Birkbeck Bank and Building

Society (Offer, 1977). More moderate opinion within the Law Society accepted that the profession needed to streamline the system of private conveyancing if it were not to lose most of the business altogether by registration. However, the Society opposed compulsory land registration throughout the Conservative administrations of 1895-1905.

With the imminent threat of the subsequent Liberal administration (see Chapter Fourteen) to introduce land registration as a preliminary to site value 'taxation', in the face of the Law Society's opposition, a Royal Commission on Land Transfer was established in 1908. The desire of Asquith's government (with Lloyd George as Chancellor of the Exchequer) to introduce compulsory valuation, registration and 'taxation' of site values encouraged the Land Registry to press its case. In his evidence to the Royal Commission, Sir Charles Brickdale stated:

> ... there is one feature that we have not here which is no doubt of assistance to registration in Germany – that is the Cadaster. The Cadaster is a 'land tax' from which the government takes a very great revenue, and it is worth their while to keep a very accurate book of the ownership of land all over the country and its value, and an accurate description of land, and its valuation for mortgage purposes and for duty on deaths and successions is greatly facilitated by the government Land Tax Registers and maps which are established everywhere and kept always up to date under the well-known name of the Cadaster.... (Royal Commission on Land Transfer, 1909, q 1454)

The German *Kataster* in fact was not the 'land tax' but the register of land first introduced by Austria in 1719 as the *Censimento Milanese*. Taxes based on the Kataster are termed 'Katastersteuern' (Schomburg, 1992, p 189). The eventual outcome of this episode is described in Chapter Fourteen.

The royal demesne

There was a time when, in addition to Rent forthcoming from tenants-in-chief in services and incidents, the Crown drew Rent directly from lands kept by the king as his royal demesne. In 1086 this vast estate comprised what had been the Crown lands under Edward the Confessor plus much else forfeited after the revolt of the English following the Conquest. The demesne consisted of untenanted lands known as the forest, land farmed by rural tenants, and land in the urban centres. The forest comprised lands set aside under a special law to preserve game for hunting. In the 13th century the forest law was relaxed and what was cultivable was turned over to farming with acquiescence of the Crown. Stephen and Henry II were great wasters of the royal demesne, 'pawning the family silver' to meet the costs of war and secure support. In 1130, alienated land of the royal demesne was valued at a little more than £40, but by 1154 the figure stood at almost £2,500 and it continued to increase thereafter.

This was the pattern of the royal demesne over the centuries, expanding as forfeitures, escheats and wardships were aggressively pursued, diminishing to pay off debts and to secure favour. The Yorkist kings and Henry VII added to the demesne in every part of the country. Henry VIII appropriated the estates of some 800 religious communities, worth in all about £200,000 a year, together with the forced bequest of the vast estates of Henry Percy, Sixth Earl of Northumberland, on his death in 1537. As other prominent families toppled – Henry Courteney in 1538, Thomas Cromwell in 1540, Edward Seymour in 1552 – so their lands too came into the royal demesne. Much of what was acquired was sold almost as quickly to pay for warfare, but under a law of 1536 all such royal grants were to be held in tenure by knight service to the Crown (Hurstfield, 1955-56, p 53), thus bringing the holders within the reach of the Court of Wards and Liveries. In addition, should the holder wish to sell the land granted, he needed to purchase a licence for this purpose from the Crown.

In 1760, George III surrendered the revenues from most of the Crown lands and the Hereditary Excise in return for a fixed annual stipend or Civil List of £900,000. Queen Victoria's Civil List was £385,000 a year. Until 1972 the annual allowance was set for the period of the reign. Since then allowances have been adjusted for inflation, the Queen and close family receiving about £9 million annually. The Prince of Wales derives his separate income, about £6.4 million in 1999 before tax, from the ancient Duchy of Cornwall. In 1999 the Prince arranged the sale of the Duchy's stockmarket portfolio to buy 22,000 acres of land from the Prudential Financial Group, bringing (if the Treasury approved) the total holding to 147,000 acres. The Prince owns land only, being forbidden to touch the Duchy's capital.

Privatisation of Rent: an unjust institution

Consideration of the nature of Rent has shown that there is no conformity with political morality in any arrangement whereby what is produced by nature or communal effort ends up in the pocket of private individuals without due compensation. This and the previous Chapter reveal absolutely nothing in the historical record to lead any right thinking person to reverse this conclusion. But the lawyers tell us that possession is nine counts of the law (used, for example, to justify the sale by the Hudson's Bay Company of Rupert's Land to the Dominion of Canada in 1869 for $1.5 million, while retaining title to 5% of land within the so-called fertile belt).

If the thread has been hard to follow, that is because the conveyancers ravelled it that way. The great moral and political philosopher John Stuart Mill had more wisdom to offer than the land law when he wrote:"Nothing is implied in (private) property but the right of each to his (or her) own faculties, to what he can produce by them, and to whatever he can get for them in a fair market: together with his right to give this to any other person if he chooses, and the right of that other to receive and enjoy it" (Mill, 1876, p 135). Those who have received property have legitimate and exclusive possession only when the transfer to them has been by gift or fair exchange, without force or fraud. Mill continued:"The foundation of the whole (concept) is, the right of producers to what they themselves have produced. It may be objected, therefore, to the institution as it now exists, that it recognises rights of property in individuals over things which they have not produced."

In another passage in the same chapter, Mill had an especially important statement to make: "No presumption in favour of existing ideas on this subject (private property) is to be derived from antiquity." In other words we must think for ourselves. Simply because an arrangement or understanding has been handed down to us from our forefathers, that does not mean that it is necessarily right or just. On possession he had this to say:"Wrongful possession of property should not be pressed upon an individual when through lapse of time witnesses must have perished or been lost sight of, and the real character of the transaction can no longer be cleared up" (this today is embodied in the Limitation Acts). "Even when the acquisition was wrong, dispossession ... by revival of a claim which had been long dormant, would generally be a greater injustice ... than leaving the original wrong without atonement. It is all a question of balance of hardships." But Mill then went on to stress: "It is hardly needful to remark, that these reasons ... cannot apply to unjust *systems* or *institutions*; since a bad law or usage is not one bad act, in the remote past, but a perpetual repetition of bad acts, as long as the law or usage lasts" (Mill, 1976, p 135). Clearly, the institution of private property in Rent has no moral justification, and, as Mill pointed out, simply because it is a legalised custom handed down through the ages makes it neither right, the law notwithstanding, nor for that matter necessarily of any use whatsoever for Welfare Capitalism.

TEN

From the Dane-geld to direct taxes: parliamentary representation and taxation

... we've proved it again and again,
That if once you have paid him the Dane-geld
You never get rid of the Dane.
(*Dane-geld AD 980-1016*, Rudyard Kipling)

Rent now securely in private ownership, tightly bundled up with the rest of that complex of rights, privileges and benefits called land, governments made good the public's loss by taxing wages going to labour and interest going to capital. As explained in Chapter Three, insofar as an uncertain proportion of Rent finds its way into dividends and commercial rents as profit, and insofar as governments tax investment income and wages above subsistence, added to which there are death duties and capital transfer taxes, some Rent does find its way indirectly to the Treasury. The vast remainder, however, and it must be vast (but no one bothers to measure it), is vested in private monopoly. Inheritance tax raised considerably less than 1% of revenue for government in 1987-88.

There can be no gainsaying the perversity in political economy, the violation of political morality, when what is rightfully public is privatised and what is rightfully private is nationalised. This wrong-headedness, the privatisation of Rent and taxation of wages and interest, generates the very forces that perpetuate inequities in wealth and health across the socio-economic classes. Though taxation can therefore hardly be used to ameliorate injustices, this is exactly what 20th century governments tried to do, thereby creating a vicious cycle that caused taxation for Welfare to spiral upwards without ever narrowing the gap in lifespan between richer and poorer. Age-old political and social forces tied up in land have warped Britain's fiscal structure of public finance to the lasting detriment of its Welfare State. As public expenditure on Welfare mounts, it exacerbates the anomalies responsible for the social problems governments strive to ameliorate.

Historically, it was the cost of warfare rather than Welfare that was met through central taxation. Financiers and economists were only too aware of the damage such taxes inflicted on trade and commerce, but such distortions appeared petty compared with the destruction of warfare itself. In the aftermath, however, the nation suffered the burdens of debt, death and destruction. For these reasons the high taxation of wartime had to be retained in the peace.

Early forms of direct taxation

The Dane-geld was a tax imposed in Anglo-Saxon times in order to raise tributes to buy off the threat of Danish invasion. In 991 the king's council of thegns, lay and ecclesiastical, took the advice of Archbishop Sigeric and raised £10,000 to bribe away the invaders. Such large sums could be collected quickly because of the administrative organisation of shires and hundreds with their courts, together with the coinage issued by the royal mints (see Chapter Eight). Every court knew the hidage assessment of each manor in its jurisdiction, and knowing the centrally decreed rate (between one shilling (1s) and 4s per hide as circumstances demanded), the appropriate amount of geld could be imposed on each landholder. In the burghs, the geld was probably assessed on income from trade. The system was a godsend to the Normans after 1066, who continued to raise Dane-gelds for another hundred years.

England, therefore, both before and after the Norman Conquest, was familiar with rounds of taxation. Initially the king entered into separate negotiations with the several sectors of the population: with London and the royal demesne, with the feudal lords from magnate to knight, and with the representatives of those in the shires beyond the royal demesne and below feudal status, the freemen and villeins of the manors. Taxation of the first was known as tallage, the second as scutage, and the third as hidage or, later, carucage. From 1188, however, the concept of unified national taxation gained ground, and the older forms of taxation decayed and gradually faded away. Importantly, the rounds of national taxation were assessed on rents and 'moveables'. They represented, to varying degrees of penetrance depending on what was requested and what was granted, an impost on income and wealth.

First there was the wealth of the royal demesne itself, a traditional source of revenue for the regular support of State and Crown in peacetime dating back to the times of the Anglo-Saxon kings. The *Domesday Book* shows William's demesne to have consisted of 1,022 manors, plus lands in Middlesex, Shropshire and Rutland. The tenants of these rural manors supplied the royal table and pantry, following the *feorm fultum* of the Anglo-Saxons. Repeated complaints persuaded Henry I to commute these services in kind into money payments for deposit with the Court of the Exchequer. Most towns and boroughs lay within the royal demesne and they too were exacted for rent. Collection was the sheriff's responsibility through his officers (bailiffs), except when the rents had been granted to a magnate in which case the task was left to the manorial court. Tenants of the royal demesne were obliged to accept 'purveyance', the right of the king to take horses and carriages for transport; 'pre-emption', the right to purchase at an appraised value; and 'prisage', the right to take casks of wine from ships berthed in a royal port. It was also within the king's prerogative to negotiate occasional rounds of tallage with the towns and manors of the royal demesne. Negotiations would generally commence with London, the settlement setting the standard of tallage for the provincial parts of the royal demesne.

Scutage was a frequent source of conflict with the magnates, and as time went by it became increasingly difficult to collect. Repeated enquiries into knights' fees were needed, and a flat refusal to pay in 1214 was one factor leading to the Magna Carta. Scutage fell increasingly under the control of the landholders in parliament, and its last vestige disappeared after 1322 when Edward II marched against the Scots. In all, only about 40 scutages were levied over two centuries. Although in later years the obligation to pay scutage remained upon tenants holding in knight service, it was never demanded.

Hidage was rooted in the Dane-gelds which ended in 1163. In 1194 Richard I based a similar tax on the carucate, the area of land that could be ploughed by a team of eight oxen in a season. The carucate was fixed at 100 acres for the levy of 1198, a year before Richard's death. It too was difficult to collect and disappeared after 1220.

The beginning of the English parliament

To gather intelligence medieval kings would travel with their court, but this was arduous, time-consuming and risky. Rather than travel themselves, however, they could delegate the task to commissioners or justices. Even better, the king could call in nominated representatives of the scattered communities to meet in a common place. In this last option is to be found the rudiment of parliament. At first those called in were selected according to necessity, but in August 1212 King John responded to a baronial plot of assassination by issuing a general writ to all shires summoning representatives to meet him as soon as possible. This was followed by another summons in October 1213 which took the process a step further: an instruction for all to meet at one and the same time at the same place (Oxford). It was to be another 20 years before the records began to refer to such meetings as parliaments, but already there was the essence of tripartite parliament of monarch, magnates (House of Lords) and representatives of the shires and boroughs (House of Commons). Before long the representatives of the community *expected* to be summoned to receive instructions and advice. They would then return to their communities to enact what had been resolved, especially on matters relating to taxation. Representative knights were elected at the shire court from the beginning, but senior men from the towns and boroughs were not summoned until 1265 (Holt, 1981, pp 5–28).

The beginning of national direct taxation

What proved increasingly popular with king and council as a way to cover the expenses of extraordinary events, instead of the old tallage, scutage and hidage, was a national income and wealth tax. The precedent was set in 1188 when Henry II taxed all 'moveables', reaching all sectors of society from magnate to villein. The purpose of this tax was to help finance the second crusade to expel Saladin from Jerusalem. After Henry took the cross, the national council met at Geddington in Northamptonshire to approve a levy of one tenth of the assessed value of all rents and moveables of all except crusaders. Collection was made in the parish churches, witnessed by the clergy and others. Frauds risked excommunication.

Taxation by grants of fractions of assessed wealth and income continued intermittently for about 150 years, the rate ranging from one fortieth to one fourth. The tax of a fourth of moveable wealth, imposed for the ransom of King Richard I in 1193, was borne by every person in the kingdom. Sometimes poverty was acknowledged, as when Henry III exempted the arms, household utensils and food of villeins, as well as the provender of their livestock, from the fifteenth of 1225. Sheriffs, bailiffs and elected knights were responsible for assessment and collection, taking sworn statements of worth not only of each family's belongings but on occasion those of their neighbours. Stewards of the manor swore to statements of worth on behalf of the feudal lords.

With the expulsion of the Jews in 1290 a rich source of finance for the Crown was lost, as a result of which taxation became more frequent and severe: in 1294, for example, a tenth of assessed moveables beyond the royal demesne, and a sixth within it. The taxation process commenced by issue of a writ for each shire. Knights serving as commissioners of the shire were not to belong to that shire or hold lands there. The commissioners appointed tax assessors in each borough and town, hundred and parish. The assessors were to take into account all rents, monies, stock in trade and moveables except what was specifically exempted such as armour, clothes and jewellery of knights and their families, or the belongings of anyone worth less than a stated amount. Schedules for the Borough of Colchester included in the parliamentary records of 1295 and 1301 showed just how detailed these assessments could be. All money, silver buckles, clothing, linen, beds, towels – even pots and pans – were listed and valued. Wealth was liable for taxation whether kept exclusively for pleasure or used as capital.

National taxation by fixed quota

In 1332 a grant made to the Crown, of a tenth on the boroughs and royal demesne and a fifteenth elsewhere, appeared to have been exacted with unusual severity, raising about four times the previous fifteenth and tenth. To overcome this problem, for the next round of 1334 the commissioners were requested to negotiate with each borough and shire a fixed sum to be paid in lieu of assessment and appropriation of a portion. The townships and shires were then to collect from their communities as they saw fit. The quota fixed for 1334 was then used as the basis for future rounds of taxation which became known colloquially as 'fifteenths and tenths', though there was no way of knowing how close to or distant from true fifteenths and tenths of income and wealth they were. Nationally these fifteenths and tenths raised about £39,000, and each borough, shire and division of borough and shire knew what proportion of this total it was expected to raise. Sometimes the call might be for half a fifteenth and tenth, sometimes double.

Parliament's increasing business in the realm of taxation led to a strengthening of negotiating powers for the representatives of the shires. The members of the Commons served as 'petitioners', bringing the concerns of the shires and boroughs to the attention of the lords who sat to give judgement and to counsel the king. The king would reach a decision in the light of political realities, though he retained extensive prerogative powers. Monarch and House of Lords eventually began to seek approval from the Commons for taxation, and by the end of the 1300s grants were being made "by the Commons with the assent of the Lords" (Brown, 1981, p 125). Lords and Commons were summoned on 50 occasions between 1371 and 1422, usually to Westminster Palace but occasionally elsewhere (for example, to Gloucester in 1378). In return for taxation, the Commons sought and obtained concessions from the monarch and sometimes stipulated how the money was to be spent, especially in times of crisis. As the Commons grew in confidence, the petitions (or Bills as they became known) would not only request but also propose an acceptable remedy.

The poll tax, 1377-80

In 1377, fearing more war with France, the parliament of Edward III granted a poll tax of fourpence (4d) to be taken from every man and woman in the kingdom over the age of 14 years, excepting genuine beggars. Then, with the French attacking along the length of the south coast, parliament granted a graduated poll tax in 1379. Dukes were charged £6 13s 4d, earls and countesses £4, judges £5, and so on down to the poorest (excluding beggars), 4d for each married couple and the same for every single man and woman over 16 years (giving an assessment ratio of richest to poorest of 800).

Finances went from bad to worse owing to continued fighting with France, and in 1380 parliament agreed to raise another £100,000. The Church, holding a third of all land in the kingdom, was to raise a third of this amount. To speed collection, a graduated poll tax was again imposed to raise the remainder, this time from a high of £1 on a magnate to a low of 4d for man and wife. Those in villeinage were already seething with discontent under the harshness of the justices of the peace and the manorial system after the great plague (the Black Death), and this poll tax precipitated what became known as the 'Peasant's Revolt'. Chastened, parliament reverted to the fifteenth and tenth.

Land taxation, 1404-31

In 1404, with Henry IV once more desperate for cash, no one dared propose another poll tax. With the French threatening again and Welsh rebellion at its height, the lords temporal imposed a tax of 5% upon all large landholders with rental values of about £300 a year or more. A similar tax of 1411 covered all landholders with rental values of at least £20 a year, the rate being 0.66%. Care was taken to ensure, however, that these taxes were not treated as precedents (Dowell, 1965, vol 1, p 107). In 1428, still stressed by war with France, yet another tax on land was tried at a rate of 6s 8d on the knight's fee. In 1431 this tax was extended to all holders of land whatever the nature of feudal service, and a new form of taxpayer was introduced. In addition to all freeholders of land, those receiving rents because they had a charge on land by deed were made similarly liable to the land tax. However, an attempt to create a new register of taxpayers based on income from land did not succeed. Commissioners were called in to enquire into who these taxpayers were, what they held that was taxable in land values, and to put this information on record. The landholders objected strongly, so in 1432 the system was abolished and the records destroyed (Dowell, 1965, vol 1, pp 109–10). Once again taxes of a fifteenth and tenth on moveables of the general community were imposed. After 1435 the practice developed to include tax allowances for towns and districts that were impoverished through natural disaster such as flood, or deterioration in trade.

The development of parliamentary representation

By repeated summons to successive parliaments, landed members of the Lords acquired a 'track record' for their families and out of growing custom the list of members became standardised. Older families expected seniority, and rank became an important issue – a question of distance from and closeness to the monarch. By contrast, no standardised list evolved for the Commons. When the king wished to call an assembly of the Commons he sent his writ to his sheriff in each county, commanding that two knights were to be selected from the shire and two burgesses from each borough. Elections were accordingly held in the county court, the assembled electorate consisting of the knights, squires and 'better people' who were resident in the county on the date of issue of the writ of assembly.

The House of Commons as a body of knights representing the shires, with representatives of the boroughs, continued to evolve into a second chamber with considerable influence. Rising enthusiasm to sit in the Commons prompted an Act of 1430 which restricted the county franchise to knights as defined in 1247, that is to freeholders with land worth an annual rent of £2 (40s) after all charges. A statute of 1445 stipulated that only those with land worth £20 a year could take a seat in the Commons (Myers, 1981, pp 165-6). In the middle of the 15th century Thomas Kirkby, clerk of the rolls (records) of parliament, confirmed that passage of any Bill required the consent of the king, Lords and Commons. Should the Lords wish to modify the scope or intent of a Bill from the Commons, it had to be returned to the Commons for endorsement. The Bill would not be enacted if the Commons disagreed with the Lords.

A graduated income tax, 1435

There was more innovation in 1435 when parliament added a graduated income tax to the fifteenth and tenth on moveables. The charge commenced at 2s 6d on incomes of £5, taking a further 6d on each additional pound up to £100, 8d in the pound on the next £300, and 2s in the pound from £400 upwards. During the commotions in the reigns of Richard II and Henry IV much of the land of the realm had been conveyed to feoffees to use for the benefit of the cestui que use (see Chapter Nine). Thus parliament declared that this new tax was to be charged to all persons seised of manors, lands and rents for their own use or to the use of any other persons (Dowell, 1965, vol 1, pp 112-13).

A similarly graduated income tax was imposed in 1450 at a time when poverty appeared too widespread to grant another fifteenth and tenth. Care was taken to make clear that this measure was not to be taken as a precedent, but only as an exceptional measure for an exceptional situation. The nation was in the final throes of its Hundred Years War with France. Frustrated with misrule and heavy taxation, the men of Kent rebelled, occupied London, and beheaded the king's treasurer, Lord Saye and Sele. For his trouble their leader, Jack Cade, was pursued and killed near Heathfield in Sussex (there is a nearby village of Cade Street).

Parliament acquires powers to overturn common law, 1492

In 1492 the judges held that statute law from parliament was superior to the common law (Myers, 1981, p 146), a decision which showed how powerful the assembly of knights and borough gentry had become by this time. Parliamentary control of taxation by the landed was now firmly established and extra-parliamentary sources of revenue for the Crown through services and death duties (incidents) served increasingly as a source of irritation. Feudal incidents could be imposed, so the argument ran, but only by statute signifying consent of a united assembly of landholders and not simply by royal prerogative. More and more this land-owning assembly was strengthening its option of shifting the State's revenue from Rent attached to land on to other forms of income.

Taxes were of course imposed on the landless by the landed all along, but the landed saw no imposition in what they did. The feudal belief was that the magnates truly spoke faithfully for the whole community. Back in 1232 a writ for taxation had ended with the statement that "... knights, freemen and villeins conceded to us an aid (tax)". Another writ of 1237, on which was granted a thirtieth of all moveables down to corn, ploughs, sheep, cows, horses and carts, stated "... knights and freemen, on their own behalf and on behalf of their villeins, have conceded to us an aid'. Yet the assemblies granting this taxation consisted entirely of tenants-in-chief (Holt, 1981, pp 25-6).

The subsidy in the days of the Tudors: the tax shelter in land

Owing to changes made in the 15th century, the Tudor fifteenths and tenths raised about £29,000 for government. In essence the system was still that of 1334, and the fifteenth and tenth survived well into the 17th century. In addition, Tudor parliaments re-introduced the medieval practice of individual assessment, the 'subsidy', charging persons valued at more than a threshold as laid down by statute. Those who qualified paid a proportion of their wealth according to a scale determined by parliament. The taxpayer was taxed only once for each subsidy, being assessed on all land and goods wherever they were. Importantly, however, he paid tax on *either* land *or* goods, whichever would bring in the greater sum to the Exchequer. This arrangement meant that land served as a 'tax haven' for merchants with wealth predominantly in the form of stock merchandise, harvested crops, or debts that were likely to be repaid as part of business transactions. Suppose the rate on taxable wealth was 5%. A landowner with an estate worth £1,500 at 15 years purchase of Rent would realise a yearly rent of £100, on which he would pay tax of £5. A merchant worth £2,000 in goods might convert £1,000 of his capital into cash and put this into purchase of land raising an annual rent of £66. He would now pay £50 on goods still held, instead of the threatened £100 on his original capital, and no tax on his landholding (Hoyle, 1998).

With frequent subsidies to support the Tudor wars, plus requests from government for loans and benevolences from 1522 onwards, repeated demands on the merchants' wealth were a powerful incentive for tax avoidance. The Amicable Grant of 1525, for example, demanded 12.5% of wealth between £20 and £50, and 16.6% of wealth above £50 (Hoyle, 1998). As described in Chapter Nine, more than once Tudor governments considered putting a stop to the practice of transferring wealth from capital to land in order to stem the drain on the productive side of the economy and limit tax avoidance. No action was taken, however.

Customs and excise: regular, indirect taxation

In 1610 the royal demesne (Crown lands) and the feudal services and incidents raised £144,000, or almost a third of a total revenue of £461,000. A single round of a fifteenth and a tenth, plus a tax of 4s in the pound on the clergy, produced a further £70,000 of the total. The remainder, over half the total, came from the State's third major source of revenue, the Customs. As mentioned earlier, in 1660 the latter sources were augmented to make good the abolition of the first; hence the Hereditary Excise of 1660 on the people's beer. Land taxation remained an option, but collected only when and in what way the land-owning classes accepted self-imposition.

Customs pre-date Norman times, their origins being shrouded in history. The officers of the Norman kings took a toll from every ship carrying ten casks of wine or more on arrival in port. Similarly, between a tenth and a fifteenth of the value of merchandise for export was taken (Dowell, 1965, vol 2, p 76). The practice was regulated by the 41st article of the Magna Carta of 1215: "Let all merchandise have safety and security to go out of England, to come into England, and to remain in and go about through England, as well by land as by water, for the purpose of buying and selling, without payment of any evil or unjust tolls, on payment of the ancient and just Customs." (Holt, 1992, pp 461-2). Thereafter the Customs formed a permanent revenue of the Crown, though always riddled with fraud.

The Excise was introduced into England in 1643 by John Pym, shortly before his death. Taxes on articles of consumption (the name stems from 'excision', meaning 'to cut out from') had long been imposed in Continental Europe, but resisted in England. Nevertheless, though despised, much to the relief of government they soon became accepted and paid. By 1644 Excise duties had been imposed on ales, beer, cider, meat, salt, hats, hops, saffron and silks, to name but a few items. Then came the Hereditary Excise of 1660. On some goods such as tobacco the Excise was imposed at a rate per quantity (pound weight, gallon etc), while on others such as drugs and silks it was imposed *ad valorem*, that is as a percentage of the price, the forerunner of the modern value added tax (VAT).

Robert Walpole began to undo what his predecessors had created when from 1721 he pursued a policy of stimulating trade by repealing import duties on timber from colonial plantations, material for the production of paper, silk when for the production of articles for export, and other goods. Virtually all export duties on goods and merchandise manufactured at home were also repealed. The high duties on imported tea, coffee and cocoa nuts had sustained a thriving profession of smugglers, to counter which Walpole introduced warehousing. In order to raise yet more revenue, Walpole responded to Sir John Cope's report on smuggling for the wealthy by seeking to extend warehousing to wine and tobacco. He made the mistake of naming his Bill as one for the collection of Excise rather than port duties. As taxes on consumption, Excises were still detested, and after 12 years in office Walpole had many political rivals who made the most of this mistaken choice of words. They claimed that this was the thin end of the wedge, paving the way for an army of snooping Excise men enforcing the tax on everything consumed. When at one point he narrowly escaped from physical assault in the Palace of Westminster's Court of Requests, Walpole prudently decided to back down. Future ministers remained very wary of talk of either poll taxes or Excise. In 1748 Henry Fox declared that as a trading nation Great Britain ought no longer to meet the public expense by taxes that affect commerce. He wished to see ports relieved of all import and export duties to create more freedom of trade. This proved far easier to say than achieve, however; it took only the threat of war to force fresh impositions.

When George III came to the throne in 1760 there were about 800 Acts of Parliament relating to port duties. No wonder then, that when Adam Smith reviewed the tax systems of Britain and other countries in his *The wealth of nations*, published in 1776, he concluded that port duties should be kept to a minimum to free trade, limit monopolies, and lower the price of labour at the subsistence wage. Smith pointed out that Excise duties on articles of common consumption such as salt, leather for shoes, soap and candles were impediments to economy. He also claimed that the Excise on beer was unfair in reaching only that brewed for sale, to which Lord North responded by imposing more duty on malt! (Dowell, 1965, vol 2, pp 167-70).

In the Great War with France after 1793, expenses soared as Britain's allies were defeated one by one, and government was forced to raise port duties and the Excise wherever it could. Thus, by the accession of George IV in 1820, 1,300 Acts relating to port duties had been added to the 800 that had existed 60 years previously. This ludicrous state of affairs created by successive Tory administrations desperate for revenue was ultimately exposed by the Import Duties Committee of 1840. Over 85% of Customs revenue was paid on only nine articles. The remaining 1,200 tariffs on other articles served little purpose other than to waste time and labour and provoke numerous complaints.

The policy now was to get rid of what previous administrations had imposed, again to liberate trade. In 1842, Sir Robert Peel reduced the duties on 750 articles at an estimated loss of revenue of about £1 million. Further revisions up to 1860 reduced Customs receipts by another £10 million, the deficit being made up by raising income tax and taxes on tobacco, alcohol and tea. In that year Gladstone continued the process of substituting income tax for Customs duties when he raised the former by a 1d to 10d in the pound (4%) while abolishing import duties on all manufactured goods. By 1880 the list of articles incurring Customs duties was down to 14. Income tax remained a minor source of revenue, however, amounting only to about £11 million in that year. In contrast, although many Excise duties were repealed, taxes on common articles of consumption such as alcohol, tea, tobacco and dried fruits raised over £40 million out of a total revenue of £71 million. Not until 1909 did income tax begin to evolve into the major revenue-raising device that it is today.

The 18th century 'land tax': a lesson in realities of taxation

The 18th century property tax, more commonly known as the land tax, is considered at some length to dispel any idea that it resembled in any way an efficient collection of Rent for central revenue. This was in fact nothing more than another attempt to tax comprehensively all sources of income and wealth (with a few exceptions), an attempt which failed spectacularly but which nevertheless was renewed annually for a century. Its predecessor, the fifteenth and tenth, had ended with the last grant of 1623.

Seventeenth century parliaments had been hard-pressed to fund the civil warfare between 1642 and 1648, Cromwell's campaigns of 1649 to

1651, and the three wars with Holland between 1660 and 1674. In 1662 parliament had imposed a house tax of 2s on all hearths and stoves except those of cottages (Dowell, 1965, vol 2, pp 26-7). The revenue, known as hearth money or chimney money, was apparently introduced to compensate the State for revenues lost following the confiscation of Crown lands during the interregnum (Chandaman, 1975, pp 78-9). Payable by the occupier, it proved insufficient, and so extra duties were imposed on wines and beer. The old Commonwealth parliament had collected taxes on income and wealth not annually but monthly because the need for ready cash was so pressing, and these were continued after 1660. Poll taxes were added in 1660, 1666 and 1677. In 1685 duties were imposed for the first time on tobacco and sugar, adding to the earlier port duties, Hereditary Excise and what were called 'temporary Excises'. Parliament's fiscal problems were exacerbated when William III of Orange and his wife Mary, both of them grandchildren of Charles I, acceded to the throne of England in 1689. Revolution proved expensive and so another poll tax was imposed that year. From then on England was drawn into William's Grand Alliance of powers to combat the growing might of France, but the resultant participation in the French wars up to 1715 proved disastrously expensive. More revenue was desperately needed, but William had repealed hearth money on his accession and sugar duties were repealed in 1693 after protests from refiners for the export trade. The most serious effort to raise the extra revenue was the property tax of 1693 (Ward, 1953).

The Property Tax Act named commissioners of taxation for each borough and county, men who were to supervise assessments of personal income and wealth and the collection of the tax in their assigned districts. There were 250 commissioners appointed for Devon, for example, mainly drawn from local gentry. In an age when patronage rather than competitive examination secured a place in the civil service, to criticise the decision in 1698 allowing members of parliament to appoint commissioners for their own constituencies would be rather pointless, but surrender of power by the king allowed political influence to corrupt the system from the outset. Although assessors determined what was taxable in each parish, their assessments could be revised by the commissioners who had the final word in appeals. Hence political foes could be heavily assessed and friends lightly assessed. Another problem was created by the method of remuneration of staff. Assessors were not paid but the collectors were, which often meant that both tasks were undertaken by the same person. The rates for the collector and clerk were 3d and 1d in the pound, respectively. Thus pay fell when the tax rate was reduced, leading collectors to seek alternative ways of making their effort worth the candle.

The assessors were to value all goods, merchandise and personal 'moveables' or personalty, assuming that each £100 of value could raise £6 in income. They were also to record all income derived from offices and employment, exempting the stipends of masters and fellows at Oxford and Cambridge Universities and money set aside for the poor. The rental values of land, houses and mines were also to be assessed, exempting colleges, halls and hospitals as public institutions and all sites worth less than £20. At the rate of 4s in the pound (20%) granted in 1693, the property tax raised almost £2 million. London, Westminster and Middlesex contributed 15%, Yorkshire almost 5% and sparsely populated Lancashire 1%.

The tax was collected quarterly and sent to the receivers for remittance to London. Their pay was 2d in the pound. Unlike local commissioners, receivers were appointed by the Treasury which generally drew its nominees from families having long connections with the collection of hearth money, Excise and Commonwealth assessments. Remittance either by guarded convoy or bill of exchange was an expensive business which the receivers paid for out of their own pocket, although they received an allowance from the tax office when each account was closed (a practice discontinued in 1728). Receivers were also to send copies of the assessments into the tax office and their accounts were submitted to the auditors of the land revenue.

Because it was reimposed annually following approval of the Land Bill by parliament, this property tax broke down the old distinction between regular revenue and extraordinary additional taxation at times of crisis. The Land Act of each year declared that "all and every person and persons, bodies politic and corporate, guilds and fraternities ... having an estate in ready money, or in any debts, or having an estate in goods, wares, merchandises, or other chattels or personal estate whatsoever ..." were to pay so much in the pound of the yearly value (Dowell, 1965, vol 2, pp 117-18). However, enthusiasm soon waned and partly out of favour, partly owing to the sheer amount of work involved, assessments of personalty became increasingly deficient. Consequently the tax of 1697 produced about 13% less revenue than that in 1693. Parliament stopped the rot by re-imposing the old quota system. To devise these quotas the returns for the tax of 1693 were taken as the standard. Thus a rate of 1s in the pound was expected to raise £500,000, each locality contributing the proportion of the total collected in 1693. This system led to constant dissatisfaction because many believed that the North and West of England had been under-assessed in 1693 relative to the South and East.

By convention the maximum rate of taxation settled down at 4s in the pound in war and 2s in the pound in peace, though rates of 1s or 3s were granted in some years. Whatever the rate, however, assessment and collection were of very variable quality and the brunt of the taxation fell arbitrarily on those landholders who failed to evade the levy.

Amateurish by modern standards, the system was riddled with flaws. As already explained, it was a general tax which became more or less an inefficient tax on landed property by default. Hence it became known as the land tax. The land component was supposed to be paid by the tenant who would then deduct the payment from his rent, but tenants complained that land stewards were shifting the tax on to them by raising rents. Tradesmen rationalised their evasion by claiming that to tax their uncertain income as heavily as the certain income from land was unfair. Landholders complained of ruination. The Treasury had a chronic problem with receivers who withheld their balances rather than remit promptly. They invested the balances in order to make a profit to supplement their income, sometimes in their own businesses, and bankruptcies lost revenue to the Treasury. In 1699, for example, Morgan Whitley, receiver for North Wales, was more than £43,000 in arrears (Ward, 1953, p 49). Even after a committee of inquiry in 1709 had prompted a flood of payments, arrears still exceeded £1 million. Though responsible for annual Budgets by 1715 (Rosveare, 1969, p 80), the Treasury had limited powers of enforcement, resorting time and time again to beseeching and threatening letters. Receivers also delayed their submissions of the copies of assessments, thereby thwarting prompt action by the central authorities against defaulting taxpayers.

Commissioners all too frequently did what they liked, for under-assessment was an easy way to gain local popularity. There was a double tax on Catholics and non-jurors (those refusing to take the oath of allegiance to William and Mary), and some commissioners disliked being used as tools of religious persecution. The quota system led to numerous arguments whenever commissioners relieved an economically declining district of its burden, for the remaining districts of the county or borough were expected to make good the deficit. Around general elections such arguments could assume a distinctly political complexion.

In 1731, there having been no war for almost ten years, Robert Walpole as First Lord of the Treasury and Chancellor of the Exchequer reduced the land tax to an all-time low of 1s in the pound, with several untoward consequences. First, the payments of collectors, clerks and receivers fell to a minimum, encouraging even more diversions of revenue for personal profit. Walpole was forced to raise taxes by other means to make up the deficit. Secondly, landholders became nervous of complete repeal, knowing that subsequent re-imposition for further warfare would very likely mean a revaluation to replace the quotas of 1693. It was a case of 'better the devil you know than the devil you don't know'.

England suffered war or rebellion for 46 years between 1689 and 1788. The associated expense combined with non-compliance and inefficient collection meant that such low rates were impossible to maintain even in peacetime. Even the magnates practised evasion. The Duke of Bedford quite flagrantly failed to comply, using the rents from his London estate to build his mansion near the village of Woburn on land granted in 1547 to John Russell, first Earl of Bedford. In 1763 Sir John St Aubyn manipulated the local land commission to prevent his property on St Michael's Mount being rated for either land tax or window tax. The records showed that the Earl of Plymouth, Lord Cardiff and Sir Herbert Mackworth paid no tax for 10 to 25 years (Ward, 1953, p 88). The War of the Spanish Succession, the War of Jenkin's Ear, the Seven Years War and the War of American Independence had together cost more than £270 million, quite beyond a defective tax system which at best raised under £2 million a year.

The invention of the national debt

The 'solution' to the dilemma was proposed by financiers, particularly that wizard of their kind, Charles Montagu. William III was £20 million in debt and unable to pay his soldiers. The bankers' answer was that old trick of the moneylender, the fictitious promissory note (paper money), issued in bulk with a total face value far in excess of the bank's ability to redeem. William Paterson offered gold from his own vaults to the Treasury, topped up with paper money, on the understanding that he would be sole banker for the moneyed and landed to the State. Montagu, commissioner to the Treasury from 1692, accepted Paterson's plan, and so was born the Bank of England by charter in 1694. In this charter is the proclamation that: "The bank hath benefit on the interest on all monies which it creates out of nothing" (Rowbotham, 1998, p 189). The Treasury first issued its IOUs, or Exchequer bills, in the following year, for which it got paper money, confirmed as legal tender by statute in 1704.

A market quickly evolved around Treasury bills, otherwise gilt-edged securities or 'the funds', operated by men such as Henry Contigno and

Benjamin Nunes out of Jonathan's, Garraway's and similar coffee houses in London's Change Alley (demolished in 1866). Governments have never since been able to break the habit of borrowing from savings institutions and banks, even though they knew they could never clear their debts. The simple fact is that to raise taxes in an attempt to do so would have a disastrous effect on the economy, as explained in Chapter 3. Hence the national debt has grown and grown to stand at £400 billion at the commencement of the third millennium, leaving Prime Minister Tony Blair to complain that his government had paid out more in interest payments than on the entire schools system in England.

Theories abound as to what national debt means; how the richest economies in the world are at the same time, at least on paper, the most indebted; and to whom? It seems likely that there is no real debt at all, if debt refers to the nation as a whole. Rather, the national debt is a perpetual indebtedness of the public sector to the unproductive sector of the economy. As explained in Chapter Six, banks can purchase ownership of Rent through the mortgage system by creating electronic money for this purpose. They also loan electronic money to the government, backed by the security of their Rentholding in real estate, taking interest on the Exchequer bills. The startling possibilities were recognised by financiers right from the start. In 1705 John Law called, in his *Money and trade considered, with a proposal for supplying the nation with money*, for a commission authorised to create and lend paper money on the security of landownership, "the debt not to exceed half, or two thirds of the value: and at the ordinary interest". Because land was fixed unlike gold and silver, reasoned Law, the community could not lose the reserve of wealth against which it raised money (Rowbotham, 1998, p 191). The magnitude of national debt merely correlates with the pool of national wealth tied up in privatised Rent.

It has recently been written: "The ... people generally own the Treasury securities that make up the public debt ... So, as any business executive should know, a liability that is offset by an asset of equal value should not be viewed as a burden" (Cavanaugh, 1996). So we take out of the left pocket and put into our right! Here is the half truth again, because the pockets do not belong to the same suit.

For financing the war with France, Montagu was raised to Earl of Halifax in 1714. By 1715 the national debt stood at £37 million with an annual interest charge of over £3 million. Alarmed, Walpole created the Sinking Fund in 1717 as a way of reducing the interest, but to no avail. After the American War of Independence the debt stood at £230 million, by which time it was recognised to fall essentially as a burden on the masses. The prosperous classes were investing in the funds, while their profits were met out of taxation serviced largely by duties on articles of popular consumption (Ward, 1953, p 124). In 1792 the interest paid out amounted to over £9 million, more than half of all revenue from taxes, with only £2 million of the £17 million of revenue coming from the land tax.

The Great War with France forced Pitt to reform the taxation system. His measures included the abandonment of the land tax on 21 June 1798. Landholders could then settle once and for all with the government by capitalising the land tax at 4s in the pound over 14 years. Many did so, viewing the expense as a better investment than government stock, at that time in a very depressed state owing to the war. However, three in four of those eligible had not taken up Pitt's offer by 1799, so they continued to be taxed yearly by the commissioners at what became a fixed charge.

Pitt died in January 1806 from complications of an attack of gout, broken in spirit by Napoleon's victory at Austerlitz one month earlier. He was therefore spared the knowledge of the duration of the war that changed his political career. The bill for hostilities between 1793 and 1815 was £831 million, adding £622 million to the national debt. In 1818 government collected £56 million in taxation but paid out £54 million in servicing this debt.

The land tax assessment continued to be used to meet the property qualification for the political franchise, and from 1781 until the Reform Act of 1832 the value of the freehold was verified at the time of voting by production of the certificate of payment. Other remnants of this tax, on moveables and income from public office, withered to absurdly low levels and were eventually repealed in 1833 and 1876, respectively. Amazingly, the last remnant of the tax on land itself was not abolished until 1963. Of course, the national debt rumbled on, swollen by £20 million in 1833 to compensate owners for the abolition of slavery. John Gladstone, for example, father of statesman William Gladstone (see below), received £75,000 for his 1,609 West Indian slaves. Between 1822 and 1830 the average price of a slave in British Guiana was £114 11s 5¼d. Compensation averaged £51 17s 1½d. In 1842, of a total government expenditure of £52 million, the interest on the national debt accounted for nearly £30 million.

Landed wealth and parliamentary representation, 1698-1838

The period between 1698 and 1715 was one of high friction between Whig and Tory. More general elections took place in these years than at any time since the medieval period (Plumb, 1967, p xv). Many newly landed men desired the social prestige of parliamentary membership, but elections and electioneering cost money. Sums of several hundred pounds laid out every few years were a sore test of means. Furthermore, the cost often extended beyond the election, for defeated candidates regularly petitioned parliament to have the contest declared null and void or over-turned in their favour. This meant paying the transport and boarding costs of witnesses going up to London. Almost invariably the richest man was victor, though often through access to funds loaned by supporters including the tax receivers. Members of parliament were not paid for the job.

The need for wealth and property for membership of the House of Commons was emphasised by the Property Qualifications Act of the Tory-dominated parliament in 1710. Representatives of the shires were required to show an annual income of £600 from land, and borough representatives £300 a year similarly from land. The Act was not repealed until the introduction of the general property qualification of 1838. A blatant attempt to retain the monopoly of political power within the bundle of the landed class, the property qualification was not wholly successful, largely because men of non-landed wealth devised bogus qualifications (Cornfield, 1996, p 10). Of 5,034 members of parliament between 1734 and 1832, 51% had commercial and professional interests, although many of this majority were simultaneously landholders (Cornfield, 1996, p 10).

Eighteenth century wealth taxes and assessed taxes

Land tax, Customs, Excise and national debt were not enough to meet the expenses of late 17th and 18th century governments. All suggestions for raising revenue were welcomed, and many schemes were circulated in pamphlet form. Stamp duties were first imposed in 1694, another import from Holland. Taxes were placed on births, marriages and deaths in 1695. Many of these new taxes required elaborate organisation, entailing a massive increase in the personnel employed for collection. In 1718 there were 561 full-time and more than 1,000 part-time employees in the

Customs in London alone, and 400 men were employed on the Excise of salt (Plumb, 1967, p 116). The Treasury expanded at an unprecedented rate; since Sir George Downing (1667) it had steadily secured control over Customs, Excise, the Mint and Tax Office (Roseveare, 1969, p 62). Consideration of its business by Cabinet was rare in Queen Anne's reign (Plumb, 1957). Only when the Treasury had been commissioned was its first lord summoned to Cabinet; otherwise it acted with independence.

A house tax was imposed in 1694. The origin of 'daylight robbery' for any blatantly excessive charge, the rate was determined by the number of windows, leading to argument as to what was a window and what was not, plus bricking up when assessors were in the neighbourhood. In 1747, the Whig Prime Minister Henry Pelham placed a small standard tax on all houses combined with a tax of 1s on each window in excess of 20. In response to Adam Smith's suggestion in his *The wealth of nations*, in 1778 the house tax was shifted to a levy on the annual rental value. The result was farcical, because the great houses of the rich were assessed absurdly lightly. Their lordships conveniently assumed that the annual value of a house such as that belonging to the Duke of Devonshire was next to nothing. If he wished to let Chatsworth, or the Marquis of Bath, Longleat, the prospect of finding a tenant with the money would be infinitesimal. Hence the annual rental value was fatuously taken to be, relatively speaking, next to nothing (Dowell, 1965, vol 2, pp 303-4).

As an alternative approach to the taxation of wealth, attention turned increasingly to expenses for the affluent such as newspapers, pleasure carriages and servants. Such taxes required detailed knowledge of the taxpayers' circumstances, so in 1785 Pitt withdrew responsibility for their collection from the several government departments, placing them under a common board of taxes. They became known collectively as the assessed taxes.

The Stamp Act of America

A most catastrophic adventure was the attempt to impose taxes on the American colonies. Quoting back the maxim 'no taxation without representation' at the post-Revolution House of Commons, the colonists argued that they could not be taxed by London because they had no voice in Britain's parliament. Grenville did not accept this argument and was determined to lay certain duties on the American ports, together with several internal stamp duties for remittance to London. The colonists accepted the port duties as regulations of trade, and these were imposed in 1764. The Stamp Act of America became British law in 1765 but met with virulent hostility in the colonies. American traders refused to settle their debts or renew orders with British traders. When the British attempted to recover in the American courts the lawyers refused to act, rather than purchase stamped paper as demanded by the Act.

Grenville was dismissed and the Stamp Act repealed, but in 1766 London passed a declaratory Act asserting the right of parliament to impose binding legislation on colonists. This only raised hackles in America, and colonists began to refuse importation from Britain of dutiable articles. The resultant loss of trade forced London to repeal the import duties, but to make the point and save face the duty on tea was retained. This assertion of the right of colonial taxation led to the Boston Tea Party of December 1773. Britain responded by closing the port of Boston, to which the colonists replied with their opening shots at Lexington in April 1775 and Declaration of Independence on 4th July 1776. Written by Thomas Jefferson, the Declaration was clearly shaped in content and style by Thomas Paine and his electrifying pamphlet *Common sense* which had appeared in Philadelphia in the previous January. Paine not only attacked the British monarch's insistence on the right to colonial taxation; he attacked the monarchy itself as an institution contrary to nature and logic (Paine, 1976). The War of Independence raised Britain's national debt from £126 million to £230 million, and after eight years of hostilities the colonies were lost.

William Pitt introduces 'self-assessment' for taxation

Like the land tax, the assessed taxes could not bear the strain of war with France, the limit coming with the imposition of the 'guinea pig' tax on hair powder in 1795. Nevertheless in 1797, desperate for money, Pitt increased the rate of the assessed taxes enormously, creating a fiasco. His desire was to realise what the land tax had failed to realise. He made a calculation: land rentals, tenant rentals, tithes, mines and canals, professional fees, overseas income, business profits, pensions and annuities probably represented an annual national income of £102 million. He wanted to capture 10% of this income for central revenue, without disturbing Customs, Excise or the assessed taxes.

Extraordinarily, the authorities claimed that the collection of income tax could be achieved without any 'unnecessary' disclosure of what was taxable. When Pitt introduced income tax in 1799 he arranged for its collection to be supervised by commissioners, assisted by an official called a surveyor of taxes. The taxpayer made out his own return of income, but if the surveyor suspected an inadequate self-assessment the commissioners could then examine the taxpayer on oath. Should the taxpayer be uncooperative the commissioners could impose whatever assessment they chose. It was then up to the taxpayer to disprove the assessment. Through the sheer amount of work involved, many slipped through the net, and not unusually those returning dishonest assessments escaped with under-taxation even when challenged by the surveyor.

Henry Addington and 'pay as you earn'

The Tory Prime Minister Henry Addington (soon to become Viscount Sidmouth) repealed Pitt's income tax following the Peace of Amiens in 1802, stating that such a tax should be reserved for war purposes. When hostilities resumed in 1803 he was forced into re-imposition. The Property and Income Tax Act of that year differed from Pitt's system in that it required details of income from particular sources rather than a general return of income from all sources. This tax for central government revenue was divided into separate schedules. Owners of land including houses were taxed under schedule A; farmers' profits under schedule B; and income from investments in government securities, whether British (imperial), colonial or foreign, under schedule C. Schedule D contained the 'sweeping clause', covering income from all other sources. Under schedule D all residents were taxed on profits from property anywhere in the world, and on income from any profession, trade, employment or vocation carried on anywhere. Non-residents were taxed on profits from property and on income earned in the country. Finally, schedule E covered incomes of employees of the State and public companies: a sort of 'pay as you earn' because the tax was to be collected at source by all 'public offices or employment'. The schedules were examined by separate inspectors, thereby obliging the taxpayer by not revealing the total income to any one official. Incomes of under £60 per year were exempted and there was an abatement for incomes between £60 and £150. An allowance was also made for families with three or more children. At a rate of 1s in the pound, or 5% on taxable income the yield totalled almost £4.5 million in the first year of the Act (Dowell, 1965, vol 3, p 102).

After conclusion of the peace in 1815, income tax was continued at half rates, though with great unpopularity. A letter in *The Times* of 1816 denounced "the despotic spirit of this inquisitorial impost" (*Daily Telegraph*, 9 January, 1999, p 22). Lord Liverpool's Chancellor of the Exchequer,

Vansittart, was forced to abolish the system, burning all records ceremoniously in front of the Palace of Westminster. Not that the debate faded thereafter. There was sufficient general interest for the public educator, Harriet Martineau, to produce six stories illustrating the principles of taxation as advocated in her day. Confidential material was sent to her by the Home Secretary and the Chairman of the Excise Commission so that the themes of her tales should illustrate current thinking in official circles. As Harriet put it: "I owe to preceding writers on the science of which I have treated.... Great men must have their hewers of wood and drawers of water; and scientific discoverers must be followed by those who will popularise their discoveries" (Hoecker-Drysdale, 1992, p 44). Written between 1833 and 1834, the stories advocated direct taxation on income and painted the pleasures of life in a world free of the iniquities of tithes, duties and the Excise.

Those favouring income taxes won through by 1842. Under various Acts thereafter, beginning with Peel's Property and Income Tax Act of that year, the general system adhered to that established by the Act of 1803. In 1853, the income assessment for Great Britain for tax purposes was £262 million, which at a rate of 7d in the pound produced nearly £6 million for the Exchequer after abatements and allowances. In 1884–85 the nett income charged under schedules A ('Land') and D (other income) was £175 million and £251 million, respectively.

Thomas Paine and Rent for social purposes

Into this age of land tax, window tax, Customs, Excise, stamp duties and national debt was born Thomas Paine, one of the great political visionaries. Having played an active role in the American and French revolutions, it was while recuperating in the Parisian home of United States ambassador James Monroe, after imprisonment in the Luxembourg, that Paine wrote his last important work. Published in 1797, *Agrarian Justice* decried the tendency for the rich to become richer and the poor to become poorer in relative terms as wealth accrued in society. Paine opened with these words: "To preserve the benefits of what is called civilised life, and to remedy at the same time the evil which it has produced, ought to be considered as one of the first objects of reformed legislation ... Civilisation ... has operated two ways: to make one part of society more affluent, and the other more wretched, than would be the lot of either in a natural state." (Paine, 1987). Poverty in the European nations was perceived not as an absolute state of primitiveness or under-development, but rather a relative state expressing location in the order of society between the centre and the margin. Paine was in no doubt that socio-economic marginalisation had its origin in the method of land tenure in Europe: "As it is impossible to separate the improvement made by cultivation from the earth itself, upon which the improvement is made, the idea of landed property arose from that inseparable connection; but it is nevertheless true, that it is the value of the improvement, only, and not the earth itself, that is individual property. Every proprietor therefore, of cultivated lands, owes to the community a ground rent ... for the land which he holds ..." (Paine, 1987, p 476).

Paine went on to say: "Cultivation ... has given to created earth a tenfold value. But the landed monopoly that began with it has produced the greatest evil. It has dispossessed more than half the inhabitants of every nation of their natural inheritance, without providing for them, as ought to have been done, as indemnification for that loss, and has therefore created a species of poverty and wretchedness that did not exist before" (Paine, 1987, p 477). To remedy this injustice, Paine suggested the collection of Rent as a death duty to fund old age pensions, disability allowances and a one-off payment at the age of 21 as part-compensation for the loss of natural inheritance. "It is the practice", wrote Paine, "... to make some provisions for persons becoming poor and wretched only at the time they become so. Would it not, even as a matter of economy be far better to adopt means to prevent their becoming poor?" So the idea of Rent being returned to the public domain for social purposes, and dismissal of private ownership of all natural materials, forces, and opportunities as wrong, has a prestigious pedigree. Paine's concept of a Welfare State funded through Rent to prevent social exclusion has yet to be grasped by government as a 'third way', 200 years after it first appeared in print.

Paine died in June 1809. In 1819 a man was thrown into prison for selling 'the words of Tom Paine', and there he would have stayed had not a gentleman written to the Home Office to point out an unfortunate mistake. The magistrate had seen the name of Paine on the offending pamphlet and looked no further. However, the work had been published by the Religious Tracts Society, with the intent of defaming Paine rather than praising him.

Paine's logic was too much for many politicians and men of religion to contemplate. His *The age of reason* (1794) had to be discredited for its re-statement of the intellectual defence of Deism in words for ordinary comprehension (Paine, 1948). His *Rights of man*, which ridiculed claims for the inviolability of a hereditary monarchy and (in part two published in 1792) dealt with themes of poverty and inequality later developed in *Agrarian justice*, also had to be put down. The strategy employed was to attack the man rather than his ideas. Corrosive propaganda was put about of his immorality, drunkenness and lust for vice, stories which entered English folklore. Not until 1909 did the persecution of the man and his defenders fade from the English scene. Even as late as 1963, when the Town Council of Thetford, Paine's birthplace, decided to erect a statue in Paine's memory, a Conservative councillor promptly resigned in protest. Yet according to Lady Hester Stanhope, Prime Minister William Pitt's niece and private secretary, though her uncle instigated the trial of Paine for seditious libel, he had commented to her: "Tom Paine was quite right when he wrote *Rights of man*, (but) what am I to do as things are? If I were to encourage Paine's influence we shall have a bloody revolution" (Williamson, 1973, p 191).

Reaction to Paine's reforming logic has a long and bitter history in England, and he could with justice have levelled at many the charge he levelled at Edmund Burke in *Rights of man*: "Mr Burke does not attend to the distinction between *men* and *principles*; and therefore, he does not see that a revolt may take place against the despotism of the latter, while there lies no charge of despotism against the former" (Paine, 1969, p 69). Paine died in obscurity in Greenwich Village near New York, and his ideas for tax reform survived only in his published works.

The continuing struggle of landed wealth to evade death duties

More bewildering than any death duty proposed by Thomas Paine were those on the personalty or 'moveables' of the deceased, so lacking in any common principle and so full of anomalies that few could ever understand them. The authority for the administration of the goods and chattels of a deceased person, but excluding land, or goods and chattels settled on some other person such as a wife, was called the probate of the will. Originally executors had to produce the will and swear to its authenticity. The will was then deposited in the registry and a copy given to the executor with a certificate. This certificated copy was the probate. In 1694, a stamp duty of 5s was imposed when the value of the estate was assessed at over £20. Later, following the Dutch system, a rough sliding scale was introduced which had the unfortunate effect of taxing more heavily the smaller the value of the articles in the will. Great estates worth £1 million or more were virtually untouched. This was the Probate

Duty. By 1850, numerous calls for its reform were being heard; the tax was higher for some unknown reason when the deceased died without leaving a will; freehold land and freehold houses were exempt; and settled property (as arranged in the strict settlement) could not be touched by the Inland Revenue.

The second form of tax upon death was the Legacy Duty, introduced in 1780 when Lord North placed a stamp duty on the sale value of gifts of goods and chattels received by the legatee. By the tariff fixed in 1815 widows were exempt and children were taxed at 1% of the value received, while unrelated persons paid at 10% of the value. This tax also came to be seen as in need of reform because it did not affect land and touched only property passing by will or intestacy, exempting what passed by prior settlement.

William Gladstone viewed the tax system as in need of major reform during his time as Chancellor of the Exchequer in Lord Aberdeen's government of Peelites and Whigs. Income tax was falling more heavily on the productive side of the economy ('intelligence and skill') than on the unproductive side represented by landed property. Added to this, the Probate and Legacy duties were weighted distinctly in favour of the landholder and his real property (Dowell, 1965, vol 2, pp 339-40). The assessed taxes on wealth were 'overgrown' with exemptions. The old system of local assessment and collection, still in place, was riddled with corrupt practices. Thus, in his Budget of 1853, Gladstone attempted to produce a tax system that treated the social classes in a more equitable manner. One result was his Succession Duty on both realty and personalty, that is land, houses, goods and chattels.

The Financial Reform Association called for 'differentiation' so that income tax would fall more heavily on 'unearned' than 'earned' income. Gladstone thought this a recipe for class war. Indeed on several occasions during the 1860s he sought to abolish income tax, but conditions never seemed right. As second best, he argued that income tax would be more acceptable if accrued unearned wealth was taxed at the point of succession, that is at the time when the legacy duty was paid. The succession duty was therefore designed to bring in for tax all that was untouched by the legacy duty, but Gladstone had immense difficulty in carrying through the measure, not least because he proposed that the new duty should include land passing by strict settlement. The tax seems to have passed the Lords partly because, unlike other land taxes, it occurred only once in a lifetime, and according to Gladstone few could follow its complexities (Daunton, 1996, p 141). However, because land and houses formed the base of local taxes (the rates), Gladstone believed that the successor should pay a lower death duty on real estate than on other types of property. Hence the tax was imposed on the 'life interest' of what was inherited in land rather than on its full market value.

Suppose the land in question was worth £5,000 and that the annual rent which could be obtained for it was £300. The life expectancy of the person succeeding to the land was available from actuarial life tables, and if this was, say, 12 years, then the life interest was £3,600. This was less than the market value by £1,400. To Gladstone's disappointment, there proved too many ways of avoidance of the succession duty, one major method being that taxes were not paid on property in mortmain, that is owned by ecclesiastical or other corporations that cannot sell or otherwise 'alienate' land. As a result, in the mid-1880s taxes on goods and chattels contributed as much as 83% of death duties, while taxes on real estate amounted to only 17% (Daunton, 1996, p 144). Today, more than ever, financial planning consultants abound who, for a fee, will advise on how to slip through the loopholes to minimise the impact of Inheritance Tax. The exercise is part of what is called 'tax planning'.

William Gladstone as landholder

Not that Gladstone's purpose in the succession duty was to weaken the landed order – far from it. He was a prominent landholder himself, though not through inheritance. The origin of Gladstone's landholding was his father's slave-holding, coupled with a good marriage. John Gladstones (he dropped the terminal 's' in 1787) left Leith for Liverpool to set up in the family business as corn merchant. He was most successful, Liverpool being a boom town in those years, and in his final decade as a merchant he did what many were doing by investing in land and slaves in Jamaica and British Guiana. John was pro-slavery. After abolition in 1833 he persuaded Lord Glenelg to issue an order in Council permitting the West Indian plantocracy to import indentured labourers from British India on terms drawn up, not by Westminster or the Viceroy, but by the planters themselves. On his death in 1851 John left an estate worth £600,000.

William Gladstone was born in Rodney Street, Liverpool, in late December 1809. He entered parliament as a Tory in 1833, just in time to express his opinion on the Abolition of Slavery Bill. On 25 July of that year he breakfasted with the great abolitionist William Wilberforce, who was within four days of his death. Taking his leave, Gladstone went to the House of Commons to vote unsuccessfully against the Bill, which passed its third reading next day. In January 1836 Gladstone paid his first visit to Hawarden Castle in Flintshire, the estate of Sir Stephen Glynne, ninth and last baronet. In a double marriage in July 1840 William took Catherine Glynne as his bride and Lord Lyttleton took her younger sister Mary. That same year William's father transferred his plantations in Demerara to his sons.

The mother of Stephen, Catherine and Mary was Mary Neville, granddaughter of George Grenville (see the section on the Stamp Act of America above) and first cousin of Pitt the younger (see the section on self-assessment for taxation above). The Glynne estates fell deeply into debt following the banking crisis of 1847, and to preserve the estate Gladstone purchased about one third of the lands with money provided by his father. In 1865 he purchased the reversion of the estate, which thereby came into his ownership on Sir Stephen's death in 1874. Expressing full confidence in his eldest son's abilities as a landed proprietor, William transferred the freehold of Hawarden Castle to him the following year. In 1882, father transferred to son the lands purchased in Flintshire in 1847. Whatever the purpose of these arrangements, for father was certainly heavily committed in parliament with little time for estate management, they certainly would have avoided the succession duty on Hawarden for Willy. The Succession Duty Act of 1853 charged all property devolving from one person to another as a consequence *of death*. By private arrangement Mrs Gladstone had possession of the castle and contents for life, '*as if*' a life tenant, but she was never life tenant in law.

In 1875 Gladstone wrote to his son Willy: "I ... regard it as very high duty to labour for the conservation of estates, and the permanence of families in possession of them, as a principal source of social strength, and as a large part of true conservatism, from the time when Aeschylus wrote 'A great blessing are masters with ancient riches'" (Morley, 1905, p 348). No wonder that in 1878 Gladstone made some scathing remarks about Henry George and his proposals for Rent reform (Douglas, 1976, p 114) (see Chapter Thirteen). Tragedy struck in 1889 when Willy suffered a severe stroke brought on by a brain tumour. When he died in 1891 the estate was re-settled on his six year old heir, William Glynne Charles.

The abolition of assessed taxes: introduction of Licence Duty

Gladstone removed some exemptions on assessed taxes and simplified their collection. In 1869, when Prime Minister, his Chancellor Robert Lowe repealed many of the assessed taxes, introducing licence duties in their place. Licences were now needed for carriages, manservants, dogs and horses, as well as coats of arms. Together they produced about £1.3 million for the Treasury in the early 1880s.

The inhabited house tax was reformed in 1851. Its assessors were appointed from among the parishioners by the commissions for the land tax, and collection was also local. All inhabited dwellings worth an annual rent of £20 or more qualified. The rate was 6d in the pound for shops, 'liquor houses and farmhouses' and 9d in the pound for all other dwellings. In 1884–85 the 1.2 million qualifying dwellings were valued at a total annual rent of £61 million, and the tax on this yielded about £2 million. The tax was charged upon the occupier, not the owner, and houses of the royal family were exempt (Dowell, 1965, vol 3, pp 186-92).

This hotchpotch of taxes for central revenue persisted well into the late 19th century, politicians and civil servants doing their best to convince the gullible that the muddle distributed the burden of taxation across the social classes in a fair and equitable manner, bearing in mind that local taxes were paid only by those occupying the qualifying amount of real estate. The reality was an obsolescent mess that the emergent land reformers wished to sweep aside and replace by the collection of Rent. But that was not to be (see Chapters Thirteen and Fourteen).

The concept of proportionate taxation

Sir William Harcourt was Gladstone's Chancellor of the Exchequer in his Liberal administration of 1892-94. He inherited from Gladstone the notion of proportionate taxation, by which all classes including the poorest were to pay the same proportion of their total income when all their taxes were added together. Gladstone himself had received this wisdom from earlier Chancellors. Spencer Perceval, Chancellor of the Exchequer for the Tories, said in 1811: "The principle of the graduation (of taxation) was not recognised and, as for laying a higher income tax on the richer classes, that would be a complete subversion of all principles of justice by which the property of all men should be protected by law" (Dowell, 1965, vol 1, p xl). The tax system of 1860-89 continued to be based on the principle:"everyone, including the poor man, should pay taxes; taxation should be distributed in direct proportion to incomes; the roughly satisfactory method of achieving this result is by a compensatory system of taxes, each of which is distributively unfair, but in such a way that the unfairnesses cancel one another – on the one side the income tax and certain minor taxes which fall only on the rich and middle classes, and on the other the Customs and Excise duties upon a small number of imported and native (local) commodities of very general consumption, to which the poor man pays more in proportion to his income than richer people" (Kennedy, 1964, p 6).

Chancellors and the Treasury received ample support in this faith in proportionate taxation from economists of the day. Their theory was that the marginal utility of money, that is the usefulness of each additional pound added to an individual's fortune, remained constant (unlike the marginal utility of commodities, such as bread with each additional loaf). Thus an additional pound meant exactly the same to the rich man as to the poor man. Though largely steering clear of debate about the distribution of wealth, insisting that this was a social and political question rather than an economic one, by their utterances the economists provided strong support against attempts to *re-distribute* wealth (a basic function of a Welfare State). Stanley Jevons stated: "The more carefully and maturely I ponder over this question of taxation ... the more convinced I return to the principle, that all classes of persons above the rank of actual paupers, should contribute to the State in the proportion of their incomes" (Jevons, 1905, p 235). Professor Henry Sidgwick of Cambridge University held the same opinion (Sidgwick, 1883, pp 412-19). His colleague Alfred Marshall went against dogma, however, when in Ipswich in 1889 he stated: "I myself certainly think that the rich ought to be taxed much more heavily than they are, in order to provide for their poorer brethren the material means for a healthy physical and mental development" (Pigou, 1925, pp 228-9) – amazing words for his day.

According to Victorian economists (Marshall excepted), the loss of a pound to a rich man had the same consequences for him as loss of a pound to a poor man. But economists change with the times. Arthur Pigou, Professor of Economics at the University of Cambridge, wrote in 1920 in his *Economics of welfare*, that as long as re-distribution did not create economic inefficiencies (total production was not reduced) then the total sum of utility (ie the nation's overall satisfaction) was raised when the gap between the rich and poor was narrowed. In other words an additional pound to the poor man *did* give him more utility than the loss experienced by the rich man who had it taken from him. Suddenly, a Welfare State made economic sense (provided that it did not disrupt the economy) (Pigou, 1920; Galbraith, 1987, pp 212-13).

Though Jevons' analysis for the Treasury in 1869 seemed to say otherwise (Roseveare, 1969, p 191), proportionate taxation could never be realised by governments continuously stretched to finance preparations for war, a monarchy, social improvements, poor relief and public order. Land reformers were well aware of this situation, arguing that despite the local rates, death duties, income taxes and the remnant of land taxes, the landed monopoly was still shirking its responsibilities. Too much of what landholders were supposed to pay was avoided with the purchase of assistance from conveyancers and tax lawyers.

As already explained, in these years, taxes on goods and chattels made up 83% of death duties, while those on land and houses contributed only 17%. George Goschen therefore introduced a fourth form of death duty, the Estate Duty, in 1889, when Chancellor of the Exchequer in Lord Salisbury's Conservative and Unionist government of 1886–92. He imposed a tax of 1% on the capital value of estates worth £10,000 or more, believing that persons with large fortunes had been paying the least in taxes in proportion to total income. However, he made a mess by charging the duty on goods and chattels at their full value before these were divided between the successors, whereas that on landed property was paid only on a restricted value of the land and then only when an individual successor inherited land worth more than £10,000 (Daunton, 1996, p 143). This increased charges that the landed classes were yet again being favoured, legally dividing their estates in ways to avoid the intentions of the Estate Duty.

Harcourt thought that further reform of the death duties was the best way to meet demands for more equitable taxation. If carefully designed this would raise extra funds, possibly appease the Radicals if land was to pay more, soothe landholders by leaving untouched their income from Rent, and reassure the middle classes by not disturbing income tax. The great fear in 1894 was that the Budget would drive those with wealth further into the lap of the Conservative Party. Said Lord Rosebery, the leading Liberal peer, his enthusiasm for politics already sapped by the death of his wife Hannah (Rothschild) from typhoid fever in 1890: "We shall lose all the monied mercantile classes and what shall we do then at the Election? And how can we find the money to fight it?" (Daunton, 1996, p 153). This dependency of political parties on financial backers remains a thorn in the side of Democracy.

Graduation and differentiation in taxation

Harcourt had to deal with the re-emergence around 1890 of demands for a graduated tax system, first proposed by Tom Paine in *Rights of man* a hundred years before. The idea was also pressed, just as in the days of the land tax, that the income from labour, by its dependence upon the survival of the labourer, was far more precarious than that deriving from the interest on capital and rent, which would continue forward to the inheritors at the owner's death. Therefore wages should be taxed more lightly than interest and rent. As long as all were taxed equally, the labourer would find it relatively difficult to set money aside as savings and investment for his family. Harcourt started to plan for a graduated income tax (Daunton, 1996, p 155), encouraged by many in his own party who wanted the tax system revised on the principle of 'ability to pay'. If death duties and income tax were graduated, it was argued, it would be possible to remove the 'breakfast table' Excise and Customs duties on tea and cocoa that hit the poor so hard. Harcourt's difficulties were compounded, however, by Alfred Milner at the Inland Revenue.

Alfred Milner at the Inland Revenue

Born in Giessen, Germany, in 1854, Alfred Milner qualified in Law and was called to the bar in 1881. Work being scarce, he embarked upon a career as a journalist with the ultra-Liberal *Pall Mall Gazette*. By 1883 he was assistant editor to the imperialist William Thomas Stead. In 1884 his paper ran the headline on the prominent land reformer "Mr (Henry) George and his Crusade of Plunder" (Lawrence, 1957, p 55), and proposed Joseph Chamberlain as having "the best chance of being President of the British Republic" as a result of giving the people the vote (Lawrence, 1957, p 99). Disliking journalism, in 1885 Milner turned to party politics but was defeated as a Liberal candidate for Harrow. Instead, he became private secretary to George Goschen. In 1889 he went to Egypt as Director General of Accounts under Lord Cromer (Evelyn Baring). In 1892 he moved on to Chairman of the Board of Inland Revenue, where he remained until 1897 (he was knighted for his services in 1895). Milner then was appointed High Commissioner in South Africa and Governor of Cape Colony, to become deeply involved in events leading up to the Boer War of 1899. Known as a brilliant but highly inflexible administrator, it was largely Milner's refusal to make concessions to match those of

Kruger at the Conference of Bloemfontain in May 1899 which led to Chamberlain's ultimatum to the Boers.

Little wonder that this rigid man of the *Pall Mall Gazette* found calls for tax reform along the lines proposed by land reformers in the 1880s and after as amounting to 'plunder'. As Chairman of the Board of Inland Revenue when the Liberals were in power between 1892 and 1895 he made life awkward for Harcourt, at that time under pressure for land reform from the Radicals in his party. Milner did not want any erosion of the principle of proportionate taxation. He believed that those with high incomes would otherwise conceal their true worth, and to overcome this difficulty the Inland Revenue would require inquisitorial powers which would create great resentment among the honest majority, just as William Pitt had argued. Milner claimed that the costs of reform would be enormous and the political damage immense. He considered graduation of the income tax a 'financial revolution' which was financially unnecessary; the extra money needed could come instead from graduation of the death duty and the inhabited house tax (Daunton, 1996, p 162).

Milner would have known full well the long history of tax manipulation by those with wealth. The trick was (and still is) to find a lawyer who could devise a way in law for tax avoidance, guarding against illegal tax evasion. What else was the feoffee to use, other than to free the landholder of the old common law insistence that land values were the property of the State and not the private individual, for values which the State had the legal right to collect in services and death duties? Milner would have known of the report by the commissioners of the Inland Revenue in 1871 which disclosed that of a total of 358,000 persons assessed under schedule D (the sweeping clause), the 'curious fact' was that more than 80% of them claimed incomes of under £200. Also, of the entire number of adults in trade and professions, only about 1,200 reported incomes above £4,000. As one contemporary observer remarked, these figures "are hard to believe, but if they are correct then all I can say is that it is a wonder that we are so rich a country as we are" (Ilersic, 1960, pp 237-8).

Even back at the beginning of the 19th century the board of the Inland Revenue had stated that "it is notorious that persons living in easy circumstances, nay, even in apparent affluence, have returned their incomes under £60" (the threshold for taxation in 1803) (Griffith, 1949). So many were the returns coming in just under £60 that in 1806 the threshold of taxation was lowered to £50, and this to apply only to income on wages. This problem has not yet been solved. In 1951 the Committee of Public Accounts reported that "evasion was serious and widespread"

(Dowell, 1965, vol 1, p viii). Modern methods of avoidance are numerous, and a very lucrative source of income for the legal profession and accountants. Evasion also remains a major problem. The Institute for Fiscal Studies estimated Britain's 'Black Economy' to amount to between 3% and 5% of Gross Domestic Product (Smith and Wied-Nebbeling, 1986, p 88). There can be little doubt that attempts by some to sweep collection of Rent under the carpet as a realistic concept stem from the inability to conceal the unimproved site value of land and thus the lack of any opportunity it affords for avoidance and evasion.

Milner was equally reactionary on the subject of differentiation of taxation (different rates on different sources of income). Writing to Lewis (Loulou) Harcourt, son of Sir William, in March 1894, Milner was adamant: "It is conceivable, that some day income tax will be abolished and a property tax substituted. Perhaps this will be better, but it means a financial revolution of such magnitude, that it could not possibly be attempted at present. The idea that tinkering with the income tax will meet the difficulty is wholly misleading. Nothing else will meet the difficulty but sweeping the income tax right into the Thames and starting afresh" (Daunton, 1996, p 163). In other words, measures of the type proposed by land reformers *may* have been rational, but half measures would achieve nothing in return for an immense administrative effort. A complete shift to a property tax would be completely impractical, so leave things as they are until some more favourable future time.

Milner was not sure that property taxes were more fair than income taxes. He simplistically and misleadingly asked whether a widow on an income from property of £500 a year and five children to educate should be taxed at a heavier rate than, say, a barrister on his professional income of £5,000? What would this barrister do with his large income other than invest in Rent through property, stocks and shares? The barrister and widow would of course be potentially eligible for collection of Rent, but in ways that cushioned the transitional effects on persons such as this widow. To the argument that income from labour should be taxed more lightly because it was 'precarious', forcing the labourer to save for an uncertain future while that from land was secure, Milner replied that the State could not know what proportion of income a labourer should spend or save, and so income tax could not be calculated on this basis.

Harcourt had to act. He decided to raise the abatements on low incomes of under £500 per year (accounting for 90% of electors). He also gave concessions to landholders by allowing a deduction of 10% on income from land before tax under schedule A, balanced by introduction of a death duty of 8% on landed property. For this last measure he received a personal admonition from Queen Victoria, who forecast that his Budget "cannot fail to cripple all landowners", thereby destroying social order (Daunton, 1996, p 138). Nothing of the such happened, of course; the extra demands were usually so modest that they could be met out of the annual income or with insurance policies. Alfred Milner, facing the new Conservative government of 1895, went so far as to defend Harcourt's Budget as affording *protection* to the landowner, arguing that the extra cost of £600,000 a year would buy a strong case for relief of local taxes on land, which the Conservatives accepted and acted upon (Daunton, 1996, p 139).

The laissez-faire principle of the 19th century, minimal regulation of the economy by government, accorded nicely with the age-old use of central or 'imperial' taxation only for the defence of the realm and its economic ambitions. Only after 1894 did income taxation evolve into an instrument for effecting the creation of Welfare Capitalism with its emphasis on caring for the disadvantaged and the protection of all citizens against the misfortunes of unemployment, disability and ill health. In earlier times local taxation had been preferred to central taxation for Welfare, mainly because the citizen as ratepayer had greater control of the level of the tax fund and the *use* to which it would be put, than he had as taxpayer to the Exchequer. Local government was equated with *self-government*. Since the local rates were assessed on property, it is to local taxation that we must turn next, especially in relation to the Poor Laws.

ELEVEN

The dearth and the dole: the State and the able-bodied unemployed

The history of those born without a silver spoon in their mouths, that is without a legal entitlement to Rent, is one of hardship. The Poor Law bowed out in 1929 after more than 300 years, though its spirit haunts the Welfare State with ideas of 'less eligibility', the 'deserving' and 'undeserving' able-bodied poor, and the age-old dilemma summed up by John Stuart Mill:

> ... in all cases of helping, there are two sets of consequences to be considered: the consequences of the assistance itself, and the consequences of relying on the assistance. The former is generally beneficial, but the latter, for the most part, injurious; so much so, in many cases, as greatly to outweigh the value of the benefit. And this is never more likely to happen than in the very cases where the need of help is the most intense. There are few things for which it is more mischievous that people should rely on the habitual aid of others, than for the means of subsistence, and unhappily there is no lesson which they more easily learn. The problem to be solved is therefore one of peculiar nicety as well as importance: how to give the greatest amount of needful help, with the smallest encouragement to undue reliance on it. (in Fletcher, 1971, p 330)

When the privatisation of Rent is allowed to violate political morality by impoverishing Peter to endow Paul, and when the Welfare State then attempts to ameliorate Peter's distress through a political economy which only increases his dependence on Welfare through taxation of earned income, it can be seen that we are nowhere near to finding Mill's solution of peculiar nicety and importance. 'Help' is offered in lieu of entitlement.

The Church and the poor

Long before the old Poor Law Acts of 1597 and 1601, the relief of poverty was traditionally supervised and administered by the Church and monastic foundations. The Canon Law required that at least one quarter of ecclesiastic income should go to the relief of poverty. This income was derived largely from land. Until the intervention of Henry VIII in 1535, the monasteries held between 20 and 25% of landed wealth in England (Youings, 1967, p 307), and as such were large employers of labour. However, the succour they offered to the destitute amounted only to about £6,000 a year immediately before Henry's confiscation of their great wealth for the aristocratic laity (Slack, 1988, p 13). Parish clergy were meant to reserve one third of their income for the same purpose, but the admonitions of men such as the 14th century reformer John Wycliffe, that the Church was mean to the poor, fell largely on deaf ears. Thomas Cromwell, director of government policy under Henry VIII, was equally critical, commenting on how little of the income from glebe lands and Church tithes reached the poor of the parish (Youings, 1967, p 225).

With the dissolution of the monasteries, and the closure of chantries and hospitals which followed, attempts were made to compensate or make some alternative arrangements for the sick and infirm, but with very limited success. Also, under a policy to help the poor initiated by Cardinal Wolsey as Lord Chancellor after 1515, Tudor and Stuart governments attempted to regulate the supply and price of corn in times of bad harvests. The objective was to prevent hoarding designed to drive up prices. Again, there was little success (Slack, 1992). Nevertheless, the surveys conducted as part of this policy, and increasing recognition that Church and charity were overwhelmed by destitution through unemployment, led to the Poor Laws of the late Elizabethan era. There had been food riots necessitating martial law in London in June 1595, grain prices reached their highest of the century the following year, and the harvest of 1597 was the fourth disastrous one in a row.

The concept of the able-bodied poor

The old Poor Law, which survived until 1834, introduced into law the concept of the 'able-bodied poor': those willing and able to work if only work could be found. After a series of brutal experimentation with branding, flogging and execution, the Elizabethan solution for begging was the house of correction, not necessarily residential, where the unemployed would report for work financed through local taxation (what we would call today 'workfare'). Those who refused 'the house' continued to be punished. The non-able-bodied poor, the aged, the infirm and the mentally ill, were to enter almshouses or receive a pension for relief. However, most parishes were too small and the proceeds of the local tax for this purpose (the poor rate) too little to support separate institutions for the separate classes of officially destitute (the pauper), and so arose the common or general poor house.

The poor rate

Under the law, each parish was to appoint an unpaid official, the overseer, to assess the rateable value of each property or hereditament in terms of what it could fetch in rent, and then impose a rate on each poundage of value as set by the officers of the church vestry. The poor rate was to be paid not by the receiver of the rent for the property but the payer of the rent, the occupier (unless they were one and the same – the owner-occupier). Whoever had control of the front door to a property of sufficient rental value was generally regarded as liable for the poor rate.

The overseer was generally appointed for a term of one year from among those parishioners who could carry the financial responsibility. Some preferred to pay a fine rather than serve. The poor of the parish would sometimes call at his door for relief, and there were times when he had to pay out of his own funds pending re-imbursement from the revenue of the poor rate. Knowing that repayment could take months or even years, overseers would frequently vary what was paid out in accordance with their understanding of the parish's financial position. The poor if dissatisfied might then appeal to the vestry or the justices of the peace.

Initially the bulk of poor relief went to the infirm, elderly, widowed and orphaned. Gradually, however, relief for the 'casual' poor, extraordinary relief as it was called, assumed increasing importance, to assist the petitioner through a difficult period and back on to his or her feet. Certain conditions were laid down for those in receipt of relief. First, they were not to stray from the parish to seek relief elsewhere. Second, they were to accept the loss of property rights. What little they owned they were not to sell. Instead it became the practice to take a pauper's inventory and have these items made over to the parish by bill of sale or will. The parish might then sell these belongings on the death of the pensioner. Third, paupers were put on good behaviour.

Settlement and removal

The period immediately after the restoration of the monarchy in 1660 was in many ways disastrous for English legislation. There were the momentous but obscure Tenures Abolition Act and Act for the hereditary excise, parliament re-introduced the poll tax, the persecution of Non-conformists commenced in earnest in 1661, and to cap it all there was the Act of Settlement and Removal of 1662. The Act of Settlement allowed any newcomer to a parish the right to establish the process of 'settlement' there, and hence the right to poor relief if need be, but only after he or she had negotiated a 40-day probationary period without challenge. During probation, the newcomer could be ejected from the parish on request to the churchwardens and with the approval of the justices of the peace, unless property had been rented at £10 annually or more. Thus labouring families could be sent away before they had had a fair chance to find work.

Initially, probation started on the day the parish boundary was crossed, but in 1686 the law commenced the count from the day the overseer of the poor was notified of the new arrival. Then in 1692 probation was dated from a public declaration in church that strangers were in the parish. Was the alien family to hide its status in order to gain time to find work, or notify the authorities and risk immediate eviction? Even if work was found, 'settlement' status was not granted until the newcomer had worked for the one employer for a full year. Contracts of engagement were therefore frequently limited to 364 days, making eviction a continuous threat. In his *The wealth of nations* of 1776, Adam Smith was condemnatory: "To remove a man who had committed no misdemeanor, from a parish where he chooses to reside, is an evident violation of natural liberty and justice.... There is scarce a poor man in England ... who has not, in some part of his life, felt himself most cruelly oppressed by this ill-contrived law of settlements" (Smith, 1986, p 245).

In later years the law of settlement and removal was gradually softened. From 1795 no one could be evicted until actually a charge on the parish, the unmarried mother excepted (how terribly vulnerable was the young maid). From 1809 eviction was deferred if there was sickness in the family, making travel hazardous. Parishes often fought tooth and nail with each other, the pauper family being pushed hither and thither while lawyers engaged by the authorities made a thriving living out of the disputes. Even in poor parishes legal costs could run into hundreds of pounds in a disputed case. In 1815 there were 4,700 such cases costing

£287,000 in legal and removal expenses. The law was again amended in 1846 to forbid the eviction of a widow within 12 months of her husband's death.

The Act of Settlement and Removal remained in force well into the 20th century. Only in 1864 did Viscount Palmerston's administration grant permanent settlement of the nation's citizens in Britain's parishes after one year's residence, irrespective of employment history. There the law was held, and even in the early 1900s more than 12,000 people suffered parish eviction each year (Longmate, 1974, pp 17-22). As recently as 1927, the Poor Law Act (Part III, para 121) reiterated the old law: "Upon complaint made by a board of guardians that a person has become chargeable to the Poor Law union, two justices of the peace ... , if satisfied of the truth of the complaint and that the person is not settled within ... the union, may order him to be removed to the Poor Law union in which his parish of settlement is situated ...". Just as in 1662, the probationary period for settlement was 40 days.

Containing the costs of pauperism: guardians of the poor

The growth of dependence on the Poor Law during the 17th century can be seen in the records of the wealthy and fashionable parish of St Martin's in the Field in London's West End (Boulton, 1997). Of almost 52,000 parishioners in 1680, 4,000 occupied properties rendering them eligible for the poor rate of roughly three pence (3d) per week on average. This collection supported approximately 400 pensioners on the vestry list, each receiving about 17d per week. Overall, the overseers were spending annually over £2,500 in the parish in these years, most coming from the poor rate, but this wealthy parish was exceptional. Nationally the average yield of the poor rate across parishes was under £42 a year. After 1680 an increasing proportion of the poor rate went to relieve the 'extraordinary poverty' of the casual poor, the able-bodied pauper. In response to the growing demands on the Poor Law system an Act of 1691 ordered that no pension be awarded on the parish without the approval of the justices of the peace.

Occupiers eligible for the poor rate were keen to contain costs, partly by economising and partly by ensuring that paupers were a charge only on the parish of their legal settlement by birth, marriage or apprenticeship. To keep beggars within their own parish and to distinguish the parish's own poor from the vagrant, those who went 'on the parish' were frequently badged, a practice sanctioned nationally under an Act of 1697. An Act of 1722 empowered small parishes to seek permission by specific Act of parliament to join together in the construction of general poor houses. The Act ordered that "no poor who refused to be lodged and kept in such houses should be entitled to ask or receive parochial relief". Here was the progenitor of the deterrent 'workhouse test' of the 19th century. So effective was this ruling that despite the growth of population, by 1750 the cost of the Poor Law was £130,000 less than in 1698. Thomas Gilbert's Act of 1782 facilitated the formation of these Poor Law unions, as they came to be known, by doing away with the need for specific local Acts of parliament. Importantly, this same Act responded to a changing climate of opinion when it encouraged 'outdoor relief' as more cost effective than admission to the poor house. It was also in this year that justices of the peace were empowered to appoint officials called guardians, to 'oversee the overseers' of the parishes.

The family income supplement and welfare dependency

The national situation in the 1780s and 1790s was not unlike that of the 1590s. High prices, unemployment and infirmity, legacies of several disastrous harvests and war with Europe and America, threw enormous stresses upon poor relief. The unemployed flocked into the parishes of the emerging industrial urban centres. By this time parishes and unions had developed wide variations on the general theme of the Poor Law, and local ingenuity flourished in crises. Parishes were faced with honest, hardworking but poor families in which the working wage of the breadwinner could no longer support a basic diet for the wife and children. Some guardians therefore began to subsidise the wages of local labourers to tide them over the hard times, the forerunner of the modern means-tested family income supplement or family credit. The fear induced in some authorities and ratepayers by this growing practice was largely the same as that later expressed by John Stuart Mill and is essentially the same today: the risk of a permissive policy encouraging employers to pay unrealistically low wages subsidised by the taxpayer, and at the same time inculcating a 'why work?' mentality in the unemployed – today's 'Welfare dependency'.

Early thoughts on long-term unemployment: the undeserving poor

The 'sturdy beggar' or 'able-bodied pauper' has always proved enigmatic for designers of Welfare policy. When the Inter-Departmental Committee for Physical Deterioration met in 1903, very little was known even then about the causes of unemployment and low pay or the social and economic characteristics of the victims. Instead of understanding, there was much prejudice and false reasoning. That the labourer took the best wage on offer was obvious, as were patterns of seasonal unemployment with lay-offs in the winter. Also obvious were temporary unemployment when men were between jobs, and mass unemployment when a major employer withdrew from the market.

Yet these were temporary phenomena, ripples in the labour market which settled when the season changed or another entrepreneur came along. The economy, it was believed, simply did not accommodate any such state as long-term unemployment; David Ricardo's contemporary, Jean Baptiste Say, had said so (Galbraith, 1987, pp 74-6). Not long before the reform of the Poor Law in 1834, Say had laid down his law of markets which claimed that in the long run, the production of goods generated a demand sufficient to purchase the totality of goods supplied to the market. Thus in the long term there could be no such thing as over-production or its partner, unemployment, due to lack of demand. Periodic economic booms and depressions were short-term oscillations about a longer-term identity of supply and demand; things soon corrected themselves even if there was no adequate explanation for the ripples. Hence the longer a man was out of work the more suspicious became his status. He who was originally 'deserving' was slowly relegated into the 'undeserving' class as his unemployment continued. The market system was incompatible with any long denial of the opportunity to work, so the long-term unemployed or repeatedly unemployed (casual labour) must in some way be held to account for their condition. This was the point at which philosophers and social reformers had their field day.

Malthus and the fertility of the poor

Thomas Malthus was by all accounts a kind-spirited and generous man. Like the later Alfred Marshall, he studied mathematics at Cambridge before turning to political economy in the 1790s. Another noted philosopher, William Godwin, had recently acquired fame and impressed Malthus' father with the publication of his *An enquiry concerning political justice* in 1793, in which he argued that the growth of population could only improve the condition of society. William Pitt the younger was obviously in sympathy when he proposed a reorganisation of poor relief in order to pay a family allowance on the grounds that "those who, after having enriched their country with a number of children, have a claim upon its assistance for support" (McCleary, 1953, p 35).

Malthus was not so sure. His mathematical mind perceived that the size of the population would grow naturally by geometric progression owing to the sexual proclivity of men and women, whereas the ability of this expanding population to produce its subsistence would progress more like arithmetically (the law of diminishing returns). The net result of unrestrained human reproduction must therefore be poverty and nature's 'positive checks' that followed in its wake – under-nutrition, disease and warfare. Cheap and plentiful labour created by unrestrained sexual reproduction would produce a labour force desperate for work on the lowest of terms. This would encourage employers to recruit more labour, "... til ultimately the means of subsistence became in the same proportion of the population as at the period from which we set out" (Malthus, 1909, pp 14-15). Thus Malthus concluded that Godwin was wrong: "to prevent the recurrence of misery, is, alas! beyond the power of man" (Malthus, 1909, p 37). His logic led Malthus to campaign forcefully against relief under the old Poor Law, claiming that its allowances merely enabled the poor to have more children, thereby exacerbating a bad situation. This was 'Malthusianism', a philosophy that stalked the unemployed for more than a century, but one about which Malthus himself expressed considerable reservation in later editions of his work, *An essay on the principle of population*, first published in 1798. He came to believe that if a taste for the finer things in life could be inculcated in the poor, and these finer things were placed in front of them, then a desire for a better life would persuade them to postpone having children in order to satisfy these new wants. Thus the numbers of the poor did not necessarily increase in geometric progression and Malthus' law of population was reduced to something less than a law. Nevertheless, even in the face of Malthus' later writings, and the raised efficiency of labour with the industrial revolution, many clung to Malthusianism as an explanation for the able-bodied pauper. Even John Stuart Mill was impressed, writing: "The publication of Mr Malthus' *Essay* is the era from which better views of this subject must be dated" (Fletcher, 1971, p 252).

Jeremy Bentham and 'less eligibility'

Jeremy Bentham also had his own views regarding the limitations of government intervention in the economy. According to his political philosophy, collected under the term 'Utilitarianism', human beings, whether rich or poor, are motivated by the same instinctive desires for pleasure and avoidance of pain. Gifted with powers of reason, they so govern their activities when left to themselves as to maximise the totality of pleasure and minimise the totality of pain. This result did not mean that some would not experience considerable pain and others inordinate pleasure, but rather that, in an imperfect world, leaving mankind with individual independence to act in self-interest would ensure the greatest happiness for the greatest number. But man at times displaying an irrational temper, and a capacity to inflict pain deliberately on others in the pursuit of self-interest, this virtue of individualism needed to be kept within acceptable bounds by law. Being for the most part rational, however, if men were ever to find that their condition in employment caused more discomfort than their condition out of employment, then they would be "under the strongest inducement to quit the less eligible class of labourers and enter the more eligible class of paupers" (Fraser, 1984, p 44). Should the Poor Law for one moment make unemployment 'more eligible' (more desirable) than even the lowest paid form of labour, then it would spawn wilful pauperism.

The three contemporaries, Bentham, Malthus and David Ricardo, formulated their ideas as a response to conditions during the Great War with France between 1792 and 1815. They witnessed the first modern economic depression of 1795, the collapse in the price of grain in 1814, the rise in the poor rate during the years of economic crisis between 1817 and 1819, and the increasing discontent of ratepayer and hungry labourer alike. Ideas of over-population, limited land space, moral decay and 'less eligibility' formed strong currents within the contemporary climate of opinion. The problem for Poor Law reformers was that the condition of the poor labourer was highly undesirable. How could officialdom create a state even less desirable than this? Responsible officials at the parish level sympathised with neighbours and tenants known to be honest and decent but thrown into pauperism by economic conditions beyond their control. By contrast, those in the remoter corridors of central government were cultivating harder attitudes under pressure from the ratepaying electorate, fuelled by the philosophy of Malthus and Bentham. They put the experts to work.

The Royal Commission on the Poor Laws, 1832

With poor relief reaching 10 shillings (10s) per head of population in 1831, discontent fuelled by Malthusianism and Benthamism upset Whig and Tory alike. The Whigs, returned to power in 1830, announced in February 1832 the establishment of a Royal Commission on the Poor Laws. The Lord Chancellor, Henry Peter Brougham, took the cause fully to heart as soon as the Reform Bill became law that June. The nine commissioners were chaired by the Bishop of London, Charles Blomfield. Among the remainder was the first Drummond Professor of Political Economy at Oxford, Nassau William Senior, the prototype of the economist with a marked preference for objective analysis of facts and figures in a discipline stripped of concern for practical and moral issues (Galbraith, 1987, p 125). Senior had already decided that 'out door' relief had to be stopped for the able-bodied. He was certain that farmers lowered their wages given a secure supply of labour assisted by the parish system of income support and family credit, while labourers slackened their effort in response to assistance. The Royal Commission was going to say that allowances interfered with the free market system and created inefficiencies.

Bentham died in 1832, and more than any other, it was a young aspiring barrister-journalist named Edwin Chadwick who gave Bentham's philosophy practical expression. John Stuart Mill had introduced Chadwick to Bentham, and Bentham employed Chadwick as secretary. By the time Chadwick was offered a position as one of 26 assistant commissioners to serve the Royal Commission on the Poor Laws, he had fully imbibed his employer's concept of 'less eligibility'. So diligently did Chadwick apply himself to the Commission's work that by 1833 he was himself a commissioner. Chadwick was by no means the only enthusiast, however. Up north in Nottinghamshire, George Nicholls had already 'tested' the genuineness of those claiming an inability to escape destitution through their own efforts by offering relief on the hardest and most deterrent terms he could devise. He was highly encouraged by the subsequent fall in the demand on the poor rate in the parishes of Southwell and Bingham, apparently not bothering to inquire into the fate of those who had declined his terms. An influential member of Chadwick's Commission, Nicholls declared: "I wish to see the poor house looked to with dread by our labouring class, and the reproach for being an inmate of it extend downwards from father to son" (Marshall, 1961).

Assistant commissioners were dispatched throughout the nation, visiting about 20% of the 15,000 parishes and townships to interview all connected with local administration of the Poor Law. The information submitted amounted to 13,000 pages in 26 volumes, totally overwhelming Chadwick and Nassau Senior. Recent analysis of these data has shown that had the Commission time to digest completely what was presented, it would have realised that the allowance system it so disliked was already in marked decline (Blaug, 1964). Guardians and overseers were supporting large families through child allowances far more than they were making up the wages of low-paid labourers, and this had been a long-standing practice. However, government needed a report quickly to assuage the landed electorate. Bentham's 'less eligibility' was by then highly popular in these circles, and an authoritative economic argument for the abolition of allowances was needed urgently.

Harriet Martineau was both journalist and social educator. Born in 1802, by age 30 she had read widely, including Adam Smith, Malthus, James Mill and Dugald Stewart. Having discovered her gift for writing, she decided to use her talents to convey the principles of political economy as then understood through the medium of fiction. While being entertained by her characters and narrative, her readers would subconsciously absorb the lessons which would help them to understand a changing world. Harriet believed strongly that education in political economy for the general public could only promote social progress. The thirst for knowledge must have been immense, for her series of 25 *Illustrations of political economy* sold at more than 10,000 copies per month between 1832 and 1834.

Lord Brougham became aware of Harriet after five of her *Illustrations* had appeared. He called upon her in London, requesting six stories on the Poor Law as it functioned in 1832. Harriet agreed to write four tales on this theme, a task she completed within two years. *The parish, The hamlets, The town,* and *The land's end* were written with the aid of confidential material sent to her by the assistant commissioners. They taught that recipients of allowances invariably came to a bad end, that the labourer subsidised by excessive charity or outdoor relief was iniquitous and bad economy, and that evasion of the poor rate was all too frequent and too easy. Harriet was clearly being used by Brougham for propaganda, but she believed in what she was saying and genuinely considered the old Poor Law to be a "gangrene of the State" (Martineau, 1877, p 219). She wrote mainly for the middle and labouring classes. For the great and serious minded of the day there were the extracts of the commissioners' reports, leading up to the Report of the Royal Commission on the Poor Laws in March 1834.

The Report of 1834 made absolutely clear that its target was the able-bodied pauper and the system of allowances to make up his wages. Hardly any attention was focused on the non-able-bodied pauper destitute through illness, old age, infirmity or orphanhood. Nor was there any mention of the general problem of able-bodied destitution, how it happened that the nation let the productivity of so many fit and willing persons go to waste, or what number of families in this position were being helped by friends, family and charity. The Royal Commission's remit seemed to be confined to those able-bodied persons whose destitution brought them to the local Poor Law authorities. There were no statistics on unemployment or rates of pay, no consideration of trade cycles, no discussion of what are now termed frictional, seasonal and structural unemployment. Instead, the evidence was gathered largely from the Poor Law institutions, and focused heavily on proof of the belief in the waste of wealth that the allowance system had fostered in the agricultural districts. It was not able-bodied destitution which was damaging to the economy, the Report claimed, but able-bodied pauperism.

The offer of the workhouse

The official registration of the destitute as in need of relief under the Poor Law was what countenanced wage subsidies and allowances. To set the labour market right, the commissioners determined to deprive the employer of labour for which he did not pay at the free market rate, and to prevent the labourer receiving any income not wholly earned in employment. This meant that whereas the non-able-bodied destitute could continue to receive domiciliary or 'outdoor' relief in cash or kind, the able-bodied destitute were to be 'offered the workhouse' and nothing else. Obviously, this policy provided considerable motivation for the unemployed to find ways to qualify as 'non-able-bodied' (a forerunner of what might be termed today 'benefit fraud', pseudo-incapacity benefit being a more generous form of unemployment benefit). The Report declared "that except as to medical attendance ... all relief whatever to able-bodied persons or to their families, otherwise than in well-regulated workhouses ... shall be declared unlawful, and shall cease, in manner and at periods hereafter specified ..." (Poor Law Commission, 1834, XXVII, 228, 261-2).

To unify policy across the country the old hotch-potch of poor houses and parish overseers had to be swept away. In its place the Commission recommended that parishes be amalgamated into Poor Law unions encompassing populations of about 10,000 and covering areas of roughly 20 square miles. Each union would be run by an elected committee to be known as the guardians of the poor, each parish sending at least one delegate. The official linking the community to the guardians would be the relieving officer, and supervising the guardians would be a central board of Poor Law commissioners. The essential feature of each union was to be its purpose-built workhouse.

In offering the workhouse, Bentham's rule of less eligibility had to apply, using the methods devised for Southwell and Bingham. To test the genuineness of the distress claimed, what was offered by the State had to be sufficiently harsh to ensure that if there was the remotest possibility of securing work at minimal wages, the latter would be in every way preferable. If the man and his family accepted the workhouse, their pitiful state was taken to be proven and the threat of starvation was removed simultaneously, claimed Edwin Chadwick. It did not matter to the State how the family had been reduced to destitution, only by way of the workhouse test would the State intervene in the labour market. The basic ingredients of the workhouse were to be hard work at tasks which did not compete with the free commodity market, separation of the wife from her husband and children (except for breastfeeding), confinement within the building, and a subsistence diet.

The Poor Law Bill was introduced by Lord Althorp as Chancellor of the Exchequer on 17 April 1834. It had an easy passage through both the Commons and the Lords, but met some resistance from the press. *The Times* condemned the Bill, probably sensitive to the feelings of the justices of the peace who disliked the centralisation of authority. William Cobbett's *Weekly Political Register* attacked the Bill on behalf of the working class, but on 13 August it became the law of the land (Longmate, 1974, pp 58-9).

Chadwick was dismayed when Lord Melbourne appointed Thomas Frankland Lewis, John Shaw-Lefevre and George Nicholls as the new Commission and Chadwick as secretary rather than commissioner. Very soon, however, commissioners and secretary saw to it that workhouses were being erected and staffed in all southern parts of the country. By August 1836, almost half the population had been assigned to 351 unions covering 8,000 parishes, and outdoor relief had been banned in 94 unions. By late 1839 the task was nearly completed, 12 million people and 14,000 parishes having been gathered in under the Poor Law Amendment Act.

Following a further series of orders after 1845, the Commission was able to issue its General Outdoor Relief Prohibitory Order in 1847.

Amalgamated into unions though they now were, parishes still behaved as though they were self-governing entities when it came to setting the poor rate. Each parish was separately chargeable and liable to defray the expense of its own poor. In those parishes where the landholder's grip on the land gave him the power, a common practice was to keep the stock of habitable cottages for agricultural workers at a minimum. The fewer the cottages, the lower the likely demand for relief and the lower the poor rate of the parish. This policy not only discouraged house building but also meant that the central costs of the union in administration, running of the workhouse, burials and vaccination charges were often distributed unfairly across the parishes. Therefore, by the Union Chargeability Act of 1865, parish overseers were instructed to collect on the basis of a standardised pound rate on the annual value of each rateable property, for deposit in the union's common fund.

The Poor Law and the registration of births, marriages and deaths

Opposition to the workhouse movement was strongest in the north of the country, where Lord John Russell advised the Commission to move carefully. But the 1830s were reforming times in more ways than one, and three other innovations fortuitously arrived to strengthen the government's powers of imposition of the Poor Law system on recalcitrant towns such as Todmorden and Bradford. These were the introduction of regulations for the national registration of births, marriages and deaths. Michael Sadler's campaign on behalf of children led to the prohibition of employment of those under nine years of age in all textile mills except those making lace or silk. Hours of labour were also regulated for those between nine and 18 years, which immediately highlighted the need for documentation of age.

When the nation's children reached the age of maturity they were subject to Lord Hardwicke's Marriage Act of 1754 (Nissel, 1987, pp 9-11). This stipulated that all marriages were to take place in the parish church, with solemnisation by clergy of the Church of England only, Jews and Quakers excepted. Roman Catholics, Baptists and Presbyterians were denied legal marriage by their own rites, and hence the legitimacy of their children if they did not submit. In the parliamentary speech from the throne at the start of the 1836 session, it was announced that early attention would be given to certain "grievances which affect those who dissent from the doctrines or discipline of the Established Church" (Reid, 1895, p 106). Lord John Russell brought forward two such measures, one legalising marriage in the presence of a registrar in places of Non-conformist worship, and the other providing for a general civil registration of births, marriages and deaths. Russell's original proposal was that marriage in church or chapel should take place only after due notice had been given to the office of the registrar. The bishops objected and the House of Lords supported them, with the result that the registrar's services were dispensed with in parish churches. Central registration of deaths had long been advocated by the growing business of life assurance for its actuarial calculations.

With the passage of the Registration Act of 1836, Lord John Russell as Home Secretary appointed his brother-in-law, Thomas Lister, as the first Registrar General. However, as with the national programme for smallpox vaccination current at that time, the only system in place and capable of national administration of the Act was that of the Poor Law with its unions and boards of guardians. Hence the ability to insist on acceptance of the system in the northern counties, noted for Roman Catholicism and child labour in the mills. Unions were divided into registration districts, each with its clerk, the superintendent being the clerk to the board of guardians (who conducted the civil marriages). From June 1837 all births were to be registered within six weeks, while deaths could be registered at any time. Soon after, by the Population Act of 1840, the Registrar General was also given responsibility for the decennial national Census which had been established in 1801 (again by household inquiry by the parish overseers of the poor).

The establishment of national vital statistics: medicine with political undertones

This same legislation, administered through the Poor Law organisations, coincidentally provided the data with which to quantify the impact of material deprivation on health. Joining the General Register Office as 'compiler of statistics' soon after its establishment was Dr William Farr. Born in Shropshire in 1807, Farr's guardian had willed him sufficient money to study medicine in Paris and at University College London. He had a natural inclination toward statistics, being fascinated at the way disease rates varied with age, sex, climate, locality, occupation and so on. His analysis of the registers set a tradition for research in medicine and public health that continues to this day. Lister retired in 1842, but the second Registrar General George Graham remained in office until 1879. To Farr's disappointment, it was not he but Sir Brydges Powell Hennicker who then got the job. Farr therefore decided to take his leave in 1880, dying in retirement three years later. His great achievement was to demonstrate the power of national vital statistics, nowadays based on more than 260 million records stored by the Office for National Statistics in Birkdale, Merseyside (Nissel, 1987, p 14).

Lord John Russell's administrative arrangements fomented an interesting early example of political medicine and its limited power to confront political economy. Dr Farr was interested in the causes of death, which he immediately pursued by applying his skills in statistics to the reports coming in from the clerks of the Poor Law unions. His room in the General Register Office and Edwin Chadwick's at the Poor Law Commission were both located in Somerset House in London's Strand. Here in 1839 both men were trying to make something of themselves and their posts. The new workhouses under the Poor Law were meant to serve a dual purpose. On the one hand they were supposed to offer conditions harsher than the bare subsistence of the lowest paid labourers in employment, yet on the other they were intended to provide a safety net to protect poor families thrown upon the mercy of the State by unemployment. The diet, while scanty and insipid, had been tested on prisoners and was believed to be adequate for preservation of life. So when some death certificates coming in from the Poor Law institutions and elsewhere recorded starvation as the cause, and when Farr publicised the fact in his summary tables, Chadwick was alarmed at the political implications for a system to which he was devoted.

Death in the workhouse

Death certification may well have been to a better standard for the poor than the rich, because those dying in workhouses came more often to post-mortem examination. Eighteenth century England had witnessed a growth of private schools of anatomy for surgical training; London alone had at least 25 establishments. An Act of 1752 had permitted sale of the bodies of executed murderers for dissection to advance the science of anatomy, but such bodies were few. To supply the needs of students a new trade emerged – the resurrectionist or 'body snatcher'. In order to undermine this practice, in 1782 William Hey, a surgeon in Leeds, persuaded William Wilberforce to introduce a Bill for extension of dissection to the bodies of those hanged for burglary or robbery. The House of Lords rejected the measure, believing that the prospect of dissection was a deterrent to murder, and that Wilberforce's proposal would only increase murder in cases of rape or theft. It says something about the laws of property in England when it is recalled that in those days to take a body from the grave was not a crime, but to take a shroud worth more than 2s 6d was a hanging offence.

Overwhelmingly, bodies going for anatomy were taken from paupers' graves; funerals of the wealthy were guarded. A patent coffin of 1818 was marketed as 'resurrectionist proof', and fashionable cemeteries offered to guard the corpse until unfit for dissection. By contrast, the pauper could be buried coffinless. In 1828 a Bill to stop body snatching was passed by the House of Commons but bitterly opposed by the Archbishop of Canterbury and others in the House of Lords. Then within months came sensational news from Edinburgh. Over a period of one year William Burke and William Hare had murdered 16 beggars by luring them with the offer of a meal. The bodies were sold to Robert Knox whose school of anatomy operated next door to the Department of Anatomy of Edinburgh University. Hare turned king's evidence but Burke was hanged before a crowd of 30,000 in January 1829. Despite the trial, the Lords still threw out the Anatomy Bill in March. In 1831 a similar crime was committed in London. A boy called Carlo Ferrari was murdered and his body sold to King's College Hospital. The perpetrators were caught, two were hanged, and the third transported. The Bill of 1828 was now quickly re-introduced and passed as the Anatomy Act of 1832. One result of the Act was that over the following century, more than 99% of bodies for medical schools came straight from workhouses.

In London, 10 to 15% of all deaths occurred in the workhouse in the mid-1850s, and death certificates had to be signed by the attending doctor or apothecary. Farr took certificates stating starvation as the cause of death to be the 'tip of the iceberg', and said so, believing that under-nutrition and malnutrition were contributory but unrecorded causes of death in many cases among the poor. Despite Chadwick's embarrassment, Farr insisted that he had to take note of what the registrars of deaths were recording. Chadwick accused Farr of speculation and the challenge to the political economy was deflected as doctors were increasingly persuaded to describe cause of death by pathology to the exclusion of environmental or social origins.

Deaths among the poor

While there may have been dispute about the causes of death among the poor, the data from the Registrar General's office soon confirmed that the total from all causes was grossly excessive (see also Chapter One). In the annual report of 1841, Farr published graphs comparing the expectation of life at birth for the people of Surrey, London and Liverpool. Coincidentally, Dr William Henry Duncan's famous survey of Liverpool in that year revealed the horrors of life for the city's poor. Of a population of 286,000 at the national Census, about 56,000 (20%) were crammed into little courts, with 20,000 (7%) living as cellar dwellers. In some cheap lodging houses there were families sleeping 30 persons in a space of 2,100 cubic feet. Even the penal code of the day recommended not less than 1,000 cubic feet for each prison inmate. Of every 100 children born in Liverpool, Farr showed that only 51 were able to survive for five years, and the average expectation of life was no more than 24 years. In Surrey by contrast, 79 of every 100 children were alive at five years, and the average life expectancy was 45 years. These contrasts paralleled the filth, over-crowding and lack of ventilation of Liverpool's slums and the open air of Surrey. The city fathers soon got busy, introducing the Liverpool Building Act of 1842 and the Liverpool Sanitary Act of 1846, under which Dr Duncan was appointed as the nation's first local medical officer of health (see also Chapter Six). Here was the power of vital statistics in operation. The contrast between localities led to this opening statement in the Act:

> And whereas the health of the population, especially of the poorer classes, is frequently injured by the prevalence of epidemical and other disorders, and the virulence and extent of such disorders, is frequently due and owing to the existence of local causes which are capable of removal but which have hitherto frequently escaped detection from the want of some experienced person to examine and report into them, it is expedient that power should be given to appoint a duly qualified medical practitioner for that purpose. (Fraser, 1984, pp 262-3)

Similar moves were afoot in London. In 1838 an outbreak of fever occurred near a large pond in the East End's Whitechapel. The parish council sought the advice of Edwin Chadwick as Secretary to the Poor Law Commission. He suggested to the Poor Law commissioners that they appoint a medical committee of inquiry. Chadwick was well aware that the powers that be wished to see the new Poor Law reduce the poor rate paid by occupiers of property. As Lord Althorp had remarked, "The landed interest were looking for immediate relief" (Fraser, 1984, p 49). But Chadwick was also aware that epidemics of sickness among the poor threw them upon the mercy of the Poor Law, and that therefore prevention of disease made economic sense for the ratepayer. When, however, the Poor Law guardians in Whitechapel attempted to remove some 'nuisances', the government auditors disallowed the expense. The commissioners therefore wrote to Lord John Russell to advocate Chadwick's views on disease prevention. Soon after, Bishop Blomfield rose in the House of Lords to call for an inquiry into the causes of ill health in the labouring population. The government accepted this recommendation, and the job was passed back to the Poor Law Commission, and in turn Chadwick.

The Commissioners appointed three doctors, James Kay, James Arnott and Thomas Southwood Smith. The doctors were asked to prepare a medical report on the causes and effects of fever in 20 metropolitan boroughs and unions. This survey led in July 1842 to the publication of the famous *Report on the Sanitary Condition of the Labouring Population of Great Britain* (Chadwick, 1842). Chadwick did not confine himself to the 20 boroughs and unions, using in addition the new Registrar General's records and the responses to questionnaires put to Poor Law medical officers around the country. Motivated initially by the socio-economic cost of disease, Chadwick found himself confronted with socio-economic causes of disease. These data showed how strongly high death rates were linked with poor housing, insanitary conditions and over-crowding. The findings convinced him that much of the attendant evil in poverty was the result of insanitary conditions. The drunkenness of the poor, their criminal behaviour, their apparent shiftlessness, their ill health were, he concluded, the result of the conditions under which they were obliged to live, not the other way round. Here was the groundswell of public health, the emerging sanitary movement.

Local boards of health, 1848

The enormity of Chadwick's vision for the political economy frightened the Poor Law commissioners. They refused to sign the Report, which was therefore printed over Chadwick's name alone. He could openly accept insanitary conditions as a contributory cause of death because, unlike starvation, they were not within the ambit of the Poor Law system. Far from lowering the poor rate, however, it looked as if the improvements implied in the Report would raise the taxpayers' expense considerably. It took another Royal Commission of 1843 under the Duke of Buccleuch, the campaigning of Southwood Smith's Health of Towns Association, and news of a fresh epidemic of cholera closing in from the East to pave the way for the momentous Public Health Act of 1848, guided through parliament by Lord Morpeth. The Act empowered boroughs to create local boards of health to provide town improvements in water supply, cemeteries, drainage and some other public health measures without the need to resort to a private Bill in parliament as had Liverpool a few years earlier. Elsewhere it was once again the poor law boards of Guardians, already given limited powers to deal with insanitary conditions in 1846, who were made responsible for the provisions of the Act (Richards, 1975, p 17).

Under the Public Health Act the central department, the General Board of Health, could compel the establishment of a local board only when the local death rate over the previous seven years had averaged 23 per 1,000. This figure was not plucked from thin air, but was based upon the annual reports of the Registrar General, especially that of 1843 in which the meaning of the rate had been discussed at length. The average death rate for England and Wales (all ages, sexes combined) was about 23 per 1,000 from 1838 onwards (remaining so until about 1875) (Wrigley and Schofield, 1989). With local death rates ranging around the country from 17 per 1,000 to 40 per 1,000 there was little need for concern about minor statistical errors due to differences in age and sex distribution or movement between localities. Those areas with a mortality much above the average were obviously needing priority of attention. Even so, local boards had no direct powers of action – all they could do was to identify nuisances and report to the justices of the peace who would prosecute offenders. There was tension between the local justices, tenacious in their resistance of central authority, and the General Board, seeking national improvement through central direction. Chadwick's proposal to standardise the national practice of burial, for example, made in 1851, by prohibiting burials inside churches and opening mortuaries, caused heated debate.

By 1853 only 182 local boards of health had been created, only 35 towns had applied for appointment of a local medical officer of health, and Chadwick and Shaftesbury were to watch bitterly as the House of Commons voted by 74 to 65 not to renew the General Board of Health. Instead there was to be a board of ministers who were thought to be more sympathetic to the domination of local government over health affairs. For Chadwick that was the end. Tensions reached breaking point in 1854, and though his advice was sought for many years afterwards, he made no further major contribution to public administration.

Other provisions of the Act were renewed on an annual basis up to 1858, when the functions of the board of ministers were transferred to the Privy Council. The post of Chief Medical Officer, made permanent in 1855, was saved in 1859 only by the personal intervention of Queen Victoria's husband, Albert the Prince Consort, just two years before his death. This ensured for the Privy Council the continuing service of John Simon, who as medical adviser pressed for measures that would enable the 670 local boards of health by then established to make further progress. Resistance was maintained, however, owing to the dislike of raising local rates to meet the wishes of central government.

The life of the unemployed pauper

Herbert Spencer and *The Economist* heaped abuse on the poor during the 1840s, whereas *Punch,* a radical magazine in those days, took up their cause (Huggett, 1978, pp 14-28). *Punch* documented the plight of John Matthews, forced to leave his wife and child in the workhouse while he walked across England to Wales seeking work. This practice was not strictly legal, for the released father could in theory abandon his family to the care of the State, but how else was a willing man to find work? The workhouse manager would therefore sanction release on condition of return in a fixed time. Poor John Matthews mistimed his journey back, having failed in his quest. The village constable, mistaking him for a vagrant, detained him as he passed through Brinkworth in Wiltshire, where he spent two months in gaol. Put back on the road in his pauper's rags, he died of hypothermia on the open road four days later. According to the Duke of Norfolk, if he couldn't get bread and warmth in the ordinary way, John should have eaten curry! The noble Duke, speaking at the prize fat stock show at Steyning, Sussex, on 8 December 1845, amazed his audience by declaring that if the poor could not afford bread then they should try curry powder, explaining that "if a man comes home, and has nothing better, it will make him warm and go to bed comfortable".

Bitter experience proved to the Poor Law guardians and workhouse managers of the industrial cities that all too often setbacks in trade created more 'John Matthews' than the workhouses could accommodate. At such times a blind eye had to be turned to the Outdoor Relief Prohibitory Order for the able-bodied destitute. This made a nonsense of the Order, a fact ultimately acknowledged after 30 years in a letter of the Local Government Board (now in central control of the system) on 12 May 1877. The alternative measure that came to receive official approval during economic crises was not the workhouse test but the labour test, for which the labour yard had been used long before condonation that year. The test of destitution at such times was now a willingness to submit to a programme of hard labour in return for outdoor relief in cash or kind (Webb and Webb, 1974, pp 22-35). In three months alone in early 1843, about 40,000 healthy but unemployed men were put through the labour yards. In 1848, only a year after the issue of the general Outdoor Relief Prohibitory Order, a temporary fall in work in the London docks threw many men on to the Poplar workhouse in the East End, forcing the guardians to subject them to stone breaking for their relief.

The 'opening of the labour yard' became a ritual around the country when trade collapsed. Between times the able-bodied unemployed went back into the workhouse, the deterrent effects of which were raised even more by mixing the able-bodied and their families with the aged, the mentally ill, the mentally defective, the tuberculous, the tramp and the petty criminal in the same rooms (against the wishes of Senior and Chadwick). Many unions continued to find it uneconomic to maintain separate institutions for the separate classes of the poor, especially for the able-bodied destitute at times when local employment prospects were good. This mixing of all types, however, meant that the able-bodied destitute received the same (above subsistence) diet as that offered to the deserving (non-able-bodied) poor, thereby diminishing the level of deterrence. Indeed in some parishes, to enter the workhouse as a single man provided a better standard of living than the local wage on offer. Not even a 'model' union such as Tonbridge in Kent could sustain separate institutions, even though it could afford central heating and a benign regime under the watchful eye of the workhouse reformer Louisa Twining, by then retired in neighbouring Tunbridge Wells (Coomber, 1996).

Charity comes to the workhouse

Some of the most squalid streets in London were in the shadow of the beautiful 18th century Somerset House where Farr and Chadwick worked. Not far away lived the Twining family, famous importers of tea. In the 1840s Louisa was regularly visiting the poor of this area, and was dismayed to discover that she could no longer care for them once they had been admitted to the workhouse of the Strand union. The Poor Law authorities feared that visits by charitable workers to the workhouse would compromise 'less eligibility'. Louisa took up a long campaign in the cause of workhouse visiting, leading in 1859 to the foundation of the Workhouse Visiting Society. Many others like her were also seeking to ameliorate for the pauperised what an economising ratepaying constituency had inflicted on the poor. In that same year, for example, the Liverpool merchant William Rathbone (father of Eleanor: see Chapter Five) founded a district nursing service for the sick poor with advice from Florence Nightingale. Just as Louisa Twining had shown compassion for the workhouse inmate, so did William Rathbone as an honorary visitor for the district Provident Society. He found 1,200 sick paupers crammed into the workhouse infirmary, tended by unskilled female paupers. After a six-year battle with the authorities he and Miss Nightingale managed to secure the establishment of 12 nurses under matron Agnes Jones in the Liverpool workhouse infirmary from May 1865. Rathbone covered the cost. Over-worked and exhausted, Miss Jones contracted typhus during the workhouse epidemic of 1868 and died on 19 February.

Patients and nurses alike were daily exposed to the dangers of the workhouse, yet the authorities refused to budge. At the time of Agnes' death Miss Nightingale wrote: "What makes workhouse nursing such an awful strain on all one's faculties is what made the war hospital nursing so. It is not the hardship and the misery, but it is the struggle with all the authorities of justice – and the struggle with corrupt officials and the old masters who are all more or less in the power of the paupers who know of their malpractices" (Woodham-Smith, 1982, p 465). The scandalous death of Timothy Daly amid the filth and neglect of the Holborn workhouse persuaded the President of the Poor Law board, Charles Villiers, to enquire into the state of the sick in London's metropolitan workhouses. Horrors beyond denial were exposed. Florence Nightingale insisted that the term 'non-able-bodied pauper' was a contradiction of terms. One could be either sick poor, or pauperised, but not both at once. She asked: "Why do we have hospitals in order to cure, and workhouse infirmaries in order *not* to cure?" (Woodham-Smith, 1982, p 467).

The medical journal the *The Lancet* established its own enquiry, out of which came the Association for the Improvement of the Infirmaries of London Workhouses. Relentless agitation eventually secured the Metropolitan Poor Act of March 1867, generally acknowledged as an important early milestone on the road to State-administered healthcare. A Metropolitan Common Fund was established from central government revenue in order to unify standards of care for the sick poor of the capital city and overcome the disadvantages of those in poor parishes. This fund provided for the placement of the mentally ill and those with fever in separate institutions, placement of children in Poor Law schools, and the salaries of Poor Law medical officers and nurses. Louisa Twining retired aged 70 to open a children's nursery in Tunbridge Wells. Florence Nightingale devoted her life to the cause of nursing up to the age of 74.

London's treatment of its unemployed poor, 1871-1908

From 1871 onwards the central authorities impressed upon the boards of guardians the need to go to the extra expense of separate workhouses for the able-bodied poor, and in that year the Poplar board of guardians in London's East End made a serious attempt to isolate the able-bodied pauper from the sick pauper. Separation meant that the workhouse test could be rigorously enforced. To increase the financial viability of the initiative, arrangements were made for other unions in London to send their able-bodied paupers to Poplar, which thereby came London's specialised institution for such cases. Pauperised unemployed and their families were no longer offered the general workhouse, but instead were 'offered Poplar'. As Mr Corbett of the Local Government Board put it, Poplar "was essentially a House of Industry" (Webb and Webb, 1974, p 41). Married women worked at picking oakum (old rope), and failure to complete the day's task led to an appearance before the local magistrate, followed by gaol. Men were given a daily task of not less than 10 pounds of beaten oakum or five pounds of unbeaten oakum to pick, or up to 10 bushels (a volume measure equivalent to 80 gallons) of granite to break.

Paupers, children included, walked across London in all weathers with their admission orders, and Poplar quickly became a house of terror. So deterrent was the regime that, to the guardians' satisfaction, for most of the year only 25% of its capacity of 788 persons was occupied. Many found Poplar unendurable. Of 3,745 admissions from 25 unions in 1877, the number of inmates at any one time never exceeded 200, making the average stay about 19 days. The distress of these people was reflected in the fact that 30% were re-admissions. Despite the terror, a large proportion were forced by conditions outside to re-submit themselves. As with all inhuman treatment, the inmates frequently rebelled, and it says much that local magistrates would at times refuse to prosecute, much to the dismay of the Local Government Board.

Poplar became the route by which other metropolitan unions attempted to get rid of their non-able-bodied paupers. The aged would be offered Poplar, and even the physically handicapped, to get them off the books. Poplar responded by asking for a medical certificate from 1876 onwards. But it was the non-able-bodied of the Poplar locality who eventually had this 'Bastille' closed. The building was always at least half-empty, while the neighbouring workhouse at Stepney for the aged and infirm was frequently overflowing. To keep the poor rate down, the overflow eventually found its way into Poplar, destroying the management's ability to maintain its harshness. Poplar reverted to a general workhouse in February 1882, but in its place the Local Government Board quickly opened Mary Place, Kensington, for the able-bodied pauper. Mary Place was functioning when the Inter-Departmental Committee on Physical Deterioration sat, and when the Poor Law Commission of 1905-1908 was dwelling on its problems. The masters of the metropolitan workhouses referred to those who refused the offer of Kensington as 'able-bodied loafers'. Their refusal was proof for the masters that the men had employment outside but were too idle to work until confronted with the grim alternative facing their wives and children in Kensington. Mary Place suffered the same fate as Poplar, with referrals of men with an inguinal or femoral hernia, for example, and others with undiagnosed disease causing debilitation mistaken for idleness. So frequent was this practice that Kensington was forced to employ a special medical officer to oversee the inmates. When Kensington closed, disappointed but undismayed, the Local Government Board set aside Belmont Road workhouse, Fulham, for the same purpose in September 1908 (Webb and Webb, 1974, pp 40-54).

Helping the poor stay out of the workhouse

The response to a depression in trade and rise in unemployment was not confined to opening the labour yard. Depressions were times for charities to rally to the cause, distributing food, clothing and money to the poor. Sometimes relief funds raised by a mayor's appeal would be used by the local authority to put men to work on roads and sewers. Shelters for the homeless poor would appear, some of them becoming established institutions. Huge charitable distributions took place in London's East End in the winter of 1861-62, and there were hundreds of other examples around the country over the years, helping to keep those in distress out of the workhouse. In 1878, a Mr Francis Peek attempted to coordinate these scattered efforts at relief work and philanthropy under a central committee. Sir Charles Trevelyan, the noted Treasury-reformer, objected on economic grounds, claiming that labour must be subjected to free market conditions and nothing else, either employment at the going rate or unemployment and severe privation: "when ... labour and charity are mixed up together, great abuse and demoralisation are engendered.... It was so in the Irish Famine. It was so in the Cotton Famine.... This should be left to the Guardians" (Webb and Webb, 1974, pp 103-4). In Sunderland in the early 1880s, the mayor's fund established a distress committee caring for up to 17,000 of the town's inhabitants.

Committees and agencies for the Victorian homeless preferred to help 'distressed persons of good character', and their press articles and advertisements frequently said as much. Consequently, in the 1880s the middle classes of London and the big cities were hearing more and more of the thousands of 'outcasts, weak, and fallen', left to live rough on the streets, seeking shelter in such places as brickfields. For years General Booth's Salvation Army had been caring for these unfortunates, but by 1887 the organisation realised that the Bible was not enough. Booth opened his first food and shelter depot in that year, with food sold by the farthing and lodgings at 4d a night. The Church Army opened the first of its labour homes in 1889, taking ex-convicts, tramps, old soldiers and deserted wives. For fear of being accused of interference in the labour market, however, the Church Army could offer only wood-chopping and similar tasks at a nominal rate (even this was attacked by the Firewood Trade Association). When the Salvation Army attempted to set the skilled cabinet maker to work at a rate below that set by the trade union, the Trades Union Congress objected. In desperation, these agencies opened rural labour colonies for training, often with assisted emigration in mind (Webb and Webb, 1974, pp 104-8).

Local government reorganisation: stumbling toward Welfare Democracy

Even when unionised much was inefficient about the use of the Saxon unit of Church organisation, the parish, for Victorian Welfare and other non-ecclesiastical purposes. Parish boundaries could date back to the Roman estates, and many complexities had been created over the centuries. Over 1,000 parishes were split into two or more completely separate localities (as had been the old manors). Other parishes straddled awkwardly across county or national borders. The parish of Threapwood, for example, was partly in the English county of Cheshire and partly in the Welsh county of Denbighshire. When a woman of the parish, an insane pauper, was confined to the local asylum, the question arose as to whether the Poor Law union of Wrexham, in which Threapwood belonged, should be charged the weekly rate for England (14s) or Wales (8s). The clerk of the union discovered that the patient had been born in a house sitting on the national border, but that her birth bed had been in Wales. Thus the charge was fixed at 8s (Richards, 1975, p 19). When Gladstone's government of 1870 required parishes to furnish elementary schooling wherever this had not been provided by a voluntary organisation, parishioners in divided parishes had to establish a school in the detached part even when the main part had a decent Church school. Charging a school rate on the whole parish for the benefit of the minority aroused indignation (see also Chapter Five).

As Edwin Chadwick had emphasised, the old Elizabethan parish system of unsalaried, amateur, local volunteer officials with its overseer, surveyor, churchwarden and constable was unsuited to the increasingly complex social demands of Victorian central government. Neither were borough and county wholly suitable for these purposes. The justices of the peace and officials of the borough corporations were unelected and often perceived to be using their powers for personal advancement. They were unrepresentative, not accountable to the general public, and therefore unfit to spend public revenue for social purposes.

The early solution had been to create institutions for specific purposes. Examples were the improvement commissions and the turnpike trusts, the latter having powers to charge ratepayers for maintenance of the major highways. This approach was piecemeal, however. The powers and functions of the parishes, boroughs and county officials varied considerably, as did the manner in which parliament's wishes were translated locally. Some areas had improvement commissions while others did not. Some highways were maintained by the turnpike system – others were not (Richards, 1975, pp 18-19). The first attempt to create some semblance of regularity was embodied in the Poor Law Amendment Act of 1834. Then came the Municipal Corporations Reform Act of 1835.

The Reform Act of 1832 (see Chapter Twelve) had extended the national electoral franchise in the counties, not only retaining the ancient right of the freeholder with property worth an annual rent of 40s a year according to the land tax estimate, but bringing in the copyholder and long-leaseholder with land justifying a nett annual rent of £10 or more, together with short-leaseholders and tenant farmers paying a rent of at least £50 a year. In the boroughs, the ancient voting rights continued for the lives of current holders, but with their demise occupation of property worth a rent of £10 yearly was to be the only form of enfranchisement. But this arrangement led to inconsistency. The £10 borough ratepayer was now enfranchised at national level but remained voteless at local government level.

In 1833 Lord Grey's administration appointed a commission which documented numerous anomalies at local level. Out of 237 boroughs, 186 had councils which elected themselves, while 26 had no council at all. Lord John Russell found himself Home Secretary introducing the Municipal Reform Bill in June 1835. This measure proposed to sweep away the host of antiquated privileges of corporate cities and towns dating back to feudal times, abolish the authority of the cliques of freemen, and give the local franchise to the £10 ratepayer.

Once again the House of Lords turned the exercise into a contest. The peers managed to force amendments whereby there would be a property qualification for councillors, and each council would elect one third of its own members as aldermen. These amendments left local government wide open to abuse of privilege, which they were meant to do. The purpose of the Lords was to retain a link between the reformed elected councils and the traditions of the ancient chartered corporations. The selection of aldermen was and remained based on seniority and party political affiliation. Aldermen could hold their seats for six years, so that a party losing an election could still dominate politically even though returned as a minority, because its aldermen remained to provide the power. Democracy was the victim. Aldermen did not disappear from councils outside London until 1972, from the Greater London Council until 1976, and from London boroughs until 1977.

In contrast to the Poor Law Amendment Act, the amount of central control provided for in the Municipal Corporations Reform Act was negligible. A borough's power to make bylaws was subject to approval of the Privy Council, but the total effect was weak and the City of London avoided these provisions altogether. By the 1870s, therefore, local government based on taxation of property had evolved once again into a most bizarre organisation. In some towns citizens found themselves affected by as many as six separate local authorities, which meant a vote on six separate franchises at different times and payment of six rates collected by separate officials. There were Baths and Washhouse Boards from 1846, Burial Boards, Highway Boards, Sewerage and Drainage Boards and, of course, the Boards of Health. Then came the School Boards in

1871. When in 1869 the medical officer for Merthyr Tydfil was asked by a Royal Commission to say who was responsible locally for public health, his reply was: "The local Board of Health, two Burial Boards, The Board of Guardians, the Superintendent and District Registrars, and the Inspector of Factories and his subordinates" (Best, 1971, p 56). Public health in one conscientious area could easily be affected adversely by a negligent neighbour, the two differing widely in the extent of local legislation and efforts to enforce Acts of central government. All this Edwin Chadwick had foreseen but had been unable to prevent.

The Local Government Act of 1888

By 1880 local government and local finance were again in dire need of extensive reform as parliament made increasing demands on local authorities for national Welfare. In 1888 Joseph Chamberlain and the Liberal Unionists, working within Lord Salisbury's Conservative government, succeeded in passing the Local Government Act which was to be the foundation of local government until the reforms of 1972. Among the great achievements of the Act were election of county councils by ratepayer franchise, bringing counties into line with boroughs, re-organisation of the financial relations between central and local government and the creation of the County of London with its own council. There was much argument about the size at which a borough would have equal administrative powers to a county, thereby avoiding payment of the county rate, but eventually a population of 50,000 was accepted for these 'county boroughs' (the smaller county boroughs of Chester, Worcester, Canterbury and Burton on Trent excepted).

There had always been a strong argument that whenever central government compelled local government to act, then central government should off-set the burden. The associated costs should be shouldered by the taxpayer (that is met out of income tax, Customs and Excise duties and other property taxes) rather than the ratepayer (exclusively from the rental value of land and buildings). Accordingly, the Exchequer had been in the habit of making supporting grants in respect of several services. In 1833 the Whig Chancellor of the Exchequer, Viscount Althorp, provided £20,000 to assist the education societies of that time, and many education grants followed. A grant was made in 1834 to meet the cost of criminal prosecutions. The County and Borough Police Act of 1856 enforced the establishment of police forces, supported by Exchequer grants. Some aspects of the Poor Law and highways maintenance were financed in a similar manner. The Act of 1888 consolidated these grants into a single combined grant to be paid out of a local taxation account. Even under this Act, however, in the county divisions of borough and urban district the poor rate was collected separately from the school rate and the rate for public health, an arrangement not corrected until the Rating and Valuation Act of 1925. Reformed local government was destined to assume responsibility for the unemployed poor in years to come (1930).

The Victorian middle classes and unemployment

The standards of conduct embodied in the Poor Law for the working classes were essentially those of the expanding Victorian middle classes, which by the 1850s amounted to about one sixth of the population. These were the merchants, traders and professional people whose opportunities to earn an income commensurate with middle class status had been advanced dramatically by the industrial revolution and expansion of Empire. They were not landed, mostly renting their domestic and business premises. But the family income afforded a rent that entitled the breadwinner to the electoral franchise and his wife to domestic help, even if only part-time and non-residential. Unlike late 20th century Britain, where small Rentholding distinguished the middle classes from the working classes, in mid-19th century Britain service was what separated them. Basically, the Victorian middle classes were served by the working classes.

Income permitted not only social but geographical distance between the classes. The middle classes were mainly located in the expanding suburbs beyond the urban poor but not penetrating into the territory of the rural landed classes. As a class they practised what they preached. The proper time to marry was when a young man could meet his social obligations and support a family. However, as the *Manchester Guardian* recorded in 1858: "People these days have an acute sense of the duty of not marrying without a competent support; but instead of tempering the idea of competency by habits of frugality and self-denial ... they are daily adding expensive appliances for show or comfort to the list of necessities, and so the upper surface of society rises higher and higher ... It is not generally so much the mere taste for personal enjoyment which leads to this, as the opinion that a certain class of luxuries and scale of expenditure are necessary to the maintenance of a due social position" (Burnett, 1986, p 100).

This neat summary re-inforces the validity of Dr Stevenson's use of occupational status to judge social class. The strictures placed by display of adequate income for entitlement to class membership meant that among the middle-classes of Victorian times the average age of marriage for men was postponed to almost 30 years. In 1851, 42% of women between 20 and 40 years were unmarried. Thus when, despite their moral rectitude, their thrift and dedication to work, the middle classes tasted the bitter fruits of unemployment during the economic recession of 1882–1890, the distinction between the respectable (deserving) and disreputable (undeserving) poor was sharpened. Suddenly, the study of the phenomenon of unemployment became fashionable. Men such as Dr Thomas Huxley, President of the Royal Society between 1883 and 1885, caught the mood, urging the application of the scientific method to study society.

Nothing about the Poor Law was acceptable to the social conscience of the middle and upper classes when it came to the upright family man whose small business or source of skilled employment disappeared in a severe recession, as, for example, in Birmingham in 1885. Jewellers, silversmiths and artisans by the hundreds were reduced to destitution. These were the people usually called upon to support the mayor's appeal, so the town council's Distress Committee could not cope. The Liberal politician Joseph Chamberlain had been Mayor of Birmingham between 1873 and 1875, and was keenly aware of developments in the city. In October 1885 he wrote to the Poor Law guardians in Birmingham to point out that: "the law exists for securing the assistance of the community at large in aid of their destitute members; and where the necessity has arisen from no fault of the persons concerned, there ought to be no idea of degradation connected with such assistance. Those compelled to apply have probably paid rates and taxes in past time. The payment is, in part, an insurance against misfortune" (Webb and Webb, 1974, p 116). This was of course special pleading for the propertied and enfranchised middle classes, worried by the thought of ruin and the disenfranchisement that went with pauperism.

In 1886 Chamberlain, as President of the Local Government Board under Gladstone, faced economic distress across the country. There were riots among the unemployed of London in February. The guardians were unsympathetic; they insisted that their duty was to administer the workhouse test. So, on 15th March 1886, Joseph Chamberlain issued his famous circular (Fraser, 1984, pp 274-6). After emphasising the essentially good qualities of the classes now in distress but refusing to present themselves to the Poor Law guardians, Chamberlain concluded that it was not right that such people should "be familiarised with poor law relief". The Local Government Board had no power to enforce any particular new proposals. Rather, the object of the circular was merely to inform the boards of guardians and the local authorities of the President's considered opinion. He suggested that work be found that did not involve the stigma of pauperism, that could be performed by untrained men, and that did not compete with labourers in employment. Chamberlain placed the ball firmly in the court of the local authorities, but strangely, he regarded it as necessary that men so employed should "be engaged on the recommendations of the Guardians", whom he thought could separate the deserving from the undeserving poor and steer the former to the town council's Distress Committee.

Mr Chamberlain was soon out of office, he and 92 other Liberals having precipitated the fall of Gladstone's administration by defying the whip on the (Irish) Home Rule Bill. Thereafter, however, successive presidents reissued the Circular whenever times were hard. But for another 10 years local authorities did little more than they had done prior to 1886, which was to open a mayor's fund when times called for action. The unemployed artisan was not enamoured by Chamberlain's idea either; the risk of guardians sending him the wrong way was too great. Action speeded up when a Commons Select Committee of 1896 endorsed the principle of municipal work for the unemployed. Heads of municipal departments would be instructed when necessary to take on extra men, creating work by reverting to manpower and spade and parking the machinery (Webb and Webb, 1974, p 118).

These calls for special assistance for the respectable unemployed produced a number of difficulties unforeseen by Joseph Chamberlain. First, the principle of 'less eligibility' could not apply. One could not recruit extra men from the unemployed and pay them less for the same work than the regular municipal employee. Such attempts, known as sweated labour, led to Trade Union objections and riots on the worksite. Thus after 1894 the re-issued circular made no reference to lower wages. Second, the step involving the Poor Law officers was quietly dropped. Instead, the local authority would open a register of unemployed claimants. People would 'go down to the municipal' in times of need. There were many occasions when local authorities could not find enough work to go around, so men were offered part-time work in rotation. Nevertheless, some thereby avoided 'going on the parish'.

The Poor Law moves into the 20th century

In 1905 the Poor Law of 1834 held fast, though in many unions there had been a considerable softening of the test of less eligibility. This relaxation caused consternation among die-hard officials of the Poor Law division of the Local Government Board, a body of opinion that probably persuaded the Conservative Prime Minister, Arthur Balfour, to establish the Royal Commission on the Poor Law in that year. Others have suggested that the move was an attempt by government to present itself as responsive to concerns for the welfare of the poorer classes. Recognising the complexity of the issues, Arthur and his brother Gerald (now President of the Local Government Board) decided to assemble the representatives of a wide range of opinion to decide what ought to be done (McBriar, 1987, pp 175-8). The final report in 1909 showed the Commission to have been divided. The majority concluded: "The administrators of the Poor Law are, in fact, endeavouring to apply the rigid system of 1834 to a condition of affairs which it was never intended to meet. What is wanted is not to abolish the Poor Law, but to widen, strengthen and humanise the Poor Law" (Poor Law Commission, 1909, part vi, ch 1, para 337). They blamed the incompetence of the Poor Law guardians for failing to adapt to modern circumstances. The minority disagreed, regarding the 24,000 members of the 646 boards of guardians in England and Wales as doing a stalwart job within a system riddled with inconsistency and waste; a system rapidly becoming superseded by the work of the expanding county borough councils and county councils. The minority wanted the abolition of the Poor Law, but not for Malthusian reasons.

In 1834, at the commencement of the new Poor Law, there had been no health authority, no public health service, no education authority, no salaried police force outside London, no mental hospitals in most of the country, no organised gaol system to speak of, no Distress Committee to deal with unemployment and no system of national pensions. All of this had come about by 1908. The Edwardian state was providing, usually free of charge, education from five years up to university for those young people who qualified. Local health authorities maintained more than 700 municipal hospitals, and from 1906 the education authority had a duty to examine medically the millions of children in public elementary schools and supply free school meals when needed. By 1908 every county council and county borough council had its Local Pension Committee awarding the State's old age pension to persons over 70 years. What had happened between 1834 and 1905 was that the State, at the levels of both local and central government, had found it necessary to intervene increasingly in those areas identified by John Stuart Mill as inefficiently dealt with by the laissez-faire private economy: in public health, education, care of the sick, infirm and mentally disabled, provision for the elderly and protection of the unemployed.

But the problem of able-bodied destitution, the labouring man who through unemployment or low pay could not maintain himself and his family, remained unresolved. On account of this failure, the families of such men continued to suffer under the Poor Law. In 1905 there were 50,000 children in Poor Law institutions, 15,000 of them still in general mixed workhouses alongside the mentally defective, mentally ill, the senile, tramps and adults with criminal records, in addition to the respectable able-bodied destitute. In 1905 the stigma of pauperism was still there and many guardians held fast to 'less eligibility'. The 'rubbish of society', those susceptible to 'self-deterioration' as the witnesses before the Inter-departmental Committee on Physical Deterioration (1903) called them (Inter-departmental Committee on Physical Deterioration, 1904), still lived in the shadow of the general workhouse, the labour yard and the ward for casuals.

The study of unemployment: William Beveridge

The word 'unemployment' was certainly in currency by the 1840s (Ashton, 1946). In his chapter on 'The Primary Cause of Recurring Paroxysms of Industrial Depression', included in *Progress and poverty* published in 1879, Henry George specifically used the phrase 'unemployed men' when linking cyclical economic recessions with the privatisation of Rent (George, 1979, p 273), but not until 1888 did Alfred Marshall popularise the term with economists (Harris, 1972, p 4). The first formal definition of unemployment appears to have been that of J.A. Hobson in 1895 (Hobson, 1895), the year of the first Select Committee on Distress from Want of Employment.

Caught up in this concern about unemployment was young William Beveridge as he passed through Balliol College, Oxford. He was born into a family of modestly middle class status in 1879, his father having been a district sessions judge in the Indian Civil Service. Beveridge's mother described how during a summer holiday in England in 1886 William was deeply shocked at his first sight of working class children in Epping Forest. Apparently his sister wept, while William tried to help the children wandering 'bonnetless, shoeless and in a most abject state'. His father had been moved to write on another occasion: "Poverty in Calcutta bears a much less dread aspect than it does in London or Edinburgh. There are no gin palaces ... and not so much terrible squalor" (Harris, 1977, p 15). Two years beforehand, Toynbee Hall had been established as a settlement in London's East End by Oxford University in order that its young lawyers, doctors and clergymen could 'live with the poor' and thereby 'bring the classes in relation'. Their purpose was to raise the morals and standard of education of the labouring classes. Alfred Milner, a close friend of Arnold Toynbee, was a devoted supporter of the Hall throughout his life.

Beveridge's mother suggested that he should model his career on Joseph Chamberlain (Harris, 1977, p 35), but Beveridge preferred other routes to social reform. After attending a recruitment meeting for Toynbee Hall in 1899, he eventually joined its staff in 1903. By 1900, Canon Samuel Barnett, who was in charge of the Hall, had come to accept Charles Booth's eventual conclusion that the chief cause of urban poverty was not weakness of character or lack of genetic worth, as Booth had first suspected, but quite simply low and irregular wages at the bottom of the Capitalist system. Beveridge set himself the task of raising the probability of employment at a decent wage for labouring men. Throughout his life he was to hold it more moral for a family to live on poor relief than to be victimised by an economic system which worked labourers for an unjustifiably low wage (Harris, 1977, p 414). Not that he advocated dependency on Welfare for one minute. As mentioned in the Introduction to Part I, Beveridge explained to his mother: "Granted that many parents now have the responsibility of feeding their children without the power of doing so (through low wages), the remedy is not to remove the responsibility but to give power" (Harris, 1977, p 55).

The outdoor labour test was still in existence in 1905, but was not being applied stringently in many workhouses. When the regimen was extremely punitive, some men would refuse work in the hope of a brief spell in the 'recalcitrant ward' or gaol. The labour yard was exclusively for men, many of whom were employed by local firms as casual labour (taken on a day at a time). They turned to the yard, if open, on days when they were not taken on. In 1903, the year Beveridge joined Toynbee Hall and the Inter-departmental Committee met, a group of organisers of charities devised a plan for the creation of funds to permit a better system for the provision of work for the casual unemployed of Stepney, Poplar, Bethnal Green and Shoreditch in London. William Beveridge worked for the Stepney joint committee, soon taking charge. The idea was to inquire into the background of applicants for work in order to help those of good character, and by collecting the facts to demonstrate the magnitude of the problem. Walter Long, President of the Local Government Board, promoted the extension of the inquiry to other parts of London, encouraging semi-official joint committees in the boroughs, coordinated by a central committee.

In early 1905 Beveridge and Samuel Barnett held a meeting at the House of Commons in which they outlined proposals for legislation to cover the establishment of local authority labour exchanges, emergency relief works, penal labour colonies for 'vagrants', and agricultural training colonies for the 'genuine unemployed'. On the terrace of the House of Commons afterwards, Beveridge took the opportunity to discuss with John Burns and other Liberal members of parliament the effects of unemployment on infant mortality and 'physical deterioration' (Harris, 1977, pp 113-14). His audience appeared largely ignorant of such matters, showing more interest in agricultural labour colonies, which Beveridge regarded as peripheral.

The winter of 1904-5 was yet another of extreme distress and public disorder. The Local Government Board quickly published a Bill to put labour exchanges and labour colonies on a firm basis, funded from the local rates. The measures were immediately denounced by some in the Conservative Party as a dangerous concession to the idea that men had an automatic 'right to work'. The Bill received strong support from the Liberal opposition, however, and the government, sensing public opinion, eventually passed the Unemployed Workmen Act in August 1905, allowing a three year trial period. Introduced by Gerald Balfour, the Act was to target the 'elite of the unemployed', as he put it. No man who had received poor relief in the previous year, and none who had ever received such relief on two occasions, was eligible for assistance under the Act.

The lone mother

The status of women under the Poor Law was particularly troublesome for the authorities. Guardians had always held powers to grant outdoor relief to able-bodied persons in exceptional circumstances, a provision used generally for respectable families who fell upon hard times when the labour yard was not open. But on 1 January 1907, of 62,240 able-bodied adults receiving outdoor relief, 59,712 (96%) were women. About 60% of unions classified single women as non-able-bodied, even if not ill, and all unions considered women with young children not to be able-bodied. As the Minority Report of 1909 put it, such women were:

> not free to engage in industrial employment, because they are occupied by the care of young children dependent upon them.... We have chosen so to organise the industrial world that the wife and children are normally supported by the industrial earnings of the husband and father, with the result that when women engage in industries their wages are habitually fixed at rates calculated to support themselves alone, without a family of children. If, by some mischance, the husband or father is withdrawn from the family group, the wife and mother is, with regard to self-support, under a double impossibility. She cannot, consistently with her legal obligation to rear her children properly, give her time and energy to wage-earning to the extent that modern competitive industry demands; and even if she could do so, she finds the woman's remuneration fixed on the basis of supporting one person, and not several. Hence it becomes practically indispensable, as it is only equitable, that there should be afforded to the mother bereft of the man ... suitable public assistance ... as to enable her to bring up the children whom the community ... still expects her to rear. (Webb and Webb, 1974, pp 19-20)

All too often the relief given was meagre, however, leaving at least 100,000 children to grow up malnourished.

National unemployment insurance and the dole, 1911-27

The difficulty for Victorians and Edwardians who disliked the Poor Law was to find a better, less undignified way of protecting the unemployed worker and his dependants and relieving them of the need to rely on charity. The eventual solution was a scheme of national insurance against unemployment in the shape of Part II of the National Insurance Act of 1911. A fund for this purpose needed to be created through the contributions of insured workers, which would not be too difficult given an initial long spell of low unemployment nationally. The government started by bringing in about 2.7 million workers, or one sixth of the national workforce, engaged in industries particularly prone to recession and lay-offs such as construction, shipbuilding and ironfounding. Dockworkers were not included.

Provided they had made sufficient contributions while in employment, unemployed workers received 7s per week for 15 weeks, after which they had to resort once more to mutual aid groups such as the Oddfellows, charity or the Poor Law. The Munitions Insurance (Part II) Act of 1916 extended unemployment insurance to civilian workers supplying the armed forces (and as usual there were problems of definition), in anticipation of serious disruption after Armistice Day, but by 1918 some two thirds of the workforce were still not covered by the national scheme. Serious disruption did indeed occur with the end of fighting, and within three weeks of Armistice Day Dr Christopher Addison extended what was an 'out of work donation' to uninsured demobilised troops so as to cover uninsured unemployed civilian workers. In addition to this payment out of central funds to the uninsured workers, there were allowances to cover the subsistence of their dependants. So arrived the 'uncovenanted benefit' or the modern ' dole' (Fraser, 1984, p 184).

The insurance principle was extended again in 1920 in response to rapidly rising unemployment, bringing into the scheme most earning less than £250 per year. Workers on the lowest pay had previously been excluded from the scheme on the grounds that they simply could not afford the weekly contribution of 2½d. Even so, servants and agricultural workers were still left uninsured, as were low paid workers in industries allowed to opt out because of the low risk of unemployment (such as banking and railways). The tragedy was that 1920 turned out to be the first year in which unemployment affected more than one million of the workforce, and the rate was not to fall below this figure again until the Second World War. With the Act of 1920 three quarters of the workforce were entitled to £1 per week for a limited period when unemployed and fully covered. The problem for the government was that long term unemployment exhausted the entitlement of so many men and women. Faced with an inability to pay out without going into debt (which it did anyway), but an unwillingness to admit defeat and fall back on the Poor Law, the government continued with its new tier of uncovenanted unemployment benefit sandwiched between insurance and outdoor relief from the Poor Law guardians. But uncovenanted benefit, lacking the insurance principle, was little more than poor relief paid out of central taxation.

In 1921 the government was forced to introduce 'proof of seeking work' as a qualification for uncovenanted benefit, and almost three million claims were disallowed on this account between 1921 and 1930. In addition, insurance benefit was reduced from £1 to 15s per week. In what was the start of the juggling we have all become used to, as governments seek to manage the problem of the unemployed, the short Labour administration of 1924 raised the benefit to 18s per week and announced that henceforth the genuinely unemployed should have access to benefits for unlimited duration while they needed State support. The Liberals forced Labour to accept a time limit of two years. To sort it all out the incoming Conservative administration appointed the Blanesburgh Committee to advise on future policy. Its report of 1927 annoyed William Beveridge by formally separating any claim to benefits from the payment of unemployment insurance contributions. Beveridge believed that this arrangement simply threw the unemployed of inefficient industries that employed casual labour, such as the docks, on to the backs of more efficient industries that kept their workers employed. He still believed that if inefficient industries could be made more efficient through the labour exchange scheme and re-training, plus public work schemes reserved for bad times in private industry, then unemployment would be much less of a national problem (Harris, 1977, pp 353-4). Beveridge was even more annoyed when Stanley Baldwin incorporated the advice of the Blanesburgh Committee into the Unemployment Insurance Act of 1927. Uncovenanted benefit was now called Transitional Benefit.

The Poor Law becomes Public Assistance, 1929

Local taxpayers continued to pay a poor rate throughout the 1920s to meet the needs of those who slipped through the net of covenanted and uncovenanted unemployment benefit. In England and Wales during 1923, for example, expenditure under the Poor Law amounted to £42 million, £37 million falling on the local rates and £2.5 million being met by government grants. In 1926 there were 2.5 million people on outdoor relief and 226,000 in Poor Law institutions. Economic conditions were bad. The guardians of Chester le Street near Durham were dismissed by government, under powers acquired that year, for paying outdoor relief to unemployed able-bodied miners in distress. In 1928-29 Poor Law expenditures were about £40 million out of the local rate, with another £33 million from central government (Board of Trade, 1932, table 69).

In 1928 Neville Chamberlain took the plunge. He recommended repeal of the system of Poor Law guardians, turning their responsibilities over to the local authorities who were instructed to constitute local Public Assistance Committees to take care of the able-bodied and non-able-bodied threatened with destitution. The Local Government Bill became law on 27 March 1929, Arthur Greenwood's move for rejection, on the grounds that it did nothing to prevent unemployment and poverty, failing. The 'seeking work test' now abolished, and the full cost of transitional payments met by the Treasury, the incoming Labour Party was soon to be appalled by the onset of the great depression. Watching funds ever more depleted by the costs of rising unemployment, Ramsay MacDonald appointed the Holman Gregory Royal Commission in November 1930 to look yet again at unemployment insurance. The General Council of the Trade Union Congress, which had not been consulted on the composition of the Royal Commission, objected strongly to its recommendations of increased contributions and smaller benefits.

Immediately following the financial crisis of 1931 and the establishment of MacDonald's National government, benefits were cut by 10% and limited to 26 weeks. Thereafter the long term unemployed had to turn to their local Public Assistance Committees, which subjected them once more to a stringent means-test of what the family (not merely the unemployed man himself) brought home. Like the defunct Poor Law boards of guardians and their unions, Local Assistance Committees differed considerably in their levels of generosity, and to the ordinary citizen the system appeared similarly mean, confused and unjust. These committees still ran what were the old workhouses under new colours, and even in the 1940s the communities still called them workhouses. Applications for relief still went before what were called 'guardians committees' who remained concerned to keep down charges on the local rates. Only the National Assistance Act of 5 July 1948 extinguished the last remnants of the Poor Law in Britain.

The legacy

This ill-fitting assemblage of fiscal intervention where there should be no intervention, and non-intervention where there should be intervention, placed the Welfare State of the following decades on the shakiest of historical foundations. The puzzle assembled remains an enigma. Rent was long ago privatised for reasons of no virtue for modern Welfare Capitalism, yet remains retained by a private monopoly, sequestered from the public domain and bundled up in red tape with the rest of that complex called land. On top of that, for no good reason, the best offered being that governments have taxed wages and interest since medieval times, the same approach is used to fund Welfare with all the distortions to the economy and frustration of purpose entailed.

No explicit theory has ever been forthcoming as to why income as wages and interest is preferable to take for social purposes than income as Rent. Political morality frowns on this state of affairs and political medicine condemns it. Aesthetically it is not what it could be. Its way of taking is disliked, and its way of giving is continually questioned. Added to that, the system is hopelessly bedevilled by a jumble of archaic attitudes inherited from the era of the Poor Law; handicapped by deep suspicions about what it is doing and about the 'worth' of those requesting its support. When even government ministers talk in a 'them and us' manner, and raise the bogey of the scrounger; when the system transfers the onus from the agency to the claimant, despite what the manuals might say; when the 'peculiar nicety' of distinguishing the 'deserving' from the 'undeserving' smacks of mutual suspicion: this is a kind of Welfare Capitalism that perpetuates economic inefficiencies, breeds disharmony and drives wedges between socio-economic classes.

To repeat John Stuart Mill (in Fletcher, 1971, p 330): "... in all cases of helping, there are two sets of consequences to be considered; the consequences of the assistance itself, and the consequences of relying on the assistance". Mill overlooked the consequences of the method of assistance. The lack of a well developed theory of what properly constitutes a Welfare political economy, which must be a very different political economy from the system of 2000 that mollifies Business-Capitalism, leaves the Welfare State on the defensive and vulnerable to subterfuge. Weighed against the endless heart-searching over 'the consequences of relying on the assistance', the lack of introspection regarding the fiscal system that does so much to create need reveals just how imbalanced the debate has been. But how can one justifiably criticise the giving classes? One cannot – until it is recalled that the injustices in holding on to what is rightfully public, and the nonsense of then attempting to repair the social damage by taking into the public domain what is rightfully private, were knowingly preferred to Rent reform by informed representatives of the giving classes a century ago. Their biased judgement has not been seriously questioned since that time. The next chapter describes the prelude to this episode in the evolution of Welfare Capitalism.

TWELVE

The English tyranny and the able-bodied employed

Ill fares the land, to hastening ills a prey,
Where wealth accumulate and men decay
(Oliver Goldsmith, *The Deserted Village*, 1770)

In one of his tracts against West Indian slavery, written in 1823, the Evangelical William Wilberforce referred to 'free British labourers'. The remark infuriated William Cobbett, with good reason, for the labour laws of England made a mockery of Wilberforce's turn of phrase. Here was the other side of that tyranny which ruled the life of the ordinary labourer, the laws which defined his status and condition when in work. Somewhere between 'in work' and 'out of work' was that standard of eligibility that Bentham discerned, a line drawn by the upper classes. Quack balms were also prescribed by the upper classes for the consequences of their law-making, more soothing for their own conscience than the suffering of the poor. In 1793 Archdeacon William Paley penned his *Reasons for contentment addressed to the labouring part of the British public*. The poor were mislead into believing themselves worse off than the rich, wrote Paley. Their disadvantages in this life were more apparent than real. Frugality is a pleasure. To make ends meet successfully with little to hand is an entertainment lost to those who have in abundance. All that a poor man's child requires is 'industry and innocence'. With health in body and mind, and an industrious nature, his parents need not be afraid for him. Who would be the rich, addicted to indulgences to the extent that all desire is dead? ... and so on (Hammond and Hammond, 1932, pp 232-4).

To this comforting reasoning the Evangelicals added their interpretation of the Christian purpose. Christianity taught the poor humility, patience, that "their lowly path hath been allotted to them by the hand of God; that it is their part faithfully to discharge its duties, and contentedly bear its inconveniences ...". So wrote Wilberforce in his *Practical view of the prevailing religious system of professed Christians in the higher and middle classes in this country, contrasted with real Christianity*, published in 1797 (Hammond and Hammond, 1932, pp 231-2). Common law and statute law, in defending the constitution and arranging the population into the higher orders, middle orders and lower orders, were in conformity with God's law, preached the Evangelicals. Men of a Radical turn of mind, who opposed such teachings, were therefore irreligious and anti-establishment by definition. In the troubled period following the passage of the 1815 Corn Law, parliament passed a Seditious Meetings Act which prescribed the death penalty for all who refused to disperse when ordered to leave assemblies aimed at reform of the established Church or State. At that time, Anglican churches were in short supply in the fast-growing towns of the industrial revolution. Arthur Young, Secretary of the Board of Agriculture, asked: "Where are they (the poor) to learn the doctrines of that truly excellent religion which exhorts to content and to submission to the higher powers?" (Coupland, 1923, p 426). Eventually responding, parliament voted £1 million in 1818 for church building. As Lord Liverpool told the House of Lords, the prevalence of dangerous political influences in the new industrial centres was one reason to regard the New Churches Bill as 'the most important measure' he had ever submitted for their lordships' consideration.

The more questioning among the poor of the labouring classes saw their life rather differently. To them the origin of their poverty was no theological mystery. In *The traveller* (1764), Goldsmith had written that: "Laws grind the poor, and rich men rule the law" (line 386). Rich men were by and large landed men, and economists were beginning to identify their wealth with Rent. Back in 1647 during the debates of the Council of the Parliamentary Army, it was asserted that no person had any right to a share in the determination of the affairs of England, ie a right to the parliamentary franchise, unless he was a landed freeman (Kennedy, 1913, p 92). This was still the rule in 1800. In essence, tenants and labourers who lacked any fixed interest in land were in a position similar to that of a resident alien. Though English by birth, they lived and worked for their subsistence in their native land on terms set down strictly in law by the landed class. This tyranny against the lowly born had a long history which we can pick up in the 14th century. We have examined the oppression of those without Rent when out of work. Here we examine their condition in work.

Poor labouring families knew from bitter experience the consequences of poverty, hunger, disease and death of the breadwinner, long before William Farr accumulated the statistics. In December 1834, the Society for Promoting Christian Knowledge included in its penny paper, the *Saturday Magazine*, an extract from the *Philosophical Journal* entitled 'Life Prolonged by Civilization'. Reporting that the annual death rate in England, Germany and France had fallen in recent years by 700,000, owing to 'the social amelioration in the three countries', the article explained: "The life of man is thus not only embellished in its course by the advancement of civilisation, but is extended by it, and rendered less doubtful" (less insecure) (*Saturday Magazine*, 20 December, 1834, p 238). For some less doubtful than others, retorted the poor.

The Black Death and the Statute of Labourers

A series of famines and epidemics of plague, including the Black Death of 1348, reduced England's population by about 1.5 million. The medieval economy collapsed and Rent with it, while the labour market shifted distinctly in favour of the labourer. Landholders responded by using their political power to turn market conditions back to their advantage. What they did shaped labour relations for centuries to come, leaving a permanent impression on the nation's judicial system. The Statute of Labourers of 1349 set the tone:

> Edward by the Grace of God, etc, ... Greeting. Because a great part of the people, and especially the workmen and servants, late died of the pestilence, many seeing the necessity of masters, and great scarcity of servants, will not serve unless they receive excessive wages, and some rather willing to beg in idleness than by labour to get their living; We, considering the grievous incommodities, which of the lack especially of ploughmen and such labourers may hereafter come, have upon deliberation and treaty with the prelates and the nobles, and learned men assisting us, of their mutual counsel ordained:

> That every man and woman of our Realm of England, of what condition he be, free or bond, able in body, and within the age of threescore years, not living in merchandize, nor exercising any craft, nor having of his own whereof he may live, nor proper land, about whose tillage he may himself occupy, and not serving any other, if he in convenient service, his estate considered, be required to serve, he shall be bounden to serve him which so shall him require; and take only wages, living, meed, or salary, which were accustomed to be given in places where he oweth to serve, the 20th year of our reign of England (ie 1347), or five or six

other common years next before ...; and if any such man or woman, being required to serve, will not the same do, that proved by two true men before the sheriff (or the bailiffs ...) ... he shall anon be taken by them ... and committed to the next gaol, there to remain under strict keeping, till he find surety to serve in the form aforesaid.

Item, Because that many beggars, as long as they may live by begging, do refuse to labour ... none upon the said pain of imprisonment shall, under the colour of pity or alms, give any thing to such, which may labour, or presume to favour them, so that thereby they may be compelled to labour for their necessary living. (*Statutes of the Realm*, 1826, vol 1, pp 307-9)

The Ordinances and Statutes of 1349 and 1351 attempted to freeze wages at pre-1348 levels. To refuse to work as required, if a labourer, was a crime punishable by imprisonment. To assist the 'able-bodied' unemployed to survive without labour was also a crime. To attempt to take 'excessive wages' as defined by statute was a wrongful act against the employer, for which the court devised a specific remedy.

The justice of the peace and wage bargaining

From about 1250 the king's court had accepted a class of offence called trespass, where 'trespass', as in the Lord's prayer, meant simply a wrongful act. The writ of trespass originally alleged that the defendant had performed a wrongful deed *by force of arms* against the plaintiff's person or against his land. The remedy used by the court was compensation, not primarily to cover damage done (which might be difficult to assess), but rather as the price necessary to persuade the plaintiff not to take the law into his own hands, thereby achieving the court's purpose, the maintenance of the king's peace. Many cases of trespass did not involve actual violence, however, and to solve this problem a new form of writ was created known as 'trespass on the case'. This writ described the particulars of the special case, opening with a clause beginning "Whereas ...". It was the writ of trespass on the case to which the landlords turned when the labour market went against them, and Rent of their land collapsed.

    The Statute of Labourers of 1349 made the 'taking of excessive wages' a wrongful act against the landlord, for which the remedy was a writ of action on the case. The legislation generated by the labour laws of 1349 and 1351 so overloaded the courts that a new type of official had to be created to deal with the situation, drawn from among the landed themselves. There were already local officials with policing functions known as the 'keepers' of the peace, and these were now given powers to judge offences as 'justices' of the peace; specifically they could deliver judgement and impose sentence under the new labour Laws. After 1361 these men, assisted by judges and serjeants of the central courts, were given permanent responsibility for enforcement of criminal law in the shires. The quarter sessions of the justices became the courts for an appreciable proportion of cases of felony and trespass brought in medieval England. Wage bargaining was in this way shifted from the custom of the manor court into the realm of the common law provided by the king's court (Ormrod, 1995, pp 109-15).

The new legislation, though ruthlessly applied in many cases, largely failed to prevent an escalation of wages in the years after the Black Death. Villeins refused either to resettle the lord's land as the court had ordered unless the rent was acceptable, or to work to the lord's satisfaction unless the wages merited the effort. Nevertheless, by the middle of the 14th century the landed interest had secured a firm hold on the State system of justice in order to maintain their own interests. The justices of the peace displaced the ancient right of the villagers to oversee their own law and order through the constable, the watch and the hue and cry, as formalised in the Statute of Winchester of 1285. Justice came to be seen by labouring people as guided by the self-interest and influence of the landed classes. So intense did the resentment become that the justices were repeatedly assaulted. Sir John Cavendish, chief justice of the king's bench, was decapitated at Lakenheath in Suffolk and his head paraded in Bury St Edmunds.

To add insult to injury, unlike the old system, the new commissions of the peace required money to gain access to justice, an expense beyond the reach of many. The imposition of a poll tax in 1381 brought frustrations to boiling point, the whole episode culminating in the 'Peasant Rising'. Wat Tyler led men of Kent into London on 11th and 12th June, demanding that there was no true law but 'the Law of Winchester' (Ormrod, 1995, p 116). Outbreaks of violence occurred in Essex, East Anglia and Cambridgeshire, reaching north into the Wirral and Yorkshire. The revolt was, however, soon suppressed by force and accomplished little except a place in English history as a working class rising against aristocratic oppression, rural and urban (riots occurred in St Albans, Norwich, Beverley and York, for example). The new system survived. The Statute of Labourers gave rise to countless actions on the case in subsequent centuries for breach of contract and conspiracy in labour conflicts between master and men.

Parliament sets wage rates, 1388

In 1388 further legislation set a maximum scale for agricultural wages. When this soon failed, from 1390 onwards the justices of the peace were given powers to make local assessments. In 1445 the law returned to a revised scale of national wage rates, adjusted in 1514 to allow for inflation in prices. A long term upward trend in prices created increasing pressure on wages, accentuating labour discontent. When a great influenza epidemic in 1557 and 1558 raised pressures further by temporarily reducing the available workforce, the landed classes suffered another bout of nerves and resorted once again to the powers of their parliamentary representation. They brought in the Statute of Artificers in 1563, a major piece of early Elizabethan legislation.

The purposes of the statute of 1563 were to enforce a universal obligation to work, re-iterate the law on labour relations going back to the Statute of Labourers, and emphasise the application of these principles to all workers, not merely those in agriculture. All able persons were obliged to seek employment and accept any regular work offered to them. Unmarried persons under 30 years of age were to serve any employer who had need of their labour. Justices of the peace were empowered to require men in all occupations to turn their hand to the land at harvest time, or else spend a night in the stocks. The only exceptions were children under 12 years, men over 60 years and women over 40, a 'gentleman born', and an heir either to land worth £10 a year in rent or to goods worth £40, already in employment or attending school or university.

The Statute of Artificers placed a duty on justices in town and country to fix wages by local assessment. The agreed rates were returned to the Lord Chancellor in London who arranged for printed royal proclamations to be displayed in all market towns by Michaelmas, the traditional season for hiring labourers. Hours of work in summer were fixed from five in the morning to seven or eight in the evening, with up to two and a half hours for breaks. In winter the hours were from dawn to sunset. There was to be a penalty of one penny (1d) for each hour not worked (average pay was about ½d per hour). The Act extended the requirement of apprenticeship beyond the towns (where craftsmen and traders had operated the practice for generations) into the rural areas to cover even farming (Youings, 1991, pp 291-6). Finally, a statute of 1566 confirmed the laws of 1464 and 1512 in forbidding payment of wages in kind, and the Poor Laws of 1598 and 1601 extended apprenticeship to pauper children under the direction of the parish overseers.

Under the Statute of Artificers justices tended to peg wages year after year at the old rates, giving way only when protests and agitation reached alarming levels. Nevertheless, employers would pay their workers over the odds when that was what was needed, and much rural work continued on a casual labour basis. Essentially the Act was there in reserve for the employer, should he see advantage in its application; he was not obliged to demand its enforcement if it suited him otherwise.

The justice of the peace and industrial relations

The Industrial Revolution was crowding labouring men and women together as never before, sharpening their sense of shared grievances against the tyranny in the terms on which they had been forced to work since medieval times. They seized the opportunity to associate, or 'combine', in common cause, much to the consternation of many employers. Trespass on the case did not help, because there was no clear case to answer in law against combination against the employer, though there were 40 statutes dealing with combination against the State. There had been royal proclamations and acts against combinations in specific trades in earlier years (for example, tailors in 1721), and combinations were popularly held to be illegal throughout the 18th century, but this law proved weak and its effectiveness short-lived. The legal uncertainties, taken together with fear of the spread of revolution from France, created much nervousness among the masters of the new factories. The massacre of more than 1,000 imprisoned notables in Paris in September 1792, with 260 human carcasses heaped on the Pont du Change, was still spine-chilling to recall (Carlyle, undated, p 427). All European ruling classes had been horrified at the trial and regicide by guillotine of Louis XVI that same winter.

In April 1799 the master millwrights of London petitioned parliament for help to prevent their journeymen associating in an attempt to improve conditions of work:

> ... a dangerous Combination has for some time existed among the journeymen millwrights ... for enforcing a general increase in their wages, preventing the employment of such journeymen as refused to join in their confederacy ... (T)he masters have as often been obliged to

submit ...A demand of a further advance of wages ... not being complied
with, the men ... have refused to work.... (I)n support of the said
Combination ... the journeymen have established a general fund, and
raised subscriptions ... (I)n case of non-compliance, the different
workshops (where their demands are resisted) are wholly deserted by
the men, and other journeymen are prohibited from applying for work
until the master millwrights are brought into compliance, and the
journeymen, who have thus thrown themselves out of employ, receive
support in the meantime from their general fund.... (Hammond and
Hammond, 1932, pp 115-17)

The petition was referred to a committee, who sought leave to introduce
a Bill to protect the master millwrights and give justices of the peace
powers to regulate the millwrights' wages. During the debate William
Wilberforce suggested that a measure 'to prevent unlawful combinations
of workmen' in general, not simply millwrights, would be desirable (Pelling,
1976, p 16). The readings of the Bill to restrain millwrights proceeded,
only Sir Francis Burdett and Benjamin Hobhouse opposing. Sir Francis
argued that there was seldom a combination without great grievance or
provocation. He quoted Adam Smith's summary of the situation in 1796:

The workmen desire to get as much, the masters to give as little as
possible. The former are disposed to combine in order to raise, the
latter in order to lower the wages of labour. It is not, however, difficult
to foresee which of the two parties must, upon all ordinary occasions,
have the advantage in the dispute, and force the other into compliance
with their terms. The masters, being few in number, can combine much
more easily; and the law, besides, authorises, or at least does not prohibit
their combinations, while it prohibits those of the workmen. We have
no Acts of parliament against combining to lower the price of work,
but many against combining to raise it. (Smith, 1986, p 169)

The reasoning of the opposition was to no avail. The Bill passed the
Commons but was dropped in the Lords owing to the introduction of a
more general Bill along Wilberforce's lines by William Pitt as Chancellor
of the Exchequer.

The Bill against combinations in general was passed with remarkable
haste, 24 days from introduction to royal assent. Under the Combination
Act of 1799 any workman associating with another to raise wages or
reduce working hours could be brought before a single magistrate. On

conviction the maximum penalty was three months imprisonment or two months hard labour. It mattered not if this magistrate happened to be the workmen's employer, or a master in the same trade. Justices of the peace as landholders had for centuries convicted labourers for challenging landholders. The Combination Act took this as a precedent for the industrial age. Many justices were by now both landholders and businessmen.

The same penalties awaited the labourer convicted of incitement to strike, or of withdrawal of his own labour. An involvement of any sort in a meeting called to consider wages or hours of work was made illegal (Hammond and Hammond, 1932, p 120). Petitions against the Act flowed in by the score, one from Liverpool pointing out that no workman was safe discussing his employment. Others stressed the exposure of workers to the risk of false accusations by those in league with the employer for profit. In 1805, Colonel Fletcher of Bolton, coal owner and local justice of the peace, sent his bill for £123 to the Home Office for re-imbursement. This money was in recompense for the wages of spies in his employment, used to watch a 'combination' of weavers. Numerous such bills went to the Home Office in those days for spies which it employed either directly or indirectly through officers of the local militia, clerks of the courts or the justices. To earn their living these men would often lie to the authorities, telling them what they wanted to hear, even when the sentence for the unfortunate innocent might be transportation or hanging. Spies, searches and interceptions of the mail for suppression of labour movements were not stopped until Robert Peel entered the Home Office in 1822.

Under the Combination Act appeals to a higher court were expressly forbidden, even when the justice of the peace had been the master. There was a right of appeal to the quarter sessions of the justices, but the costs incurred were beyond most working men. Another clause in the Act granted justices the power to permit an employer to take on unqualified men if the journeymen refused to work for 'reasonable wages'. This made nonsense of apprenticeship.

The oppression in the Combination Act of 1799 was abominable. Doubtless the fear of combination engendered by the French revolution had provoked some to these extremes, but parliament went too far even for its own time. For reasons not altogether altruistic, Liverpool was at the forefront of objectors. In July 1800, Tory and Whig members for the city, Colonel Gascoyne and General Tarleton respectively, introduced an amending Bill. The case for the labourer was put eloquently by the dramatist Richard Sheriden, a parliamentarian since 1780: "A more intolerable mass of injustice had never entered on the Statute Book" (Hammond and Hammond, 1932, p 125). The result was the Combination Act of 1800, which raised to two the number of justices to try the case. Justices involved in the trade in question were forbidden to sit on the bench.

In 1823 a spinner named Ryding hit upon the idea of having the grievances of his trade taken to a court higher than that of the justices. If he wounded his employer Horrocks he would be taken before judge and jury, and there he could expose Horrocks' attempt to impose a reduction in Wages. William Cobbett reported the trial in his weekly journal, the *Political Register* (30 August, 1823), highlighting two features of the Combination Act. The first was that, proof of combination for wages being difficult to obtain, under the Act the accused were compelled to give evidence against themselves or their associates. Refusal meant prison without bail. Secondly, although the Act of 1800 forbade combinations of employers, any master found guilty was treated lightly. Unlike the worker, the master could not be called upon to give evidence against himself or his associates. If convicted, the master's maximum penalty was not two months hard labour but a fine of £20, the sum needed by the labourer simply to bring his case to appeal in the quarter sessions (Hammond and Hammond, 1932, pp 127-9).

In evidence taken by the Committee on Artisans and Machinery in 1824, Francis Place, a tailor, pointed out the virtual impossibility of workmen prosecuting their employers. So little used was the law against the employer that many were not even aware that the Act forbade them to combine. Employers considered the Act there to be used at their discretion, and that was how it operated. Place's ally in parliament was John Hume, who led the Select Committee. Many witnesses stressed how the labour laws created much ill-feeling, while failing to suppress combinations of workers. The Committee was of the opinion "that masters and men should be freed from such restrictions, as regards the rate of wages and hours of working, and be left at perfect liberty to make such agreements as they eventually think proper" (Pelling, 1976, p 21). The result was the Combination Law of that year, repealing all statutes against combination going back to medieval times, and allowing combinations of labour provided they were peaceful.

Combinations came to light immediately across the country. One outcome was Chartism, a national effort by organised working men and women to secure a vote for themselves and thereby raise their standard of living through democratic means. The demands of the Chartist movement were entirely political, rooted in the belief that enfranchisement would bring to the working classes what up to then it had brought only to the enfranchised of the upper middle classes and aristocracy. The Chartists trusted in democratisation for the realisation of justice. In 1835, three years after Lord Russell's Reform Bill (see below), a committee of the General Working Men's Association of London, with William Lovett as leader, drew up the six points of the People's Charter, one of which was the abolition of the property qualification for prospective parliamentary candidates enshrined in the Act of 1710, in order that every voter should be eligible to stand (Wood, 1982, p 131). A revised general property qualification, introduced in 1838, was finally repealed in 1858.

The plight of the labourer forced his wife and young children into work. On 15 May 1830 William Wilberforce presided for the last time at the Anti-slavery Society, having been retired from parliament for five years by that time. Yorkshire County returned four Abolitionists in the general election of that year, among them Henry Brougham, and the abolition of slavery in British colonies was only three years away. Yet during Wilberforce's political career the infamous system of child labour had taken hold of the mills, prompting Richard Oastler's famous letter on 'Yorkshire Slavery' in the *Leeds Mercury* of 16 October 1830:

> Let truth speak out ... thousands of our fellow-creatures ... the miserable inhabitants of a Yorkshire town (Yorkshire now represented in parliament by the giant of anti-slavery principles) are at this very moment existing in a state of slavery, more horrid than are the victims of that hellish system 'colonial slavery' ... The very streets which receive droppings of an 'Anti-slavery Society' are every morning wet by the tears of innocent victims at the accursed shrine of avarice, who are compelled (not by the cart-whip of the negro slave-driver) but by the dread of the equally appalling thong or strap of the over-looker, to hasten ... to those magazines of British infantile slavery – the worsted mills in the town and neighbourhood of Bradford!!! (Fraser, 1984, pp 254-5)

Here was the launch of Britain's 'factory movement', though Sir Robert Peel's Health and Morals of Apprentices Act of 1802 had represented an earlier false start. This legislation referred exclusively to exploitation of pauper children in the new water-driven cotton mills, and Wilberforce's attempt to extend its cover to other manufacturers and all children proved unsuccessful.

The suffering of the unenfranchised poor in 19th century Britain was appalling by all accounts. Engel's description of the dreadful slum conditions in England's cities, published in Germany in 1845, did not appear in Britain in translation until 1892 (Engels, 1993, pp 36-86). On the Marquis of Ailesbury's estate, the steward of Savernake highlighted the horrifying conditions of the rural labourers. Their homes were thatched hovels, with in extreme cases persons of both sexes sleeping 12 or more in one room (Thompson, 1958–9). Military records of the body height of recruits indicated that the nutritional status of the working classes actually declined between 1800 and 1850, and that although significant improvement followed, by 1914 male height had recovered only to where it had been in 1815 (Floud et al, 1990, p 319).

The labourers' struggle against tyranny after 1810

Over 70 offences were made capital during the reign of George III. Even petty theft could result in transportation to the colonies or hanging. After the sentencing of a child of 10 years to death in 1800 for theft at Chelmsford Post Office, protests were such that the sentence was commuted to 14 years of servitude in Grenada, West Indies. A list of prisoners sent up from the Chester Assizes in 1818 included a boy of 14 sentenced to hanging for stealing a silver watch and two bank notes, and a cooper who was transported for life for stealing a handkerchief (Hammond and Hammond, 1932, pp 75-6). Death was the penalty for felling a tree or impersonating a Greenwich pensioner. So barbarous was the law that some judges strived to procure an acquittal, and many juries perjured themselves rather than find the accused guilty. So many were the cases brought to court, however, that numerous of the poor were hanged or transported.

Against seemingly impossible odds, the labouring classes gradually clawed their way up through emerging institutions such as the cooperative societies, mechanics institutes, Methodist chapels, trade unions, and specialist political clubs. Their leaders acquired literacy skills through the Church schools and went on to speak out against such oppressions as the Combination Laws. But the popular cheap press, such as John Doherty's *The voice of the people*, was handicapped by the newspaper tax, viewed by government as a tax on the luxuries of the upper classes. Between 1831 and 1836, 500 persons were imprisoned for failing to pay stamp duty on papers they had published and sold. These duties were gradually reduced after 1836 and repealed altogether in 1855 (Hammond and Hammond,

1932, p 250). Many in parliament were unhappy, arguing that a repeal of the tax on soap would do labourers more good than cheap newspapers.

Just how difficult was the struggle for self-betterment was illustrated by a copy book in which the secretary of a fledgling society of working men had practised the rudiments of writing. Confiscated by a justice of the peace, it ended in the archives of the Home Office, obviously considered a threat by the authorities (Hammond and Hammond, 1932, p 251). What hope had the ordinary working man for his wife, his children or himself, in the face of such tyranny? Lord Ashley was their champion in parliament, but his repeated efforts on their behalf in the 1830s and 1840s were all to fail in the face of Tory opposition. Charles Dickens was so furious at this obstructionism in the name of laissez-faire that in 1841 he fired off to the *Examiner* his satirical version of 'The fine old English gentleman', of which the following is part (Johnson, 1986, p 185):

> The good old laws were garnished well with gibbets, whips, and chains,
> With fine old English penalties, and fine old English pains,
> With rebel heads, and seas of blood once hot in rebel veins;
> For all these things were requisite to guard the rich old gains
> Of the fine old English Tory times;
> Soon may they come again!

Free trade and the landholder

'Those who have got', as Lord Salisbury described the landholders, were also seeking reforms in those years, not for others so much as for themselves; for they had got into a mess. *The Economist* of June 1868 described what had happened (*The Economist*, 13 June, 1868, pp 10-11). In the 150 years or more since Orlando Bridgman had devised strict settlement, much landed property had become encumbered by debt and placed in the hands of trustees. Under the strict settlement (see Chapter Nine) the tenant had only an interest for life, the remainder being pledged to the eldest son, born or unborn. Debts had accumulated as charges raised on mortgages at interest were taken on to support the younger children. This interest had to be met from the estate's rents, often excessive because the family had awarded itself too high an income, though deemed necessary to meet social expectations, electioneering expenses and purchase of additional land. In this way each successive generation inherited debt, the only way out being either to raise the rents or make a good marriage.

Consequently, the institutions profiting from the Rent were those who held the landholders' debts, including the banks. Through the strict settlement, landholders were boxed in because their ancestors had rendered them powerless to sell the right to Rent.

David Ricardo was at the peak of his financial career in the Stock Exchange between 1811 and 1815. The national debt was soaring to meet the cost of war with France, and war loans to the government reached nearly £50 million in 1813. Another loan brought out in 1815, 'the Waterloo Loan', made Ricardo's fortune. He had bought just before the famous battle when the price of stock was low, and watched its value soar when news of Wellington's success reached London. With this fortune he purchased Gatcombe Park in Gloucestershire, the owner of which was in mortgaged debt through extravagant building. What Ricardo bought was not simply land and buildings, but Land. The Deed of Covenant read that the owner: "doth bargain and sell all that Manor or Lordship ... of Hampton, otherwise Minchinhampton ... and all the rights, royalties, members, appurtenances thereof in the County of Gloucester ... all that building containing several rooms ... and the benefits from the tolls paid and arising from wool and yarn brought to the Yarn Market in Minchinhampton ... all the warren called Amberley ..." (etc). In all the Manor with 5,000 acres cost him £60,000. Now he had the privileges that went with land, and soon found himself High Sheriff for Gloucestershire.

Ricardo went on to negotiate his largest investment in a mortgage made to Francis Dukinfield Astley of Cheshire. Astley too had spent extravagantly, beyond the rents of his estates, and in 1819 Ricardo advanced to him more than £150,000. With that money was constructed the town of Stalybridge, sitting on the richest coal seam in the area. As the coal mines multiplied so did the Rent and the wealth of Astley and Ricardo. Finally, by advancing another Irish landholder in debt, Lord Portarlington, £25,000 on mortgage, Ricardo was able to purchase a seat in parliament for £4,000, entering the House of Commons in 1819 (Weatherall, 1976). Here he developed his views on the Corn Laws, about which he had first written in 1815.

David Ricardo and *The Economist* told landholders that they had moved from military Feudalism into a 'modern Feudalism', to the detriment of trade and agriculture, hence Rent and their rents from tenants. The attitude of the landed was completely out of keeping with the laissez-faire economics of an industrial age, as evidenced by their enactment of the Corn Laws and other misguided restrictions meant to protect their interests. Farmers had prospered during the French wars, and their landlords responded by raising rents by maybe 90% (Thompson, 1963). In 1812 and 1813 poor harvests had caused the price of farm produce and bread to soar. This profitability encouraged landholders to enclose commons and waste lands of relatively poor quality (see below), some three million acres being converted in this way between 1789 and 1815 by private Acts of parliament (Gayer et al, 1953, vol 1, p 129n). Then immediately after Napoleon's abdication in April 1814 foreign producers of corn felt safe to ship their stocks to England. The economy went into recession, and corn prices halved. Landlords who had speculated in enclosures found themselves with interest on their new loans but a severe decline in income. They refused to drop the rents despite the tenants' hardships, throwing many into bankruptcy. In response, the Tory government introduced the Corn Law of 1815 in an attempt to prop up prices and save the landholder. The lowest selling price of corn needed to survive comfortably was estimated to be £4 a quarter. Therefore the ports were closed to foreign corn for three-monthly periods when the average selling price of corn during the previous six weeks had fallen below this figure. The people had expected the peace to deliver cheaper bread. To have the price of corn fall, only to watch it forced up again by their own government, provoked outrage. For centuries laws of this type had been an integral part of the nation's mercantile system, but to be imposed in that way after so much tolerance of the adversities of war was too much. William Wilberforce was one who spoke in favour of the Corn Bill on 10 March 1815, believing that to protect the landed interest was to protect the nation's preparedness for future hostilities. Fear of reprisal after his speech was so great that a sergeant, four soldiers and an officer of the peace were immediately stationed in his house.

David Ricardo told the House of Commons that its Corn Laws were folly. By restricting the supply of corn, and creating an artificially high domestic price, landlords were encouraged to bring poor land under cultivation. Since this land would then realise Rent, all rents and land prices would rise in response, thereby reducing the return to tenant farmers and driving labour off the land and on to the Poor Law. The landholder's income would rise, tying up wealth for his own use instead of releasing it for productive purposes. The landlords and their representatives in government were unimpressed by these arguments, claiming that the commotion was simply to force down corn prices, hence the price of bread, and hence the wage that the industrialist paid to his worker. The

Corn Law's enactment ushered in seven years of Tory rule marked by terrible repression of the working classes.

The Economist and its campaign for free trade

The Economist, also titled *The Political, Commercial, Agricultural, and Free Trade Journal*, printed its prospectus and preliminary number to volume one in August 1843. It campaigned for free trade, claiming that the Corn Laws had set one class (industry and labour) against another (land). While science, capital, commercial enterprise and labour were actively seeking ways to benefit all, proclaimed the journal, the landowning class had enacted self-interested legislation through "ignorance, prejudice and short-sighted selfishness" (*The Economist*, August, 1843, pp 3-14). It praised William Huskisson for his "partial triumph over the ignorance and prejudice which ruled" when he attempted to introduce a sliding scale of duties in 1827, only to be thwarted by the Duke of Wellington.

By 1843 those in the free trade camp had had enough. A bad harvest in 1838 was followed by more than three years of economic recession, but the Corn Laws were still in place. *The Economist* blamed these laws for the recessions and their damage to the economy. Its writers claimed that high prices for corn lowered the demand for other goods and services by working people on low wages. This threw men out of work in manufacturing, wholesale and retail businesses. There was less money to import foreign goods, precipitating recession among importers and shippers. Eventually the 'knock on' effect must hit landholders, despite their protective legislation. The remedy, proclaimed *The Economist*, was to raise the demand for goods and services, which was only possible by extending Britain's markets abroad. To export, however, Britain needed to import in exchange, which meant freeing trade from the restrictions of the Corn Laws and import duties.

Robert Peel, Prime Minister of the Conservative Government of 1841-46, was gradually persuaded of the sense of these arguments, but he feared the grip of the landholders on his party. Gladstone had already decided that the Corn Laws must be repealed. Then in 1845 came news that potato blight, which had started in the United States, had struck Ireland. The Irish famine set in, but the English harvest had been poor and little corn was available for Ireland. If expensive bread forced the English into more reliance on potatoes, thought Peel, the situation would be grave. Thus amid political turmoil, Peel repealed the Corn Laws and reduced duties on many manufactured articles in 1846.

Enfranchisement and land: I

Slowly but surely, during the 19th century that bundle of rights and privileges termed land began to show signs of loosening – just a little. The incorporeal hereditaments covered by the Law of Property Act of 1925 were not altogether those which had existed in 1825. Most momentously, the red tape had been slackened sufficiently for two privileges to be released. The political franchise and the right to sit in the House of Commons came to be shared among those without a stake in land, though for many years the shares were most unequal. The Reform Act of 1832 came into being only because some among the landed were willing to acknowledge that when that bundle had been put together certain lasting injustices had been inflicted on others. Prominent among these new thinkers was Lord John Russell.

Lord John Russell, the son of a duke, was unusual for his class in his enthusiasm for reform and empathy with the middle classes. His origins illustrated well how inherited land came so frequently at the whim of a monarch's patronage. Hugh du Rozel had crossed from Normandy with William the Conqueror. Two hundred years later the first John Russell was among the landed of Dorset. William Russell was a member of parliament in 1307, and Sir John Russell was Speaker of the House of Commons in the 15th century. Sir John's son, the third John Russell, was cousin to the sheriff of Dorset, Sir Thomas Trenchard. A storm at sea in 1506 forced Philip, Archduke of Austria, to take refuge in Weymouth, leaving Sir Thomas with an unexpected guest who did not speak English. The sheriff therefore sent for Squire Russell who spoke Spanish, and Philip took a liking to him. Travelling with the Archduke to London, John Russell met Henry VII who was likewise impressed, and took him into service. In this way John Russell rose to Earl of Bedford, and under 'grants of inheritance' from Henry VIII and Edward VI, the lands of Tavistock and Woborn abbeys passed into the family possessions.

Lord John Russell was born in Mayfair in 1792. He acquired unorthodox views for his class as a result of his father's decision not to send him to Oxford or Cambridge but to the University of Edinburgh. There Professors John Playfair and Dugald Stewart shaped the young lord's ideas of justice and virtue. While travelling in Minorca, Lord John received a letter in which his father stated his intention to ensure for his son a seat in the House of Commons (Lord John was not yet 21). The House which Lord John entered in 1813 was riddled with corruption. Ninety members were returned by 46 districts in each of which there were fewer than 50 electors, and 70 members were returned by 35 places with hardly any electors at all. The Duke of Bedford himself controlled the nine electors at Camelford. Bribery and corruption in the shires was notorious.

Many had already spoken out in parliament against the level of corruption, not least William Pitt the elder. Old Sarum (nothing but a green mound which returned two members) was in the pocket of his family, and it was by this route that Pitt had entered the House of Commons at the age of 23. Even so, he championed parliamentary reform in his later years, denouncing the borough representation as a 'mortified limb' of the constitution. The Whig statesman Charles James Fox was of like mind, having declared in 1796 that: "The voice of the representatives of the people must prevail over the executive ministers of the Crown; the people must be restored to their just rights" (Reid, 1895, p 25). In 1792 the Society of the Friends of the People was formed, consisting of Mr Lambton (father of the first Earl of Durham), Mr (later Sir James) Mackintosh, Mr Richard Sheridan, Mr (later Lord) Erskine, Mr Charles (later Earl) Grey, and more than 20 other members of parliament. In the country, men of a Radical turn of mind were also agitating for reform, including Major John Cartwright, brother of Lord John Russell's tutor at Woburn Abbey, and originator of the cry 'one man, one vote' (Reid, 1895, p 26). William Cobbett was another powerful advocate of reform, stating his case through his *Political Register*.

When returned in 1819 as member for Tavistock, Russell spoke out against electoral corruption and inequalities. Manchester, Birmingham, Leeds and Sheffield had no parliamentary representation, and the landed interest meant to keep it that way, regarding the cities as hot-beds of sedition and unfit for a say in national affairs. Turbulent meetings in the cities were common, demanding political representation. Cartwright advised that the cities send eminent representatives to petition parliament. Birmingham selected Sir Charles Wolseley, and Manchester's citizens met on 16 August 1819 to initiate a similar course of action. In response the magistrates of Lancashire sent in the cavalry to disperse the 50,000 citizens gathered on St Peter's Field to hear the Radical Henry Hunt, and in the ensuing panic 11 were killed and 400 injured. Hatred around the country after this 'Peterloo massacre' reached new heights, inflamed by the Prince Regent's praise for the justices of the peace and military. The government cracked down, ruling that no meeting of more than 50 people was to be held without six days notice to a justice of the peace; even then only freeholders and local citizens were allowed to attend.

Russell repeatedly introduced proposals for electoral reform, all to be defeated. On 26 May 1826, Russell's Bill for the discovery and suppression of bribery in elections was abandoned owing to the weight of opposition. Despite defeats, the unrepresented towns were increasingly seeing him as their champion. The Tory party under Lord Liverpool was wilfully defiant, and Liverpool's sudden stroke on 18 February 1827 did little to change matters. When Russell proposed in 1828 that Manchester should be given the seats of a rotten Cornish borough, Penryn, the House of Lords once more refused; the seats were part of the bundle of land. The Duke of Wellington, head of the Tory administration of 1827, declared approvingly: "I see in 30 members for the rotten boroughs 30 men, I don't care of what party, who would preserve the state of property as it is." The first parliament of William IV assembled on 26 October 1830 and in the debate on the king's speech, a few days later, Wellington made his historic statement in reply to Earl Grey of the Friends of the People:

> "I am not prepared to bring forward any measure of the description alluded to by the noble lord. I am not only not prepared to bring forward any measure of this nature (electoral reform), but I will at once declare that, as far as I am concerned, as long as I hold any station in the government of the country, I shall always feel it my duty to resist such measures when proposed by others."

This declaration of perfection as he saw it created agitated excitement in the Lords, causing Wellington to whisper aside to a colleague: "What can I have said to have made so great a disturbance?" The reply came back: "You have announced the fall of your government, that is all." He went on 16 November and the king sent for Earl Grey, who made clear that his acceptance of office was on condition that parliamentary reform would be a priority for his Cabinet (Reid, 1895, p 61).

Charles Grey had a daughter who married the son of Mr Lambton of the Friends of the People in 1816. John George Lambton headed one of the oldest landed families in the north of England, and he too entered parliament at 21. His views on reform earned him the popular sobriquet 'Radical Jack', and he took his ideas to the Lords as Lord Durham in 1828. Grey now had Durham in his Cabinet, and Russell in the Commons. Durham and Russell worked with Sir James Graham and Lord Duncannon to frame the measures which Russell introduced to the House of Commons on 1 March 1831. The country was alive with excitement, but the opposition resorted to a mixture of ridicule, horror and despair at what they were hearing. Asked Russell: "Would not ... a foreigner be much astonished if he were taken to a green mound, and informed that it sent two members to the British parliament; if he were shown a stone wall, and told that it also sent two members to the British parliament; or, if he walked into a park, without the vestige of a dwelling, and was told that it, too, sent two members to the British parliament?" (Reid, 1895, pp 70-1).

Under Russell's Bill 60 boroughs with under 2,000 citizens would lose their seats to London, the large towns, the English counties, Scotland, Ireland and Wales. The county franchise was to include the 40s freeholders, copyholders and long leaseholders with holdings worth £10 annually, short leaseholders with holdings worth £50 annually and farming tenants at will with rents of £50 a year or more. The borough franchise went to all ratepayers of property valued at £10 annually. The measure was reckoned to enlarge the electorate by 500,000 to a total of 814,000.

The Bill was carried by a majority of one on 23 March. The nation celebrated. Then, defeated in a debate on the proposed size of parliament, the government resigned. 'The Bill, the whole Bill, and nothing but the Bill' demanded the people. In the ensuing general election Russell was returned for Devonshire and entered the Cabinet. The opposition fought tooth and nail, such that by summer Russell was ill with fatigue. Nevertheless, the Bill eventually reached the Lords, only to be rejected on 8 October by a majority that included 21 bishops. Now the people grew menacing. Nottingham Castle was burnt down. Newspapers were edged in black and church bells were rung in muffled peals. There was rioting in Bristol and Derby. The aristocracy were assaulted on the streets and the bishops were jeered. The middle classes talked of withholding taxes. The king was petitioned by a procession of 60,000.

Lord John introduced his Bill for the third time in December, and it reached the Lords in March 1832. This same month a young Charles Dickens joined the reporting staff of a new 7d paper, *The True Sun*, just in time to hear the closing debates from the strangers' gallery of the House of Commons. The Bill was mutilated by a motion carried by Lord Lyndhurst. Ministers now asked the king to create sufficient new peers to pass the measure through the Lords. As long ago as 1712 Queen Anne had used this tactic when she created 12 peers to counter opposition to the Peace of Utrecht. However, William IV and Queen Adelaide were hostile, so Grey resigned. Rumours of revolution were now so alarming that the Scots Greys were ordered to rough-sharpen their swords. Suddenly the king's nerve broke, and he urged the Lords to withdraw their opposition. That achieved more than all the rioting. The Lords relented and the Bill received royal assent on 7 June 1832. The Act did not relieve the nation of its electoral evils, but it was a start. Members of the Commons still needed to show an annual income of £600 from land in the shires, and borough members £300 from land. Furthermore, the property qualification left the poor disenfranchised.

The Economist and free trade in land

Having achieved its purpose against trade restrictions, from 1847 *The Economist* embarked upon a new cause, 'free trade in land'. A House of Lords committee had found that "the state of the law as affecting the title to land formed by far the greatest burden of which proprietors of land had to complain" (*The Economist*, 29 May, 1847, vol 5, pp 605-6). This was the law that landlords had had conveyancers design for them for their own purposes. But with families living profligately off Rent for several generations, many estates were now burdened with debt and in the hands of trustees brought in to salvage what was left. Interest on debt ate into the revenue from rents to such an extent that the maintenance of land and buildings was seriously neglected. Having made little progress, *The Economist* repeated in 1866 that: "As rules of property such laws are wholly absurd. They run counter to every economical law applicable to the ownership and use of land" (*The Economist*, 7 July, 1866, vol 25, p 796). *The Economist* was unconcerned with what was in the bundle, but fretted over the lawyers' red tape which impeded the free trade of the bundle and its use as security for loans to support commercial and industrial development.

The interference of strict settlement with the landholders' ability to sell, mortgage or lease land which was entailed on their children generated increasing resentment among estate owners, up to their necks in debt and seeing opportunities for money-making beyond their reach. The fact that the landlord held only a life estate tended to keep the leases to his tenants short so as not to over-run his own interest. This discouraged investments by tenants who could foresee their outlay falling into the landlord's hands at the end of the lease. Together these forces were running down the performance of the estates. Only when entrepreneurs stepped in, as had Ricardo for Astley, might potential be realised. Landlords decided that the power of the tenant for life to use up more of the rights and privileges in his bundle had to be strengthened. Fathers and sons with foresight had occasionally written such powers into their strict settlements, as when the Duke of Portland in 1726 included permission to lease building land in London for 99 years. This practice became quite common in the early 19th century (Spring, 1977), but left many problems unresolved. Between 1800 and 1850 there were 700 private Acts of parliament seeking powers to lease, sell or mortgage that were not there in the strict settlement (Spring, 1977, p 46). The Encumbered Estates Act of 1848 eased the sale of landed estates in debt to men with the capital. Further help came in 1849 in the form of the Board of Enclosure Commissioners, established to provide a dual service to landholders. It drew firmly into the bundle additional corporeal hereditaments – lands formerly held as 'waste' and open fields, thereby raising Rent, and from 1849 it facilitated the use of this Rent for private purposes.

Enclosure: extension of privatisation of Rent

Alfred Russell Wallace described his experiences during the 19th century enclosures of common land (Wallace, 1908). Wallace was born in Usk, Monmouthshire in 1823. William, his eldest brother, was articled to land surveyors in Kington, Herefordshire, a profession in which work was plentiful at the time owing to two Acts of parliament. Traditionally the clergy were maintained by the tithe, paid in kind. By the Commutation of the Tithes Act of 1836, however, the tithe was henceforth to be paid in cash. This meant that parishes had to be valued in preparation for the new tax. More work was generated by the private enclosure Acts which gave landholders of the parish powers to enclose the open fields and wastes.

From early in the 18th century a series of private Acts of enclosure, more than 4,000 in all and covering seven million acres, were passed before the General Enclosure Act of 1845. Almost certainly about the same area again was enclosed without application to parliament. Alfred was 22 years old when the General Enclosure Act became law, by which time most of the open fields had been enclosed (only another 200,000 such acres being enclosed after this Act – Hoskins, 1985, p 185). From about 1800, landowners had turned their attention to the wastes, high agricultural prices during the Napoleonic wars having made it profitable to bring marginal land under cultivation. More than 500 private Acts had enclosed 750,000 acres of 'waste', as this rough heath and moorland was called, up to 1801, and in the early 19th century another 1,300 private Acts allowed enclosure of a further one and a quarter million such acres. The whole operation was the brainchild of people like Arthur Young, Secretary of the Board of Agriculture from 1793, who believed that landholders had a duty to demand high rents, because according to him low rents encouraged slovenly agriculture. Thus the preamble of the General Enclosure Act started: "Whereas it is expedient to facilitate the enclosure and improvement of commons and other lands now subject to the rights of property which obstruct cultivation and the productive employment of labour, be it enacted...". These 'obstructive rights' belonged to the cottagers.

For generations poorer cottagers had supplemented their income by keeping a cow or a few geese on the waste common, by collecting fuel off it, and by a little cultivation. In many cases their rights to the commons arose solely from occupation of cottages which they rented from local landholders. When enclosure occurred the *owner* of the cottages obtained allotments of land in compensation for the extinction of the common rights, *not the tenant*, who got nothing in return. Where the cottager was the owner of his dwelling, documentary evidence had to be produced to confirm legal entitlement to the exercise of rights of common. In numerous cases the cottager, who could neither read nor write, could not produce convincing documentation, thereby losing his rights without compensation. The resultant hardship was immense. Even Arthur Young admitted that "by 19 Enclosure Acts out of 20 the poor are injured". The cottager, previously a smallholder with common rights, was reduced to a labourer pure and simple, a fact resented deeply. While the Poor Law authorities were doling out allowances to see poor families through a bad harvest or an agricultural depression, the families cried out "Give us back our commons and you can keep your poor relief" (Slater, 1913).

Alfred and his brother surveyed the parish of Higher Gobion in Bedfordshire in 1837. They then moved to other parishes in the county, and on to Radnorshire, all in connection with the Commutation Act. Later, as a result of the General Enclosure Act, they moved yet again to Llandrindod Wells. This is what Alfred had to say:

> ... there was then a large extent of moor and mountain surrounded by scattered cottages with their gardens and small fields, which, with their rights of common, enabled the occupants to keep a horse, cow, a few sheep, and thus make a living. All this was now being taken away from them, and the whole of this open land divided among the landowners of the parish or manor in proportion to the size or value of their estates. To those that had much, much was to be given, while from the poor their rights were taken away; for though normally those that *owned* a little land had some compensation, it was so small as to be of no use to

them in comparison with the grazing rights they before possessed. In the case of the cottagers who were tenants or leaseholders, it was simple robbery, as they had no compensation whatever, and were left wholly dependent on farmers for employment. And this was all done – as similar inclosures are almost always done – under false pretences.... In hundreds of cases, when the commons, heath, and mountains have been partitioned out among the landowners, the land remains as little cultivated as before. It is either thrown into adjacent farms as rough pasture at a nominal rent, or is used for game-coverts, and often continues in this waste and unproductive state for half a century or more, till any portions of it are required for railroads, or for building upon, when a price equal to that of the best land in the district is often demanded and obtained. I know of thousands of acres in many parts of the south of England to which these remarks will apply, and if this is not obtaining land under false pretences – a legalised robbery of the poor for the aggrandizement of the rich, *who were the law-makers* – words have no meaning. (Wallace, 1908, pp 79-80)

From 1845 enclosure and land drainage were supervised by the Board of Enclosure commissioners, which oversaw the expenditure of large sums of taxpayers' money that parliament had lent landholders for these purposes. In 1865, loss of land for public recreation having by then reached alarming proportions, the Commons Preservation Society was founded to stop the rot. Enclosures continued up to the passage of the Commons Act in 1876, and during these years Wallace became convinced of the need for radical land reform. Many years later he inquired about the condition of the enclosed land he had surveyed around Llandrindod Wells. The district remained unimproved for 30 years until the railway was constructed from Shrewsbury to south Wales. With Llandrindod opened to tourists, the land was immediately turned over to their accommodation and entertainment. Prices for what was previously common land soared to as high as £1,500 an acre, and a large area was used for a golf course. Here was the economics of Rent in full force, and the consequence of its privatisation blatantly obvious.

The Board of Enclosure found itself from 1849 overseeing drainage schemes funded on settled land through mortgages permitted by a new Act of parliament. This supervisory role grew as a series of similar Acts allowed tenants for life under strict settlement to borrow in order to finance agricultural development. Under the Improvement of Land Act of 1864, the tenant for life was permitted to borrow so that he could invest in railways that were to cut across his estate (Spring, 1977, p 46). These Acts took great care to ensure that the integrity of the estate as intended by strict settlement was not compromised, relying on the powers of the trustees and assurances of consent of all interested parties. Henry, third Earl Grey, realised that had not landholders devised these safety valves the only alternative would have been to capitulate to those who demanded an end to the law of strict settlement (Spring, 1977, p 48).

Enfranchisement and land: II

In 1867 the wealthier of the working classes were granted the electoral franchise. Agitation for electoral reform had led to the establishment of the Northern Reform Union in Newcastle, similar movements elsewhere, and the Manhood Suffrage and Vote by Ballot Association in London. In 1864 the National Reform Union began to campaign for the vote for householders and lodgers, while the more 'working class' National Reform League pressed for enfranchisement of all male adults mentally competent and without a criminal conviction.

When Lord Palmerston died in October 1865, Queen Victoria asked Lord Russell to carry on as Prime Minister, as 'an old and true friend'. Parliament was opened on 1 February 1866 and the queen's speech included the guarded promise of a Reform Bill. Proceeding cautiously, Russell and Gladstone separated the question of enfranchisement from that of the distribution of parliamentary seats. The Representation of the People Bill of March 1866 proposed extension of the vote to borough householders paying £7 annually in rent, and to county householders paying £14 annually in rent. Compound households (those 500,000 who paid the rates to the landlord in their rent) and lodgers paying £10 a year in rent were also to be enfranchised.

These reforms to the franchise, estimated to bring in what Lord John called 'the best of the working classes', satisfied neither Radicals nor Conservatives. Some Liberals in the House of Commons were panic-stricken by what was proposed. The Conservatives saw their opportunity, and Lord Grosvenor brought an amendment on the omission of re-distribution of seats. Although the amendment was defeated, the government moved promptly to bring in a Re-distribution of Seats Bill in May. Lord Dunkellin then brought in an amendment to substitute rating for rental in the boroughs, thus intentionally leaving many unenfranchised, including compound householders. His amendment was carried by 11 votes on 18 June (Reid, 1895, pp 329-31).

Russell's administration resigned immediately. His resignation speech alerted parliament to the dangers of alienating the common people from the Crown and the aristocracy, reminding peers that universal suffrage existed already in the United States of America and in Britain's colonies. Only weeks before, the Liberal Robert Lowe claimed that American and Australian democracy simply created opportunities for corruption, and that ignorance and drunkenness were major characteristics of the working class which Russell proposed to enfranchise. Working class men and women had their own views on these parliamentary speeches. Three days after Lord John's resignation more than 20,000 of them gathered in Trafalgar Square to hear Charles Bradlaugh, member for Northampton, deliver Russell's speech of resignation. The gathering then walked in procession to Carlton House Terrace to cheer Mr Gladstone. About three weeks later another large demonstration was announced for Hyde Park by the National Reform League. Although prohibited by the Home Secretary, the League went ahead anyway after formal protest.

Lord Derby and Benjamin Disraeli of the new Conservative administration apparently decided to steal the Liberals' thunder and propose their own reforms, knowing these would be popular in the country and more likely to be received sympathetically in the House of Lords when coming from them rather than from Gladstone and Russell. The gamble was the uncertainty about the way an expanded electorate would use the vote. The Bill eventually put to parliament in March 1867 was at the cost of loss of the right wing of the Cabinet, Lord Cranborne and others resigning. Now it was time for tit for tat. Having been defeated on an amendment to their own proposals, the Liberals embarked upon their own more extreme proposals for amendment of Disraeli's Bill. Debate raged until May, when Disraeli accepted that lodgers and compound householders should be enfranchised (the latter were to pay the rates themselves instead of as part of the rent). In the counties the vote was extended to all occupiers of property valued at £12 or more annually, plus copyholders and leaseholders with property worth £5 annually. In the boroughs it went to all householders resident for one year and to lodgers paying a rent of £10 annually (Wood, 1982, p 266).

Giving up land ever so slowly: responses to working class enfranchisement

The 1867 reforms raised the electorate in the United Kingdom from about 1.4 million to 2.5 million, bringing in some of the wealthier working classes for the first time. Both parties now considered what to do in order to attract these new voters without losing the old. William Gladstone told the House of Commons that the working classes were "our fellow Christians, our own flesh and blood". But for many, and in particular Conservatives such as Lord Salisbury, neither 'flesh and blood' nor Christianity was the issue, but that bundle called land. Salisbury described his politics as centred on "the great primeval subject matter of all human conflict" (ownership of property), which manifested itself as "a struggle between those who have, to keep what they have got, and those who have not, to get it" (Spring, 1996, p 186).

Years later, Henry Hyndman recalled a conversation with Lady Dorothy Nevil in which her remarks, for him, gave "a very true and telling statement of the attitude of the cleverest aristocratic class in the world towards social and political developments". Turning to him during a dinner party, she said:

> Besides, we shall never offer any obstinate or bitter resistance to what is asked for. When your agitation becomes really serious we shall give way a little, and grant something of no great importance, but sufficient to satisfy the majority for the time being. Our object is to avoid any direct conflict in order to gain time. This concession will gain, let us say, 10 years: it won't be less. Then at the expiration of that period you will have worked up probably another threatening demonstration on the part of the masses against what you call the class monopoly of the means and instruments of production. We shall meet you in quite an equitable and friendly spirit and again surrender a point from which we all along mean to retire.... Yet another 10 years are thus put behind us, and once more you start afresh.... Once more we meet you with the same tactics of partial surrender and pleasing procrastination. But now, remember, 30 years has passed and you have another generation to deal with, to stir up, and educate, whilst, if I may venture to say so, you yourself will not be so young nor perhaps quite so hopeful as you are today.... (Hyndman, 1911, pp 385-6)

Enfranchisement and land: III

Russell did not live to see the Act of parliamentary reform in 1884, having died on 28 May 1878 at the age of 86. He did, however, see the introduction of secret voting in the Ballot Act of 1872, which put an end to the notorious poll book, open to reveal to any interested landlord those who had and those who had not given him their vote. Lord John would have remembered George Grote's attempt to introduce the ballot as long ago as 1833, and how he (Russell) had at that time shown open hostility to the proposal. Grote, a founder of London University, and strong proponent of Athenian democracy, died the year before what he had fought for came to be realised in the Act of 1872. There were shades of 1867 when the Bill for electoral reform introduced by Gladstone's administration in early 1884 was checked by the Lords' insistence on the prior necessity for a Bill of Re-distribution. It was peers against the people yet again. In the end, however, the Franchise Act extended household suffrage into the counties, increasing the electorate to about 5.7 million. The Re-distribution Act moved seats from small boroughs, redistributing 142 in all. Up to that time the electorate of some boroughs had had the right to send two members to parliament, but by this Act almost the entire nation was divided into single member constituencies (Wood, 1982, p 320).

Up until 1885 politics in the counties had been the preserve of those with an interest in landed property, essentially in the pocket of the 40s. freeholder ever since 1430. To meddle with this in 1867 was more than Disraeli dared, for of the 172 county divisions in 1868, the system gave his party control of 127. Following the re-distribution of 1884, however, county seats increased to 234, of which the Conservatives held only 101 in 1885. This change was largely due to the shift from franchise on the basis of tenure (freehold, copyhold, leasehold) to occupation (household). Many agricultural labourers qualified as householders, as did some servants, although not all of them were eligible to vote (setting aside the few women householders who remained excluded on the basis of their sex). Householders had to occupy their house continuously for 12 months up to 15 July in order to qualify for inclusion on the electoral register in force on the following New Year's Day. Paupers in receipt of poor relief were automatically disenfranchised. In Suffolk, for example, probably only about 75% of male agricultural labourers were entitled to vote (Clark and Langford, 1996, p 126). However, when the Conservative candidate for North East Suffolk claimed in the election of 1885 that "the labourer has no more natural rights than cows and suckling pigs", he was to regret his underestimate of the power of the new franchise (Clark and Langford, 1996, p 129).

Any assumption that after 1884 the electoral system provided for universal male adult suffrage, equal electoral districts and removal of all earlier anomalies would be far from the reality. The Whig and Radical wings of the Liberal Party were far from unanimous about what was desirable, and the Conservative House of Lords was as usual reactionary. Assimilation of the county and borough franchises to produce a rational and national electoral roll was resisted by the Lords; compromise would be considered only if the Conservatives got the re-distribution of parliamentary seats they wanted. True, the household franchise applied to adult males in the boroughs and counties who owned or were tenants of 'any dwelling house or portion of a dwelling house defined as a separate dwelling', but this definition excluded many lodgers, as well as tenants holding their own keys when the landlord lived in the same building. Domestic servants living in, most sons living with parents, and soldiers and policemen in barracks also remained without the vote. The residency requirement, and the fact that the electoral register was always at least six months out of date, disenfranchised many casual labourers who needed to move at short notice to find work. In addition, those receiving poor relief were disqualified (Pelling, 1967, pp 6-8).

There were other anomalies. Most borough freeholders in England and Wales had a second vote in the county division in which their borough was located (for example, freeholders in Colchester could also vote in the county division of Essex North East). Businessmen and professional men with their work premises in a borough but residence outside could vote in both places. University graduates could also vote for nine university members of parliament. On the other hand, the lodger paying less than £10 annually for his unfurnished room had no vote. Although the aim was to achieve constituencies of equal size, boundaries were drawn to separate communities according to 'the pursuits of the people'. Thus in the larger cities with several single member constituencies, middle classes and working classes were separated as completely as possible, while county divisions gave the agricultural and industrial areas distinct representation. This manipulation strengthened the chance of the Conservative Party picking up borough seats and shielded the landed interest of the counties. Another anomaly arose because polling took place in different constituencies on different days over almost a month. When in 1895 Sir William Harcourt was defeated in Derby, he was able to persuade the local Liberal candidate in Monmouthshire West, a safe Liberal seat, to make way and thereby enter the contest there before nominations closed. Gladstone was elected both for Midlothian and Leith in 1886, and chose to sit for Midlothian (Pelling, 1967, pp 8-10).

Prospective members of parliament still had to be able to support a very considerable expense from private means, payment of members by the State still being 26 years away in 1885. All expenses of the electoral process had to be met, and a candidate had to support all sorts of local causes through financial generosity to secure favour. The church may need an organ, or repairs may be needed at the hospital. The novelist Rider Haggard recalled how standing for Norfolk East as a Unionist in 1895 cost him more than £2,000 (Pelling, 1967, p 11). Such expenses eliminated almost all potential working class candidates and made life difficult for many Liberals. Even the returning officer could view an election as a profitable enterprise, perhaps demanding the hire of the polling booth at four guineas a time (Pelling, 1967, p 12). The whole system gave enormous advantage to the Conservatives and Unionists, their ostentatious show of wealth in transporting their supporters to and from the booth sometimes arousing resentment among those struggling on foot. Nor was the ballot always strictly secret. The practice of numbering the ballot paper as it was issued to the voter meant that paper and elector could be linked at the counting tables. In the counties, the landlord could thereby gain an impression of each village's voting pattern, and if not to his liking, he could apply 'the screw', as it was called.

The shape of modern British party politics was forged in the heat of a late Victorian and Edwardian battle over Rent. In retrospect, from a political perspective the struggle from 1875 onwards to wrest Rent from the bundle called land was premature. The landed classes had finally relinquished the property qualification for prospective parliamentary candidates only 17 years previously. They were in turmoil over the erosion of the parliamentary franchise as a form of property right. Many landed estates were deeply in debt. Not surprisingly, therefore, the leading social class was deeply shocked at proposals to take Rent into the public domain, and fought tooth and nail to prevent this from happening.

Had the conflict been fought with sword and lance, deeds of noble valour, treachery on the field, and destruction of murderous dimensions, then it would have entered the annals of popular history along with the Wars of the Roses. Unlike the wars of 1455 to 1487, however, this was a war without bloodshed, with combat played out in the political arena. As such, despite its momentous significance for the Britain of today, these events have receded from the national consciousness within a span of 80 years far more than have the battles of the Plantagenets and the Tudors in 500 years. In many respects, apart from mass bloodshed, this political battle over Rent was as vicious and merciless as any of its more notorious predecessors. Despite the achievement of remarkable constitutional reforms which weakened the Lords (and incidentally paved the way for the reform of 1999), Rent was not brought back into the public domain. Hence the life and death forces stemming from privatisation of Rent, so troublesome to the Welfare State, remain with us.

THIRTEEN

The battle for Rent and Welfare
Part I: 1880-1905

It is not our business to make things pleasant all round. (Robert Lowe,
Chancellor of the Exchequer, 1871)

Charles Darwin had only a few months to live when he wrote to Alfred
Russell Wallace in July 1881, "I see that you are going to write on the
most difficult political question, the land. Something ought to be done,
but what is the rub" (Wallace, 1908, pp 234-5). It was in large part
because the bundle that we call land had been made so complex that
there was such potential for reform in those days. Some, like the editors
of *The Economist*, were unconcerned about what the bundle contained,
fretting only because the red tape and the lawyers' seals impeded its sale
and reduced its usefulness as security against commercial loans. Others
were similarly untroubled about what went into the bundle of private
landholding; rather, they feared that some bundles were too big, whereas
the number of small bundles seemed to be diminishing, to the detriment
of the small man. Such anxieties found expression in legislation to preserve
smallholdings and allotments. There was also the special problem of
landlordism in Ireland. None of these movements concern us, although
they brush against any consideration of the history of Rent. The reform
movements to be examined in this chapter were all committed to the
return of Rent to the public domain for social purposes.

The British school of land reform – nationalisation

Three schools of thought qualify for consideration, which could be called
British, American and German. In the British school were such men as
John Stuart Mill, Herbert Spencer, and (in his earlier years) Wallace, all of
whom talked of nationalisation of the land *with some form of compensation
to the landholder*. Herbert Spencer's first edition of *Social statics* had a
chapter entitled 'The right to the use of the earth'. This work, plus his
experience as a land surveyor, convinced Wallace of the need for land

nationalisation. His publications caught the eye of John Stuart Mill, who wrote to Wallace enclosing the programme of his own Land Tenure Reform Association (formed in 1869). Its objective was strictly to claim the future 'unearned increment' of land values for state revenues (ie the increase in value of the Rent between purchase and sale) as had been proposed by his father, the economist James Mill. Wallace accepted Mill's invitation to become a member of the Association's General Committee, but advised that the Association should propose for the State the power of acquiring land by purchase, in order to break the monopoly of land ownership. Mill then wanted to go even further and pay the landowner not only the market price but also a figure in compensation, a suggestion Wallace could not immediately support. This debate and the Association both collapsed with the death of Mill in 1873.

Wallace was criticised for his views, which ran counter to laissez faire in threatening extension rather than restriction of the role of the State in the land market. To some, Wallace's scheme would encourage an "inevitable jobbery and favouritism from placing the management of the whole land of the country in the hands of the executive" (Wallace, 1908, p 321). In an article in the *Contemporary Review* of November 1880, Wallace moved closer to the views of the man who launched the American School, Henry George, when he distinguished two parts to the value of land. One of these was its 'inherent value', as he called Rent, which arises quite independently of any effort or expense on the part of the holder, but which is due *solely to nature and society*. The other part is the 'improvement', essentially impermanent in nature and due *solely to the effort and expense of the holder or occupier*. Wallace stated, "My experience in surveying and land valuation assured me that the two values can be easily separated. It follows that land as owned by the State would need no 'management' whatever, the rent being merely ground-rent, which could be collected just as house-tax and the land-tax are collected, the State-tenant being left as completely free as is the freeholder now" (Wallace, 1908, p 322).

Wallace's article caught the eye of several prominent men, among them A.C. Swinton, who organised a number of meetings leading to the establishment of the Land Nationalisation Society in 1881, with Wallace as president. Unlike George, Wallace believed that, through compulsory purchase, land should gradually be acquired by the State from private owners. Compensation would be calculated on the basis of the net income derived from the land before nationalisation, and paid as an annuity limited in its duration to the lives in being (ie in the case of strict settlement, to the father and son, but not the unborn grandson) (Gaffney, 1997). The

State would then lease out the land, taking Rent in lieu of taxes on wages and interest.

The Land Nationalisation Society continued through the 1880s, and in March 1891 launched a series of promotional country tours in its 'yellow vans'. In reaction, the landlords fueled their own propaganda machine called the Liberty and Property Defence League. The Society eventually lost steam, failing to convert major politicians to land nationalisation. Wallace moved on, being attracted increasingly to British variants of German Socialism (our third school of thought), calling with Sydney Webb for nationalisation of capital as well as land.

The American school of land reform – Rent collection and Henry George

In his letter to Wallace, Charles Darwin also wrote, "I will certainly order 'Progress and Poverty', for the subject is a most interesting one. But I read many years ago some books on political economy, and they produced a disastrous effect on my mind, viz., utterly to distract my own judgement on the subject, and to doubt much everyone else's judgement! So I feel pretty sure that Mr George's book will only make my mind worse confounded than it is at present" (Wallace, 1908, pp 234-5).

Henry George (Geiger, 1939), the originator of the American and purist school on Rent, was born in Philadelphia, Pennsylvania on 2 September 1839. After trying his hand at errand boy, clerk and foremast boy on an East Indiaman, George was eventually invited to move to the American West by former neighbours. On 22 December 1857 he sailed as a steward on the steamer *Shubrick* bound for San Francisco.

In June 1858 gold was discovered on the Fraser River in British Columbia, so George sailed north to try his luck, but to no avail. Later, while browsing in the library of a small hotel in San Francisco, he came across Adam Smith's *The wealth of nations* and discovered classical economics. For a time he worked as a printer before trying again for gold in northern California, but suffering severe hardship without reaching the mines, he returned to San Francisco. These, the years of the American Civil War back East, brought George close to destitution as he struggled to support his wife and two young children. He later told how on the day in 1865 when his younger son was born, in sheer desperation he had to beg $5 from a passing stranger.

George's breakthrough came when an article he wrote on the assassination of Abraham Lincoln was published as a leader in the *Alta*

California, and by 1868 he had advanced to managing editor. This was the year he started to reflect on developments around him. In his article, 'What the railroad will bring us', published in the *Overland Monthly,* George wrote, "The truth is, that the completion of the railroad and the consequent great increase of business and population, will not benefit all of us, but only a portion ... Those who have lands, mines, established business, special abilities of certain kinds, will become richer for it and find increased opportunities. Those who chance only their own labour will become poorer, and find it harder to get ahead, first because it will take more capital to buy land or get into business; and second, because as competition reduces the wages of labour, capital will be harder for them to obtain ..." (Lee, 1996, p 27).

A visit to New York later that year impressed upon George what the railroads were bringing to California when he saw "for the first time the shocking contrast between monstrous wealth and debasing want" in that city. Back in San Francisco, another experience led him to connect poverty and private ownership in land. One day, riding into the hills, he stopped to ask a passing teamster what land was worth in those parts. The man replied, "I don't know exactly, but there is a man over there who will sell some land for a $1,000". George saw in a flash the reason for advancing poverty alongside increasing wealth. With the growth of population, land grows in value, and the men who work it must pay more for the privilege. In New York he had witnessed the outcome as it existed back East and in Europe. In California he was experiencing the evolution of the problem as it rolled westward.

The Bank of the United States had been established to finance its federal government, and since 1838 agent Samuel Jaudon had been marketing American securities in the City of London. Much on offer was pure speculation, and there was anti-American feeling in 1841 when the Bank collapsed and eight American states defaulted on loans raised in London. However, the promise of wealth offered by American expansion was irresistible. King Cotton in the South and the locomotives rolling across the prairies were propelled not only by finance from the East Coast but also from across the Atlantic, especially London. The mercantile house of Barings, founded by Francis Baring of Exeter in 1763, financed much of the cotton trade with the Southern States, opening an office in Liverpool in 1832. American finance houses such as William and James Brown and Co established branches in England for the same purpose. George Peabody, American merchant, financier and philanthropist, who settled in London in 1838, played an important part in distributing shares in the Illinois Central and the Ohio and Mississippi railroads. Barings and Rothschilds were involved in the finance of railroads in Canada and Pennsylvania. In 1865 a third of all railroad securities issued in London were for American concerns. During the 1880s Barings associated with Kidder Peabody, the New York and Boston house that specialised in the railroad business (Kynaston, 1995, vol 1, pp 258-9).

Out West, California having hardly been touched by civil war, investment looked decidedly good. Alphonse Rothschild had written in 1848, "Without the slightest doubt, this is the cradle of the new civilisation ... The new settlement of California is an event of enormous potential ... I have no hesitation in saying that a Rothschild house should be established in America". James and Lionel Rothschild chose not to act, however, deciding instead to continue operating through their agent August Belmont (Wilson, 1994, p 181). This decision cost Rothschild dearly, for it was not this family but J and W Seligman and Co that became Abraham Lincoln's principle war financier. The Seligman family, known as the 'American Rothschild', became a dominant force in American taxation policy in later years, and displayed great hostility to Henry George. The approaching might of this financial power, riding on the railroad, caused land speculators to rush ahead into California, sending Rent soaring in 1869. While it was natural for Rent to increase with development, investment of capital and an expanding population, George saw how this value was being captured by the private landholder as an 'unearned increment', with decidedly unnatural consequences.

Poverty was the common concern of land reformers and the public health movement. The land reformers saw private landholding with monopoly of Rent as poverty's major cause, while those in public health saw poverty as a root cause of sickness and premature death. George's remedy was to return Rent to the community as a 'tax' on landholders (the choice of the word 'tax' in this context was unfortunate; governments cannot tax what rightfully belongs to the State). In his pamphlet called *Our land and land policy, National and State*, published in 1871, he wrote, "Land taxation does not bear at all on production; it adds nothing to prices, and does not affect the cost of living. As it does not add to prices, it costs the people nothing in addition to what it yields the government; while the land cannot be hid or moved, this tax can be collected with ease and certainty, and with less expense than any other tax; and the landowner cannot shift it to any one else" (Lee, 1996, p 29).

Nevertheless, the notion that landholders could shift the loss of Rent on to others soon gave rise to objections to a tax on land values on grounds of effectiveness. George devoted an editorial to this misconception in his New York paper the *Standard*. This is how he explained it:

> Here ... is a piece of land ... Its Rent ... is the highest price that anyone will give for it – it is a bonus which the man who wants to use the land must pay to the man who owns the land for permission to use it. Now, if a tax be levied on that Rent ... this in no way adds to the willingness (or ability) of anyone to pay more for the land than before, nor does it add in any way to the ability of the owner to demand more. To suppose, in fact, that such a tax could be thrown by landowners upon tenants is to suppose that the owners of land do not now get for the land all it will bring; it is to suppose that, whenever they want to, they can put up prices as they please.

> This is of course absurd. There could be no limit whatever to prices did the fixing of them rest entirely with the seller. To the price which will be given and received for anything, two wants or wills must concur – the want or the will of the buyer, and the want or will of the seller. The one wants to give as little as he can, the other to get as much as he can, and the point at which the exchange will take place is the point where these two desires come to a balance or effect a compromise. In other words, price is determined by supply and demand. Taxation cannot affect price unless it affects the relative power of one or other of the elements in the equation. The mere wish of the seller to get more, the mere wish of the buyer to pay less, can neither raise nor lower prices. Nothing will raise prices unless it either decreases supply or increases demand. Nothing will lower price unless it either increases supply or decreases demand. Now, the taxation of land values, which is simply the taking by the State of a part of the premium which the landowner can get for the permission to use land, neither increases the demand for land nor decreases the supply of land, and therefore cannot increase the price that the landowner can get from the user. Thus it is impossible for landowners to throw such taxation on land users by raising rents.

What George had to say next is of fundamental importance:

> a tax on land values is not a tax on land. They are very different things, and the difference should be noted, because a confusion of thought as to them may lead to the assumption that a tax on land values would fall on the user ... tax on land, that is to say, a tax of so much per acre ... on all

land – would fall on the user. For such a tax, falling equally on all land – on the poorest and least advantageously situated as fully as on the richest and best situated land – would become a condition imposed on the use of any land, from which there could be no escape, and thus the owners of rentable land could add it to their rent. Its operation would be analogous to that of a tax on a producible commodity ... But a tax on economic Rent or land values would not fall on all land. It would fall only on valuable land, and on that in proportion to its value. It would not have to be paid upon the poorest land in use (which always determines Rent), and so would not become a condition of use ...

A tax on land values does not add to the cost of producing land. Land is not a thing of human production ... Its price therefore, is not fixed by the cost of production, but is always the highest price that anyone can give for the privilege of using a particular piece. Land ... has no normal value based on the cost of production, but ranges from nothing at all to the enormous values that attach to choice sites in great cities, or to mineral deposits of superior riches, when the growth of population causes a demand for their use.

Here, let us say, is a lot on the principal select street of a city having an annual rental value of $10,000. Such a lot would now command a selling price of some $250,000 [George was equating the Rent of land with an annual interest of 4% on its market value]. An increased tax upon land values would not reduce its rental value, except as it might have an effect in forcing into use unoccupied land at a greater distance from the center of the city. But as less of this rental value could be retained by the owner, the selling price would be diminished. (George, undated, p 4)

The proof of the pudding is in the eating; the violent reaction of landholders to the notion of collection of Rent testifies to their appreciation of the basic fact that they could not shift their loss on to others.

In September 1877 Henry George set about explaining the interrelation between land values in the private market and poverty in his work, *Progress and poverty*, completed in March 1879 (George, 1979). The manuscript was rejected by several publishers, forcing George to make the plates himself and print an 'author's edition' of 500 copies. Appleton and Co then agreed to use the plates to bring out an edition in the USA in January 1880. An important breakthrough came at the end of that year when Paul Kegan of London ordered an edition of the book, to be brought out in Britain in January 1881. The work became the largest selling book of any dealing with economics, subsequent reprints totalling more than 100,000 copies. George was a major force in British politics for some years to come.

The American school comes to Britain

The 'Irish Problem' provided George with an opportunity to become directly involved in land reform in Britain. Soon after the formation of Michael Davitt's and Charles Parnell's Land League of Ireland in 1879, Parnell visited the United States and spoke in 62 cities. As a result the American Land League was formed as an auxiliary of the Irish League. The United States poured money into the nationalist cause in Ireland. In Cincinnati Parnell declared, "None of us, whether we are in America or Ireland, or wherever we may be, will be satisfied until we have destroyed the last link which keeps Ireland bound to England" (Kee, 1982, p 126). He was followed by Davitt, who met George and was introduced to *Progress and poverty* at that time. Quickly, George wrote a pamphlet, *The Irish land question*, which gained wide circulation in the United States, Canada and Britain. His monograph criticised Parnell's advocacy of state sponsorship of a new class of Irish small landowners, with compensation to the original landlords for their loss of property. George's principal objection was that private landholding would remain undisturbed, retaining Rent in smaller but more numerous hands instead of returning it to the State for public revenue. In this pamphlet George turned his mind to the political practicalities of what he was proposing; faced with what he termed "ignorance, prejudice and powerful interests". He clearly saw the need not to rush headlong into wholesale reform: "to demand a little (Rent) at first is often the surest way to obtain much at last" (George, 1941, p 57). This statement, for all its moderation, frightened the Conservative Party into bitter opposition of a land tax in any shape or form, no matter how trifling it might appear when introduced. For them, Rent reform was extremist radicalism – period!

When the editor of the New York paper, the *Irish World*, decided to send a correspondent to Ireland to cover the 'Land War', Henry George was the obvious man for the job. He sailed in October 1881, aged 42 years. The country he entered was operating under suspension of *habeus corpus*, its jails held 500 political prisoners including Parnell, and 15,000 military constables and 40,000 troops had the task of enforcing Gladstone's Coercion Act. In this climate, with his views having travelled ahead of him, George was almost *persona non grata*, and he was closely supervised. In a dispatch of 10 April 1882 he wrote, "while there are large portions of the population that show in pinched features and stunted stature that they have been underfed, and while one reads in the papers of Coroners' juries in the heart of London returning verdicts of death by starvation, the Duke of Albany ... is voted a pension of £25,000 per annum to enable him to marry a German princelet ... what this royal prince is to get [is] wrung from the labouring classes by a system of indirect taxation which presses on them most hardly, and ... for the mere trouble of being born of a royal mother is [granted a sum] a thousand times as much as many Englishmen are able to obtain by the hardest work for the support of themselves and their families" (Lawrence, 1957, p 16). This Duke was Leopold, the eighth of Queen Victoria's nine children, who was about to marry Helena of Waldeck. George's pro-Irish, anti-English dispatches to the *Irish World* intensified English opposition to him.

In a speech in Liverpool in June 1882, Michael Davitt spoke in favour of Henry George's remedy for the Irish Land Question – restoration of Rent to the community, turning the sympathy of thousands of emigrant Irish to George's cause (*The Times*, 7 June, 1882). Consequently, through his book and Irish adventures, London was fully aware of George when Alfred Russell Wallace introduced him at a meeting in London arranged by the Land Nationalisation Society. George now was in a difficult position. His hosts at this and many subsequent meetings wished to use him to promote *their* favoured solutions to the privatisation of Rent, which by calling for public ownership of land (the British School) or, more extremely, the nationalisation of capital assets under Socialism (the German School) were proposing more than George considered necessary. Yet he needed an entrée into the English debate, and could afford neither to offend his hosts nor decline their offers. This strategy seriously blurred his message, leading to him being labelled erroneously as a land nationaliser or a Socialist.

Although largely misunderstood, by the time he returned to New York in October 1882 he was being taken seriously in academic circles and the press. The Conservative papers tended to accept George's criticism of social conditions but considered his solution little less than plunder of private property. Even before George reached New York, powerful property owners launched their Liberty and Property Defence League, complete with a parliamentary committee that included Lord Bramwell, Earl Fortesque and the Earl of Pembroke. One newspaper pointed out that 21 members of this League owned between them more than two million acres of British land (Lawrence, 1957, p 31). Joseph Chamberlain was at that time in the radical wing of the Liberal Party. Yet even he attacked George's ideas with these words, "If something is not quickly done ... we may live to see theories as wild as those suggested by the American economist adopted as the creed of no inconsiderable portion of the electorate" (Chamberlain, 1883). Economists such as Arnold Toynbee were similarly antagonistic. Toynbee regarded George's views as dangerous because he believed that their acceptance would damage Trade Unionism and Socialism. Socialists, Liberals, Conservatives: all were alarmed at the sudden entry of Henry George and the challenge posed by his ideas. The gut reaction of each was to attack and deride while playing for time to consider what he was saying. However, only the Conservatives were to persist, Liberals and Socialists modifying their stance with time as popular opinion swung behind the American.

In June 1883 land reformers of all persuasions, whether Socialists, land nationalisers, or what were coming to be called 'Georgists', united as the Land Reform Union. The movement was weak, however, with a membership of only 70, little financial backing, and only the vaguest of talk about 'restitution of the land to the people'. Among its members was Helen Taylor, the Socialist (*Justice*, 1884) stepdaughter of John Stuart Mill. The Union survived little more than a year but successfully prepared the way for Henry George's second tour of Britain.

When George reached Liverpool in December 1883, *Progress and poverty* had sold about 65,000 copies and many additional thousands of cheap editions were in circulation. Throughout 1884 and 1885 George delivered a direct and powerful message to audiences in 44 cities around Britain. He first described the appalling conditions of the inner cities, citing cases and speaking with profound conviction. Then he dismissed contemptuously the use of statistics to argue that the poor had never had it so good, as supposedly indicated by declining pauperism, higher income tax returns and a reduction in criminal convictions. Certainly, said George, wealth was accumulating as never before, but in great and rich England there were people wanting proper housing and adequate nourishment. The country was in the grip of an economic recession and the poor bore the brunt of the hardship even while, overall, wealth continued to accumulate. George identified the monopoly of Rent at the root of it all. The position of the private landholder was unnatural, and poverty was unnatural, even though society had long accustomed itself to both. Their interrelation was one of cause and effect, no matter how complex the working of the economy.

George emphasised the ways in which the state of affairs he deplored had been institutionalised in the English-speaking countries, through the law and the political system. When in 1884, warships stood off the north of Scotland, sent there with military forces by the government to intimidate the crofters who could not raise their landlord's rent, he took every opportunity to highlight the situation. Never did he advocate force or violence. 'Revolution' was to take place at the polls through a redistribution of seats in parliament, a widening of the franchise, and the return of radicals in favour of Rent reform (Lawrence, 1957, p 43). He asked, "Who is it who comes from the prisons, and are brought up for the penitentiaries and for the brothels?". When he answered himself, "Not the children of the well-to-do, but the children of the poor", he was offering the Public Health movement an economic remedy for the social problems that so taxed their efforts (Lawrence, 1957, p 46).

Newspapers continued to present Henry George as more than he was; as a nationaliser of land or a Socialist, instead of a collector of Rent. The confusion arose from his working alliance with Wallace and the Socialists – he hoping to persuade them over to his views, and they him to theirs. Many who understood the limits of his proposed measures feared that they would nevertheless be used by Socialists or Communists to push for much more, and not until his second visit in 1884 did George begin to emphasise the distinctiveness of his remedy, with its shift of the government's source of revenue from the factors of production – labour and capital – on to the non-productive accumulation of wealth in Rent. In an interview for the *Pall Mall Gazette* George suggested that Rent collection should start at four shillings (4s) in the pound, slowly rising to 20s. in the pound over time and thereby eventually restoring the full Rent to the public (Lawrence, 1957, p 56). By 1887, Socialists, no longer doubting his opposition to much in their programme, began to label him anti-Socialist. George accepted state control of education, the telegraph system and the railways, but only because, like John Stuart Mill, he saw these as activities in which the private market economy was inefficient. Unlike the Socialists, he did not see pure capital as the enemy; Rent was the element in private profit that was iniquitous. By the time of his fourth and fifth visits to Britain in 1888 and 1889, being by then branded anti-Conservative and anti-Socialist, his natural allies were the radicals in the Liberal party.

All through the 1880s George had to suffer the onslaughts of Malthusians, Spencerians and apologists for laissez-faire. *The Times* claimed that his speeches were popular because they encouraged a belief that something could be got for nothing. Unlike George, the editor believed that poverty and excessive wealth were necessarily in the nature of things. Galton would have been pleased with *The Times* of 10 January 1884 when it remarked that "Men suffering from their own idleness, vice, folly, or incompetence, or from those of their parents, would be no more contented than they are now to put up with the consequences of their defects". The *Aberdeen Journal* accused George of appealing to the lazy, improvident and worthless (Lawrence, 1957, p 67). There was much class-driven ranting. Judge Wilshere, created Baron Bramwell in 1881, called George mischievous, foolish, perverse and arrogant. Others ridiculed him as an American inventor with another wild theory. The Conservative Arthur James Balfour claimed George's arguments to be 'riddled with nonsense' (Lawrence, 1957, p 68). Such outbursts only encouraged working people to take a closer look at George's proposals.

On 28 January 1885, Balfour told his audience in the Prince's Hall, Piccadilly, "I am no Socialist, but to compare the work of such men as Mr George with that of ... Karl Marx [by then safely buried in Highgate cemetery], either in respect of its intellectual force, its consistency, its command of reasoning in general, or of economic reasoning in particular, seems to me absurd" (Pease, 1916, p 44). These were staggering words of praise to come from this philosopher and Scottish landowner for the works of a man little known in England at that time, other than as a dangerous revolutionary who had inspired the Communards during the burning of Paris in 1871. Marx had written his book *Das Capital* after settling in London in 1849, but repeated illness delayed publication of the first volume until 1867, and then in German. Henry Hyndman read the French edition while crossing the Atlantic in 1880. Even for those who founded the Fabian Society in 1884, calling it to begin with the Karl Marx Club, there was no English translation. Volume one appeared in English in 1887, a translation with revisions of the third German edition, and it was left to another German, Friedrich Engels, to assemble the remaining two volumes from Marx's notes.

Perhaps Balfour's purpose was not so much to praise Marx's high standards as to damn George, who at that time was the far more popular in England. Had Balfour been aware of the forthcoming third volume of *Das Capital*, drafted by Marx between 1863 and 1867 but not published until 1894, he might have realised that he had used George's name in vain. Entitled 'The process of capitalist production as a whole', volume three had, as part six, a section headed 'Transformation of surplus profit into ground rent', in which Marx said, "The private ownership of land -- the private ownership of some, which implies lack of private property (in land) on the part of others – is the basis of the capitalist mode of production"; and later: the "fact [is] that large property in land is a prerequisite and condition of capitalist production, seeing that it separates the labourer from the means of production" (Douglas, undated, p 9).

Marx proceeded to distinguish land from capital in a way which would have pleased George:"Capital may be fixed in the soil, may be incorporated in it either in a transient manner, as it is by improvements of a chemical nature ... Or more permanent manner, as in drainage canals, irrigation works, levelling, farm buildings, etc ...". In 1885, however, neither Socialists nor Conservatives were aware of this impending third volume, or of Marx's clear distinction of 'Land' from 'Capital fixed in land'.

So strong was Conservative antipathy that *Progress and poverty* had to be withdrawn as a textbook at the City of London College following a letter of protest from Lord Fortesque. By contrast, the Liberals took George into the National Liberal Club, and the radicals funded his visit of 1889, inviting him to speak on their platforms. In that year the National Liberal Federation passed a resolution in favour of the 'land tax' (Lawrence, 1957, p 104).

Henry George was particularly popular with the Fabian movement in its early days of 1884, for his site value taxation could be accepted as a start on the gradualist road to Socialism proper, in conformity with their preferred strategy. George Bernard Shaw was attracted to social problems and political economy by Henry George, only later moving on to land nationalisation and Socialism (Lawrence, 1957, pp 75-6). Numerous Socialists accepted George's analysis of social problems and his rejection of Malthusianism, but considered his remedy to be insufficient. Land taxation to Socialists was no more than a detail in their broad programme for taking the means of production into state ownership.

Joseph Chamberlain had set out his views for reform in a series of articles in the *Fortnightly Review* in 1885, soon assembled as a book, *The Radical Programme*. Although he considered George's views on land reform drastic, he sounded confusingly like him at times. In a famous speech in Birmingham, in January 1885, Chamberlain argued that private property (in land) had replaced the communal arrangements of the distant past, but that it was impossible to turn back the clock. Then he penned the question that horrified Alfred Milner, Milner's chief at the *Pall Mall Gazette*, the right wing of Chamberlain's own party, and the Conservatives: "But then I ask what ransom will property pay for the security which it enjoys?" (Lawrence, 1957, p 95). Yet the most Chamberlain seemed to have wanted was the right of compulsory purchase for urban development, and purchase of smallholdings for agricultural labourers. Nevertheless, Chamberlain was immediately accused by Conservatives of advocacy of plunder, blackmail and Communism. Inevitably the names of Chamberlain and George became linked. The *Pall Mall Gazette* concluded, "This emphatic passage will probably clench Mr George's conviction that, of all men now living, the President of the Board of Trade has the best chance of being the first President of the British Republic" (Lawrence, 1957, p 99). Such wild exaggeration, such misinterpretation of the views of both men, illustrated just how alarmed became the landed interest, and how anxious they and those beholden to them were for counter-propaganda. Both land reformers were abused mercilessly in the Conservative press. However, events turned the Conservatives' way when Chamberlain found himself unable to accept the efforts of Gladstone and Parnell to obtain Home Rule for Ireland. Chamberlain left the Liberal Party to form his own Liberal-Unionist Group. So weakened was the Liberal party by this development that the Conservative Party was soon back in power, where, apart from a brief interlude (1892-95), it remained for almost 20 years. Without Chamberlain, the radicals in the Liberal party moved closer to George, their London paper, the *Star*, covering his progress in full.

George's fame was now global, and he was invited to speak in Paris, Auckland and several cities in Australia. Then, in December 1890, fate dealt him a serious blow. At the age of 51 years, George suffered a stroke which caused a temporary loss of speech. However, he recovered well, and set himself the task of rebuttal of Herbert Spencer. As mentioned earlier, in his first edition of *Social statics*, Spencer had included a chapter on 'The right to the use of the earth', in which he had expressed views close to those of George on the invalidity of private landownership. Yet Spencer's reaction to *Progress and poverty* was to delete this chapter from the 1892 edition. This to George was intellectual dishonesty – Spencer was playing the man and not the ball. In *A perplexed philosopher* (1892), George attacked Spencer for his *volte-face* and the materialism behind his philosophy. Then, on 28 October 1897, while campaigning as an independent candidate for Mayor of New York, George had another stroke, this time fatal.

Standard economics was not conceived *a priori* with Welfare in mind. Rather, it pre-dated modern Welfare approaches, taking the business world at face value and reasoning *a posteriori* to explain how Capitalism worked. Welfare Capitalism is an offshoot of Capitalism, and as such its economics is something of a contrivance. Early economists, such as Nassau William Senior (1790–1864), William Stanley Jevons (1835-82) and Ysidro Francis

Edgeworth (1845-1926), sought 'scientific' respectability for their discipline in striving to model the creation and marketing of wealth. In seeking a 'pure', almost mathematical exposition, formulaic, they squeezed moral and social issues out of their discipline like juice from an orange. This coldness was especially evident in America, where a fledgling economics was over-awed by the power of the 'robber barons' – famous for their lack of scruple in pursuit of profit. It is hard to 'unsqueeze' an orange, which is what Welfare Capitalism subsequently asked of the economists of Capitalism. Far worse than that, however, was for conventional economics to be confronted with claims that certain practices of businessmen established long before the discipline emerged, and thus accepted as a major premise or 'given', may be 'convenient' to retain but a source of serious inefficiencies and inequities.

Land could be treated like any other marketable commodity when the composition of the bundle was accepted as 'given' and moral questions stripped from the economic debate. But governments as well as businessmen need revenue and so must tax wages and interest in lieu of Rent lost. Thereby massive distortions are introduced into the economy. The response of conventional economics, having accepted the demand for Welfare, is to attempt to minimise these distortions by suppressing taxation as much as possible. This, governments find very hard to do. Welfare Capitalism needs a far more sophisticated economics, one which works with the basic premise that Land and Capital are as elementally distinct in economic terms as are hydrogen and oxygen in chemistry. For the chemist to pretend that water is an element and not a compound of hydrogen and oxygen, or that the distinction is a triviality, simply because water is what consumers want, would make chemistry as incomprehensible as economics is made for Welfare Capitalism by economists who lump land and capital together as real estate for the property market. It was the desire to do just this that led to such fierce reaction to Henry George when he sought to retrieve Rent, the oxygen of Welfare.

The eruption of American business economics against George

During his lifetime Henry George received world-wide acclaim. In the USA his fame was surpassed only by Thomas Edison and Mark Twain. Yet today his name means almost nothing, eloquent testimony, even if silent, to the erasure of Rent from the public consciousness. Pure economics has never discovered an effective refutation of the proposition that public revenue is far better met by collection of Rent than taxation of wages and interest. George confronted the public conscience when he accused those in power of acquiescing in a private monopolisation of urban and rural land; a privatisation of Rent in the hands of a privileged few that created the injustice of poverty amid the affluence of cities such as New York and London. So popular became George's thesis that academic economists were thrown on the defensive and forced into public response. Most set about challenging George's claims.

Violent reaction to George's ideas from those who profited handsomely from Rent was sustained for many years after his death, on both sides of the Atlantic. In America this came largely from those making fortunes in railroads, oil, forestry and land deals, together with some in the patronage of these wealthy businessmen. In Britain the campaign was waged by landholders and their political representatives.

Business economics and Capitalism

Professor Paul Ormerod was remarkably frank about the lack of true academic freedom in university departments of economics:"The challenge of constructing an alternative, scientific approach to the analysis of economic behaviour is one to which increasing attention is being paid. The obstacles facing academic economists are formidable, for tenure and professional advancement *still* depend (in 1994) to a large extent on a willingness to comply with and to work within the tenets of orthodox economic theory. It is a source of encouragement that more and more economists are willing to look at alternatives, *despite the risks* they take in doing so" (Ormerod, 1994, pp ix–x, emphases added).

The founding fathers of the American Economic Association declared in one of their original statutes: "We regard the State as an educational and ethical agency whose positive aid is an indispensable condition of human progress" (1885). The statement was soon withdrawn, however, on the grounds that it was unfitting to an association dedicated to 'scientific' economic enquiry (Barber, 1991, p 204). Ethics was no part of economics. Yet the 'science' in this economics treated the business world as though it was a natural phenomenon, a most unscientific premise to take as a point of departure.

Capitalism as an economic system is insensitive to the condition or needs of whatever cannot command a marketable value. Productive labour is diminished to a 'human resource' with its market price. Hearts, souls, the needs of unproductive labour, under-age children, the sick and disabled, and the elderly, are outside the market formulation and therefore of no direct interest. Much of the environment, the atmosphere, seawater, and natural resources beyond the reach of the capitalist economy, cannot be captured and priced in the market. In this amoral system, aloof in its abstraction, aspects of human life and the natural environment which cannot be given a market value are treated as worthless. On the other hand, profits can be maximised by using what is beyond the market price mechanism for disposal of Capitalism's waste. Only when such behaviour begins to backfire and create inefficiencies in productive activity does the system take note. What imposes morality upon Capitalism is the enlightened Capitalist. Ways are then sought to assist the unemployed and unemployable, to raise the standard of subsistence, and to protect the environment from economic exploitation. This is the fountainhead of the Welfare State, but neglect of the power in Rent by successive governments has meant that an obvious way to protect human life and the environment from the ravages of Capitalism has been missed. In a global economy which knows no boundaries, which is 'supranational' more than multinational, this abuse of Rent by Capitalism and its insensitivity to 'externalities' are becoming massive global problems. The collection of revenue for Welfare States by taxation of wages and interest instead of collection of Rent adds injuries of its own. Modern Welfare States undermine the very defences they erect to protect the disadvantaged.

Had George been an academic economist, the holder of an endowed chair, he doubtless would have found himself dismissed for broadcasting his views. Witness the fate of academics who spoke in support. In 1915, for example, Scott Nearing published an article on land values in American cities which appeared in the Georgist journal, the *Public* (Nearing, 1915, p 1151; Gaffney, 1994, p 51). Soon after he was dismissed from the University of Pennsylvania. Joseph Rosengarten, a trustee of the university, explained that, "men holding teaching positions in the Wharton School introduce these doctrines wholly at variance with those of its founder and ... talk wildly and in a manner entirely inconsistent with Mr Wharton's well-known views and in defiance of the Conservative opinions of men of affairs" (Gaffney, 1994, p 51). Who was Mr Wharton?

Joseph Wharton was born in George's home town of Philadelphia in 1826. He studied chemistry and was remarkably successful in the production of lead, zinc, nickel and steel. The American railroads needed rails, but in 1864 their importation from England cost $162 a ton. Over the next five years home production of steel rods grew enormously, mostly coming from the Bethlehem Steel Company of which Wharton had been a founder. America was self-sufficient in steel rails by 1869, but by then the imported product had fallen to $80 a ton, undercutting Mr Wharton. Steel producers appealed successfully to Congress for an increase in the duty on imported rails. Prices of the home product then rose to $105 a ton, ensuring a workable profit margin, and Pennsylvania went on to supply America's growing industries, including shipbuilding. This experience turned Wharton into a staunch advocate of tariffs for what he called 'National Self Protection' (Wharton, 1875). Wharton was also involved in several railroads and a major owner of coal-rich land, his estates covering 100,000 acres between Philadelphia and Atlantic City.

Wharton's devotion to tariffs on trade made him a certain enemy of Henry George, a man who advocated freedom of trade and industry from all taxes, and revenue for national purposes from Rent alone (George, 1981, pp 195-6). Philadelphia was in any case a hotbed of economic protectionism, inspired by the writings of Henry Carey of that city. To promote protectionist policies, Wharton gave the University of Pennsylvania a gift of $500,000 from 1881 to instruct young men in business and the management of property. Under the terms of the gift there was no way that the Wharton School of Finance and Commerce could condone advocacy of Georgist ideas.

Late 19th century American universities were heavily dependent upon the patronage of businessmen – philanthropists. New York's Columbia University, for example, was completely reorganised and expanded by Seth Low. Mr Low was born in Brooklyn in January 1850. After graduating in the small Columbia College in 1870, he entered his father's importing business, rising to become Brooklyn's largest landowner (Fitch, 1995). His later philanthropy towards his old college included the support of several professorships. Low himself was President of Columbia University in the 1890s. In 1895, by then twice elected Mayor of Brooklyn, Seth Low was preparing to run against Henry George in the 1897 election for the new mayoralty of Greater New York. In the event George died just five days beforehand and victory went to the democratic candidate, Judge Robert Van Wyck. Low subsequently became Mayor of New York in 1902.

Columbia was also heavily funded through Wall Street, and its department of economics was well endowed by way of this connection. Sometime professor of economics in this wealthy department was Edwin Seligman of the 'American Rothschild' banking family of J. and W. Seligman. This man was another arch-critic of Henry George, waging a life-long campaign against the collection of Rent in America. In his *Essays on taxation* of 1895 Seligman devoted page after page to this campaign (Seligman, 1895), his preferred ideas coming to form the basis of much of modern taxation theory (Gaffney, 1994, p 63).

Ezra Cornell was born to the north of New York City at Westchester Landing in January 1807. In 1828 he settled in Ithaca and later associated with Samuel Morse who, between 1832 and 1835, developed the electric telegraph. Cornell constructed the first telegraph line in the United States in 1844, running between Baltimore and Washington. He was creator and largest stockholder of the Western Union telegraph monopoly and its appendage the Associated Press News Agency. Cornell had grievances against George on two counts.

In December 1868, Henry George joined the *San Francisco Herald* and went to New York to obtain a Press Association franchise for the paper. Cornell's monopoly refused him, and in an attempt to protect the *Herald* George tried to circumvent the problem by establishing an office to transmit news stories in code along Western Union's wires. When Associated Press realised what was going on it protested and Western Union refused George's business. George's protest against Cornell's monopoly was published by the *New York Herald*.

Cornell's second grievance concerned his real estate activities, especially his massive speculation in land in the western United States (Gates, 1943). His problem was that these states were raising revenue from land taxes along Georgist lines, something Cornell fought against for many years (Gaffney, 1994, pp 72-5). So having opened Cornell University with an endowment of $3 million in 1868, the year in which George began to give his news monopoly trouble, Ezra would have been in no mood to stand by and watch its department of economics promulgate Georgist ideas.

John Davidson Rockefeller was born in the same year as Henry George, but in New York State. He moved to Cleveland, Ohio in 1853, and observing the expansion of the oil industry in western Pennsylvania, he opened his first oil refinery in 1863. By 1882 his Standard Oil Company had a near monopoly of oil in the United States, and after 1890 he spent many years reorganising his business in attempts to evade the Sherman Antitrust Act (the 'trust' and the trust certificate had been invented by Rockefeller lawyers). With his immense wealth he founded the University of Chicago in 1897 with a donation of $80 million. The Chicago School of Economics became famous for its trenchant market orthodoxy. Four years later Rockefeller founded the Institute of Medical Research (later

Rockefeller University) in New York City. His lifetime benefaction has been put at $500 million.

Most leading American economists set about challenging George's claim that the private monopoly of the public's Rent was an injustice which reduced many ordinary working families to poverty. Initially the responses were rather simplistic, merely suggesting that when investors grew fat on 'interest' this was no more than testimony to the entrepreneurial talents of the managers of their capital; a justified return. A more original and damaging defence was mounted in 1887 by Francis Walker, President of the American Economic Association and Director of the US Census.

Walker taught at John Hopkins University in Baltimore, Maryland, founded on the wealth of the Baltimore and Ohio Railroad, the first length of American track to be opened, in 1830. He coined the phrase 'Rent of ability' to describe what looked to many like 'fat cat' returns (Walker, 1887). His device was to suggest a direct analogy between the differential economic productivity of land sites and the differential entrepreneurial skills of those who managed labour, land and capital in the productive process. Standard amounts of labour and capital, applied to prime sites when land was scarce and in demand, would in a free market economy generate a Rent. Similarly, standard amounts of labour, capital and land, in the hands of the best managers in an economy in which management skills were scarce and in demand, would generate a 'Rent of ability' enjoyed as high salaries for successful entrepreneurs and high returns for those whose capital they managed. Thus the wealth going to successful investors in land and their corporate managers was not an ethically unjustifiable appropriation of Rent as claimed by George, but rather, according to Walker, a justifiable return for talent. Walker's invention of 'Rent of ability' represented a novel form of income distinct from Wages, Interest and Rent. Therefore entrepreneurship needed to be elevated from simply another form of labour (albeit associated with high risk) to a factor of production in its own right. This synthetic manoeuvre ought to have been seen as flimsy and redundant, there being no valid reason to set apart the successful entrepreneur from other skilled and sought-after workers such as the accomplished surgeon or talented lawyer; all remain nothing other than qualitative descriptions of forms of labour, rewarded in wages.

Another outstanding personality among American economists was Frank Knight, who arrived at the Chicago school from Cornell in 1917. This professor said some strange things when he defended the entitlement of slave owners to their 'property', because, he claimed, there had been 'open competition' for the capture and sale of slaves (Knight, 1953). Lincoln's emancipation of slaves he had found to be 'unethical' because their owners had not received compensation. In such a climate of opinion, everything apparently having its price, a tag on Rent saying 'not for sale' was given short shrift. Staggeringly, another American economist, disturbed by George's use of Ricardo's theory of Rent, wrote in 1908, "Nothing pleases [an advocate of Henry George] better than ... to use the well-known economic theories ... [therefore] economic doctrine must be recast" (Patten, 1908).

Cornell economist Frank Fetter, President of the American Economic Association in 1913, said that the 'old lumber' of Ricardian thought should be "broken up for kindling" (Gaffney, 1994, p 78). For Fetter, "Economic theory should stop being remote from actual business usage ... Capital is essentially an individual acquisitive, financial, investment ownership concept" (Fetter, 1935). These economists had little use for labour or land except insofar as they were of relevance for Capitalism and profit maximisation of the 'firm', and no use at all for Welfare.

Richard Ely, founder of the American Economic Association in 1885, invented the sub-discipline of 'land economics' for his Institute for Research in Land and Public Utility Economics. This organisation received funding from numerous railroad companies, among them the Baltimore and Ohio, Great Northern, Northern Pacific, Atlantic Coast, Nickel Plate Road, Chicago and Northwestern, and the Chicago, St Paul, Minneapolis and Omaha. The Institute devoted itself to the companies' concerns for the protection of their land and its taxation. This land, totalling 131 million acres, or more than twice the area of the United Kingdom, had been granted away over the years by Congress. Rent of this land soared ahead of the track. One such railroad man was Andrew Carnegie, enjoying an income of $50,000 a year by 1865, with which he was able to buy into the steel industry. In his essay *The gospel of wealth*, Carnegie argued that after acquiring wealth, rich men should distribute their surplus for general welfare (Carnegie, 1962). Largesse was his antidote to Socialism. Politicians exacted enormous financial favours in return for charters and mining rights, fiercely competed for by these rich men and their companies. It was the economic counterpart of the 'wild west'.

The railways were Ely's 'Public Utilities', the very companies whose land grants George had attacked, and whose acres the Ralston-Nolan Bill was threatening to include in the land tax base. In 1938 Ely wrote, "Perhaps I am a college (economics) professor, and the street-car magnate whose rapacity I am called upon to help hold in check has endowed the chair which I occupy. Is it strange that many of us who are called upon to control others of us should simply refuse to do it?" (Ely, 1938, p 253). No statement from a senior economist could have made more clear how his discipline was subservient to its businessmen patrons, as underscored by Professor Ormerod (1994, p ix-x). In true science researchers strive to avoid 'conflicts of interest' which could arise, for example from holding shares in a company that produces drugs which they (the researchers) are subjecting to study. Some 'scientific' economists appeared by contrast to have consciences completely untroubled by the idea that 'conflict of interest' might cast doubt on the impartiality of their work. Indeed, they confessed to bias.

Ely wrote in the 1920s, "Considered as property yielding income, land and capital are on exactly the same footing ... We should not tax separately the value of land" (Gaffney, 1994, p 93). In her memoirs, Grace Jaffe, Ely's chief research assistant at Northwestern University, described how Ely became preoccupied with speculation in land. He made a fortune buying land cheaply and selling at a high price in Wisconsin real estate. This was the same man who, in 1927, was introduced to President Calvin Coolidge as the 'dean of American economists' (Gaffney, 1994, p 99). It is impossible not to conclude that some notable American economists in those years had a vested interest in land, or their patrons did, and on this account were so hopelessly embroiled in strong conflicts of interest that they could not possibly have examined competing theories of economics dispassionately and impartially. It was the businessman and Rentholder in them that threw out George, not the disinterested economist open to new ideas.

Alfred Marshall, Rent and quasi-Rent

Adam Smith wrote his most famous work, *An inquiry into the nature and causes of the wealth of nations*, to describe the mechanism of economic growth in an economy in transition between the older rural ways and emerging urban industrialism. A century later, economists, mainly American, re-wrote the discipline to accommodate corporate Capitalism and to describe the functioning of this new system. What seems inadvertently to have started the relegation of Rent was conceived in England, however. The invention of 'quasi-Rent' by Professor Alfred Marshall (Keynes, 1924) was a godsend from Cambridge to vested interest which promptly proceeded to manipulate the concept.

Alfred Marshall, the most successful British economist of his era,

Table 13.1: Quasi-rent of inelastic Labour and Capital

Labour/Capital	A Quasi-rent	B Interest	C Nett productivity
Prime quality	6	4	10
Second quality	5	4	9
Third quality	4	4	8
Fourth quality	3	4	7
Fifth quality	2	4	6
Sixth quality	1	4	5
Seventh quality	0	4	4
Totals	21	28	49 units

graduated in mathematics at Cambridge University in 1865 when aged 23. Within a few years he became attracted by the possibilities offered by his discipline to political economy. His ideas gradually took shape during the 1880s, but did not appear in print until the publication of his *Principles of economics* in 1890. Marshall realised that a model in which one factor of production is varied in productivity, the others being held constant, is not limited to one in which Land is the variable. Capital and Labour can also be considered to vary from prime quality to inferior quality from an economic perspective. Although the supply of labour and capital can be adjusted to meet demands, for example by flexible wage rates to attract people back into the workforce, and interest rates to divert income into savings for investment, the economy has an inbuilt inertia and time is needed for these adjustments to work through the system. In the short term, therefore, the supply of labour and capital can be unresponsive to demand, or temporarily 'inelastic' as economists might say. At such times we can re-label Table 3.1 to produce Table 13.1; for site we write Labour or Capital, for Rent we write quasi-Rent, and we leave Interest and Net Productivity unchanged. For example, in a world of variable Capital and standard units of Labour and Land, the productivity of prime Capital is 10 units net. By the time Capital of seventh quality is brought into the economy, the quasi-Rent on prime capital is six units. Land obtains no Rent in this model because all sites are economically identical, and it is only variation in productivity of Land that creates Rent.

Marshall was careful to stress that it is quasi-Rent and not Rent proper which temporarily goes to Capital and Labour when demand increases. In the long term competitiveness and entrepreneurship ensure that the Capital and Labour demanded are eventually supplied. The temporary advantages of superior Capital and Labour will then be diminished and with it the quasi-Rent. This sequence is not possible with the gifts of nature, which man cannot create. In the preface to his first edition of *Principles of economics* Marshall wrote, "thus ... the Rent of land is seen, not as a thing in itself, but as a leading species of a large genus; though indeed it has peculiarities of its own which are of vital importance from the point of view of theory as well as of practice" (Marshall, 1891, vol 1, p xii). These peculiarities were quietly relegated by other neo-classical economists, particularly those of the budding American schools which were soon etiolated by a burgeoning and overhadowing laissez-faire corporate Capitalism.

Profit being the bottom line, and society lacking any mature notion of social welfare, the privatisation of Rent went largely unquestioned. After all, the privatisation of Rent was nothing new. Quasi-Rent proved attractive, one important offshoot being the concept of transfer earnings, developed by the American neo-classical economist John Bates Clark, whose major work, *The distribution of wealth*, appeared in 1899 (Clark, 1925). Together, quasi-Rent and transfer earnings became the two parts of wages paid to employees. The reasoning was simple enough. Suppose a worker decided to give up self-employment and work for a wage paid by an employer. The wage needed to entice the worker and hold him or her in service was the transfer earnings, and what had been foregone from self-employment was the 'opportunity cost'. It was the difference between transfer earnings and opportunity cost that decided the situation. This was no beam of sunlight, but then came the clever twist.

Imagine there is a surplus of prime labour needed by employers. The circumstances of these workers will naturally differ, and for some will be so precarious in self-employment that the opportunity costs and the transfer earnings associated with enticement into employee status will be low, perhaps little above subsistence. Others will be in a better situation, and refuse to transfer for what is offered. The economy grows and our employer needs more labour to seize market opportunities. To attract more labour, however, and retain these workers, transfer earnings have to be raised. All workers achieving identical outputs must receive identical wages in the common labour market, and as a result the original cohort of recruits find their wages raised to the level of the transfer earnings of the new cohort. By analogy with Rent, the component of 'unearned income', raising the wages of the original cohort from their own transfer earnings to the transfer earnings of the new cohort, was called by Clark and other neo-classical economists, 'economic rent', because of a *contrived* notion of something for nothing. As the economy expands and our firm thrives, recruitment continues until the transfer earnings of the last cohort equals their productivity. Thus when the firm is operating efficiently, most of its workers will be receiving a component of what is euphemistically called 'unearned income' in their pay packets as 'economic rent'. Modern textbooks of economics teach that economic rent is the excess that a factor of production (any factor) is paid over its transfer earnings.

This logic has two important consequences. First, a major way to reduce the 'economic rent' in wages is to reduce opportunity costs to a minimum. In other words, the less eligible is the condition of the worker in self-employment or the employ of another, the lower will be the wage needed to secure his or her transfer into employee status. This encourages big business to put the small man out of business. Second, the 'unearned income' in the wage packet of most employees, so the argument ran, made them feel relatively well off and in a frame of mind conducive to acceptance of income tax, as long as the take-home pay remained sufficiently clear of their notional transfer earnings. The same reasoning could be applied to the market in capital. Capitalists induced to invest income for a small rate of interest would enjoy an 'economic rent' when operating in a market also using the capital of other cohorts enticed into the market only by the offer of higher rates of interest.

In 1880 Alfred Marshall was still five years away from his succession to the Chair of Political Economy at Cambridge University. In 1875 he had visited the USA and travelled as far as San Francisco, where Henry George earned a living as editor of the *Post*. George and Marshall did not meet on that occasion, but nine years later Marshall came to listen to George speaking at Oxford University. Marshall had lectured on *Progress and poverty* in Bristol in 1883. He criticised George at that time and was expected to do as much in Oxford. He first patronised, remarking that he "did not find fault with him (George) for getting it wrong on economic subjects without the special training that was required for understanding them". Then he attacked the book for not pointing the working man in the real direction of his salvation – thrift and industry (Stigler, 1969). Marshall asked George for proof that the people of England were in the power of the landlords. "The landlords could only get as much as competition allowed them", said Marshall, maintaining that this was "one shilling in the pound" (5% of national income). Marshall must have hated the role expected of him, for he detested involvement in controversy. Challenge George though he did, his professorial writings were more eloquent and empathetic with George than his words of 1884, his years of high ambition.

In 1899, Professor Marshall suggested to the Royal Commission on Local Taxation that a start should be made in shifting taxes off buildings and on to land, especially more highly valued urban land (Royal Commission on Local Taxation, 1899, pp 124-5). Henry George would have approved. A decade later, at a critical period when the Liberal administration's Budget proposals for a 'land tax' were being debated in the House of Lords, Marshall deliberately intervened in support of the government (Marshall, 1909). He proposed that a tax on urban land should be used for public purposes and, first and foremost in those days of urban squalor, for what might be called these days a 'green tax' to be used for improvements to the environment. Marshall suggested that landowners would be foolish to resist, since the 'clean-up' operation and preservation of green acres would only enhance the value of their properties, just as would any kind of publicly financed upgrading of their localities. Crucially, he ended by writing,

> The proposal made in the present Budget to isolate future accretions of 'public value' and to tax them ... (ie collect future growth of Rent) ... I regard ... as in many ways a great improvement ... in so far as the Budget proposes to check the appropriation of what is really public property by private persons and in so far as it proposes to bring under taxation some real income, which has escaped taxation merely because it does not appear above the surface in a money form, I regard it is as sound finance. In so far as its proceeds are to be applied to social problems where a little money may do much towards raising the level of life of the people and increasing their happiness, it seems to me a Social Welfare Budget.... (Marshall, 1909)

Arnold Toynbee was a Fellow of Balliol College, Oxford and lecturer in Political Economy to candidates for the Indian Civil Service. An inspired reformer of the 1870s, he was convinced that the plight of the Victorian working classes was a direct outcome of exploitation by their employers, the urban capitalists. Like many men of his class (his grandfather was George Toynbee, a landholder and large tenant farmer of Lincolnshire), Toynbee warmed to the traditional aristocracy. His heart overruling his astute mind, Toynbee told his audience, "An aristocracy like ours cannot be wholly base, because it has ruled for so long ... although a man may be debased by ruling a people ... the sense of responsibility may elevate him and strengthen his character". "No", said Toynbee, the debased condition of the labouring classes has arisen solely because, "Gradually capital is being accumulated in fewer and fewer hands, until at last some think we shall have nothing but a handful of stupendous monopolists, with a struggling mass of labourers at their feet". It was the responsibility of government to restrain the "disastrous and virulent greed of employers" (Toynbee, 1884, pp 22-4). This was the mast to which young Arnold Toynbee nailed his colours. Sick and dying, he declared that Henry George's 'theory is not true', without, however, providing anything in the way of refutation other than the fact that Ricardo wrote his famous book at an exceptional time when Britain's economy was in a desperate state. Malthus wrote his *Essay* in these same years, a fact that did not shake confidence in his theory of population.

Toynbee knew all about the urban landlord, but argued that as the freeholder, he was "powerless to demand a high rent for his land", because, "the mills are built either on a 99 years lease, or upon – what is practically a freehold – a 999 years lease" (Toynbee, 1884). Out of Toynbee's own mouth came the admission that as head leaseholder, the mill owner was in such circumstances the collector of essentially all Rent for the site occupied by his mill. Toynbee delivered these words, exhausted, in mid-January 1883. Nine weeks later he was dead. The following year his friends and admirers named their new centre in London at 28 Commercial Road, Whitechapel in his memory. In their own way these men and women of late Victorian social conscience looked back wistfully to a supposedly better time of social harmony and mutual respect between classes which they imagined to have been wrecked by the Industrial Revolution. They sought to re-kindle better relations by bringing the social classes back into closer geographical proximity, as had once existed on the manor. Gradually, under the leadership of Samuel Barnett, Toynbee Hall set aside this reactionary purpose and assumed a more forward-looking policy in early 20th century social reform.

The resistance to the use of Rent for public purposes within political economy in Britain and elsewhere stems not from validated objections on economic grounds, but exclusively from distorted political considerations. Had not modern economists done what Mark Blaug says they did, which was to satisfy themselves that, "In the long-run stationary equilibrium, the total product is resolvable into ... payments to Labour and Capital – there is no third factor of production" (Blaug, 1997, p 82), Welfare Capitalism and Britain's Welfare State would be much more developed than they are today. Economists threw out Land from the elements of economics like chemists threw out phlogiston; the difference being that Land is a fact while phlogiston was a fiction. Land and Rent can be deleted from economics only if fairness and equity are deleted from the discipline.

John Maynard Keynes remarked on Alfred Marshall's remarkable tardiness in publishing his ideas and opinions, which he attributed to Marshall's fear of being shown to be wrong and a tendency to be upset even by minor criticism (Keynes, 1924, pp 32-3). If so, Marshall must have felt very secure indeed in his opinion on Rent for public revenue expressed in his letter to *The Times* at such a critical time in 1909. Even more than this, he was surely very convinced of the importance of what the Liberal government was proposing with respect to 'site value taxation', for his guiding rule was always "to avoid controversial matters" (Keynes, 1924, p 45). Many years previously Marshall had written in his *Principles of economics*, "The sudden appropriation of Rent and quasi-Rents by the State would indeed have very similar effects in destroying security and shaking the foundations of society; but if from the first the State had retained true Rents in its own hands, the vigour of industry and accumulation need not have been impaired; and nothing like this can be said of quasi-Rents". Marshall went on to say: "Nevertheless, things being as they are, the distinction between land and other forms of wealth has very little bearing on the detailed transactions of ordinary life" (Marshall, 1891, vol 1, pp 670-1). Clearly, when Marshall later realised that the Liberal administration was proceeding in a way which, though shaking landed society, was not disturbing the foundations of the nation, he came out in favour of its policy on true Rent.

Marshall seemingly failed to acknowledge the argument that monopolisation of Rent in an imperfect land market has a profound effect on the detailed transactions of ordinary life by creating cyclical unemployment, cyclical poverty and cyclical exacerbations of ill health. He and his followers believed that economic cycles were a simple reflection of cycles in 'confidence' among businessmen. In the freely competitive theoretical market with its neatly arranged supply and demand, and its checks and balances, capital investment and savings were equated by the regulator of interest rates, production and consumption were equated by flexible pricing, and flexible scales of wages kept employment rates at the optimum. Capital and labour were temporarily underused when managers for some obscure reason lost confidence in the markets in which they operated. Loss of confidence was 'infectious', said Marshall, and it took time for managers to regain their composure. Other economists pursued their own theories. William Beveridge spent a lifetime assembling data in the forlorn hope of identifying the pattern of the world's climate with the strength of the economy. J.A. Hobson, forerunner of J.M. Keynes, argued that persistent attempts by managers to drive down wages created cycles of under-consumption which, for businessmen, were self-defeating. Non-economists seeking explanations for cyclical unemployment were offered the choice of a selection of unsubstantiated theories.

Socialists and rentiers

Not only the neo-classical economists were guilty of debasing the meaning of Rent, destroying its value for economic and political debate, but so also were Britain's Democratic Socialists. Sidney Webb and the early Fabians were well aware of Ricardian Rent and of Henry George's reasoning, but for them the feature of Rent with most appeal was its unearned nature (Ricci, 1969-70). In 1883 not only was Alfred Marshall discussing *Progress and poverty* in Bristol, and Arnold Toynbee doing the same in London, but so also were Frank Podmore and Edward Pease, two original members of the Fabian Society. Pease was unstinting in his praise of George: "my attention was first drawn to political economy as the science of social salvation by Henry George's eloquence, and by his *Progress and poverty*, which ... beyond all question had more to do with the Socialist revival of that period in England than any other book" (Pease, 1916, p 28). Many Fabians supported George but largely considered that his proposals would not solve Britain's social problems. True, said the Fabians, landowners exploited economic forces by appropriating Rent, thereby gaining income without labour or sacrifice. But, they continued, so did others who held in private possession large amounts of capital in great demand, acquired either through inheritance, exchange of Rent for stocks and shares, or good fortune.

To illustrate, in their Tract no 7 the Fabians referred to Sir Hugh Myddelton's New River Water Company, shares in which had reached "their present enormous value, not because [the] venture was costly, but because London had become great" (Olivier, 1896, p 6). To the Fabians, any income derived from the private ownership of wealth not produced by its owner was ethically unjustifiable, even though sanctioned in law, and all such income (not merely that from private landownership) was in this sense 'Rent'. Those who received income without labour in the production of wealth became known as the 'Rentier' class. Borrowing from John Cairnes (1874, p 32), Fabians referred to rentiers as drones, hardly less immoral in their way of getting through life than the owners of others' labour, those who had property in slaves. George Bernard Shaw wrote in 1930 (when in his mid-seventies), "a rough division of society into an upper or proprietary class, a middle or employing and managing class, and a wage proletariat is produced. In this division the proprietary class is purely parasitic, consuming without producing" (Shaw, 1930, pp 3-4). Rentiers, according to Shaw and others, were 'parasites'.

Since in its allegedly 'unearned' quality Interest was claimed to be no different in essence from Rent, Fabians were as undisturbed as the capitalists they opposed by merger of the two for their own purposes. The Fabians termed their hybrid 'Rent', the capitalist called it a species of 'profit'. Yet by corrupting the meaning of 'Rent' as others were doing, the Fabians added to confusion of thought. While claiming to be scientific in their approach, presumably because they sought to test their theories against observations assembled systematically, they were at the same time in breach of an equally fundamental scientific principle, the precise definition of terms. Fabians started to talk of such abstractions as 'rent of status' and 'social rents', incomes derived from position in society and opportunities derived therefrom (Ricci, 1969-70, pp 114-15). The consequence of this failure to retain the classical meaning of Rent was an inability of capitalists and Socialists alike to make headway against major economic and social problems that bedevilled Welfare Capitalism throughout the 20th century.

'Rent of vitality'

Scientific and technical innovations (the 'life' forces) have presented relatively few problems for the economy. Unemployment, inequitably low income, material deprivation and pollution (the 'death' forces) have by contrast remained as persistent blights on Capitalism for which no effective solutions have been put into practice. The consequence has been the persistence of wide disparities in life expectancy between socio-economic classes, even while average lifespan has steadily increased. The materially disadvantaged, having no title to land, lose what is due to them in Rent, which would come to them if collected for social purposes by government. If we were to adopt the Fabian concept of Rent, then the extra years of life enjoyed by those with considerable socio-economic advantages gained without labour would constitute a 'Rent of vitality', where vitality means power to live and capacity for survival. For this reason *par excellence* the private appropriation of Rent, no matter how engrained into society and how difficult to extract, must be corrected by the return of Rent to the public for social purposes, economic stability, environmental protection and relief of the disadvantaged. Insofar as wealth and income are major determinants of life expectancy, a Rent of vitality would represent the most pernicious aspect of modern Welfare Capitalism.

The Liberal Party and land reform

In Britain a most important figure standing for land reform was David Lloyd George. Born in Manchester on 17 January 1863, but raised in the village of Llanystumdwy near Criccieth in the Welsh Lleyn Peninsula, Lloyd George knew a Wales subjected to a domineering English culture from which it was attempting to assert its own identity. A notorious entry in the index of a 19th century edition of *Encyclopaedia Britannica* encapsulated the Welshman's dilemma: "Wales – see England" (Constantine, 1992, p 8). Lloyd George entered the land reform movement in 1886 at the age of 23, and was soon publicly attacking Tory landlords. In February of that year, Michael Davitt arrived from Ireland to address meetings in Flint and Blaenau Festiniog. At the Blaenau Festiniog assembly Lloyd George made his first noted public appearance, the *Cambrian News* (12 February, 1886) reporting his speech: "Working men acting separately, were only as particles of sand to resist the power of the landlord; but let workmen combine, firmly express their opinion, and then no opposition, however powerful, would be able to stand before them." When a Land League was started for Wales he hoped they would all join (Douglas, 1976, p 99).

Lloyd George entered local politics just at the time when the Welsh 'Tithe War' was erupting. In January 1886, the farmers of Llandrynog in Denbighshire (now Clwyd) asked the local rector for a reduction in their tithes, but he referred them to the Church's collecting agents. They, however, had not heard from the rector, and upon insisting on the full tithe the farmers withheld payments completely. When the action spread the clergy distrained the farmers' stock for sale by auction.

In September 1886 an Anti-Tithe League for North Wales was established, and Lloyd George became secretary of his local organisation. In 1887 he and his younger brother William established their own firm of solicitors, Lloyd George and George of Porthmadog. Land was at the heart of practices such as this, in a region where only 4% of farms were owner-occupied. The rest were rented from landlords, many of whom were English. Lloyd George's outspoken defence of the radical cause attracted the attention of local Liberals, and in 1890 he won a by-election for Caenarfon Boroughs, defeating the local Tory landholder by 18 votes. In the House of Commons he was soon on his feet criticising the iniquities of private landownership, demanding land reform and the disestablishment of the Anglican Church in Wales.

Henry George visited Britain for the last time in 1889, thereafter concentrating on his writing in New York. So it was up to Lloyd George and other radical backbenchers in the Liberal Party to nurture the cause for land reform in Westminster between 1890 and 1905. However, for all but the years 1892 to 1895, the Liberals had to operate in opposition. Lloyd George was as aware as anybody of the social conditions which created the crisis of 1903 and the establishment of the Interdepartmental Committee on Physical Deterioration. He also had no doubt about the connection between poverty and the private monopoly in Rent. In a very important respect, however, Lloyd George differed from Wallace and Henry George. Whereas they were agitators for a single cause, he was a parliamentarian who accepted the task of achieving the objectives of land reformers from within parliament, the very seat of power, wealth and private landholding. It was a task that broke him, though not before some memorable achievements along the way. His great compromise, the best he could wrest for the common man from the powerful grip of the establishment, was in many respects the birth of what has come to be called the Welfare State.

What burned within Lloyd George was resentment of the inherited wealth and the institutionalised privileges bestowed on the Anglican church, even outside England, and the aristocratic class with monarchy at its peak. He carried this distaste for the English landed establishment and distrust of its secretive and clannish ways through to his assumption of the Premiership in the House of Commons. Coupled with an admiration for hard working, self-made men, a genuine social conscience and a strong ambition to get ahead, this concern for issues of the land was to be a driving force in his political career for many years to come.

In August 1908, the year of his promotion to Chancellor of the Exchequer and establishment of the Royal Commission on Land Transfer, Lloyd George took a trip to Germany. There he familiarised himself with Germany's system of Social Insurance and would have been aware of its Kataster. Since 1891 the Grundsteuer had been the central tax of the general community. This was nowhere near to what Henry George was proposing, but the germ of Rent for central revenue was perceptible. There is no doubt that Lloyd George linked funding of future British welfare policy with collection of Rent, or site value 'taxation' as it was called. He knew the possibilities, but as an insider he was also acutely aware of the vested interests organised against radical reform and the need to proceed with all the political skills he could muster.

The early Labour movement and land reform

By the 1890s the Socialists were on their own tack, ever more concerned to capture both land and capital from private ownership for the State as the means of nationalised production. Alfred Wallace had by 1890 embraced the Socialist movement, having been impressed with E Bellamy's book *Equality*. An American Socialist, appalled by the grotesque debasement of the human condition in his country, Bellamy claimed that Capitalism and its enormous private wealth led directly to overwork of the labouring classes, poverty, starvation and crime. Revealingly, on election to parliament for West Ham South in 1892, as the first Independent Labour member, Keir Hardie declared his approval of "nationalising the land by taxing land values" (Douglas, 1976, p 115). This remark crystalised the way in which the treatment of land under Socialism (German school), land nationalisation (British school), and the principles of Henry George (American school) were confused in many minds (and still are). The British school wanted to nationalise land, and the American school 'tax' Rent, policies as immiscible as oil and water. Yet the Socialists could not clearly discern the difference.

In 1894, 94 members of parliament signed a memorial to the Chancellor, Sir William Harcourt, calling for site values alone to be used as the basis of local rates rather than the value of the site with its improvements. Memorials such as these revealed an increasing interest in urban land reform, with the realisation that industrialisation, high density of population and growth of civic amenities had produced a massive increase in the Rent of cities and towns. Sidney and Beatrice Webb witnessed how the "town artisan is thinking of his claim to the unearned increment of *urban* land values, which he now watches falling into the coffers of the great landowners" (Webb and Webb, 1920, p 376). The Independent Labour Party, founded in 1893, included among its objectives the proposal that "Land values, rural and urban, be treated as public property" (Mann, 1895, p 8). What it seemingly failed to appreciate was that its intention to take land into public ownership went far beyond treating Rent as public property.

Conservatives view welfare as a weapon against Socialism

On social welfare, Arthur James Balfour, now First Lord of the Treasury and leader of the House of Commons, had this to say in 1895: "Social legislation, as I conceive it, is not merely to be distinguished from Socialist legislation but it is its most direct *opposite* and its most effective *antidote*. Socialism will never get possession of the great body of public opinion ... among the working class or any other class if those who wield the collective forces of the community show themselves desirous to ameliorate every legitimate grievance and to put Society upon a proper and more solid basis" (Halevy, 1951, vol 5, p 231). In Conservative and right-wing Liberal thinking, welfare legislation and philanthropy were ways of fending off the demands of Marxists, Socialists, land reformers, and others seeking the acquisition of land, or land and capital for public purposes.

Yet surprisingly little was achieved in the field of social legislation during Lord Salisbury's time as Conservative Prime Minister between 1895 and 1901. The Workmen's Compensation Act of 1897 made the employer directly responsible for injury suffered by his employees while at work. Old age pensions faced opposition from the Friendly Societies, who did not wish to have the State take away their business. Charles Booth's experiences in London made him an advocate of non-contributory pensions, but the idea of collecting something like £16 million in taxation for redistribution in this manner found no support in any government of the 1890s. Joseph Chamberlain, when Secretary for the Colonies in Salisbury's administration, made clear his preference for contributory old age pensions but received a hostile reception from the Friendly Societies. As he said to Lord Aberdare's Royal Commission on the Aged and the Poor Law in July 1897, the Friendly Societies, "have very great parliamentary influence and I should myself think twice before attempting to proceed in face of hostility from so important and dangerous a quarter" (Wilson and Mackay, 1941, p 28). Gladstone's Royal Commission of 1893, which included Booth and Chamberlain, had similarly made little headway. Salisbury's committee of 1896 fell behind a contributory scheme. Germany had introduced old age pensions in 1889, and New Zealand's scheme, launched in 1899, prompted the appointment of a Commons Select Committee, on which Lloyd George secured a place. In part owing to his encouragement, this committee recommended a non-contributory scheme. Outside the House, Lloyd George could count on the Fabian movement, the Trade Union Congress and the Labour Representation Committee for support. During the Boer War, he attacked Chamberlain and the government for squandering money that could go towards old age pensions. As he put it, "There was not a lyddite shell which burnt on the African hills that did not carry away an old age pension" (Pugh, 1988, p 23). His seemingly anti-patriotic stance was not popular, however. At a meeting in Birmingham in December 1901 a massive crowd rioted, hurling bottles and bricks at his platform, killing a policeman and demonstrator.

The Liberal's electoral victory of 1905

Lloyd George's unbridled attacks on the government and its stand on education and the Boer War singled him out as a potential leading light in a future Liberal administration. What turned potential into reality was Joseph Chamberlain's obsession to develop the colonies for British trade. The political leaders in the colonies were looking for Imperial Preference in trading relations, and Chamberlain was sympathetic. There was at the time a temporary duty on imported corn to support the Boer War effort, and Chamberlain had the idea not to repeal this duty on non-colonial corn. This amounted to a reintroduction of trade tariffs which flew in the face of the reasoning that had led to the repeal of the Corn Laws in 1846. The issue had destroyed Peel's Conservative Party; now the same question threatened to destroy Balfour's Conservative–Liberal Unionist coalition. Balfour announced his intention to repeal the corn duty; Chamberlain, insisting publicly that duties on food needed to be expanded in order to strengthen the trading links of the Empire, resigned from the Cabinet to set up his Tariff Reform League. Sensing a unifying commitment in the protection of free trade, the Liberal opposition came together as it had not done since the 1880s. In disarray, Balfour resigned and the leader of the Liberals, Sir Henry Campbell-Bannerman, accepted the Premiership.

The new Liberal ministers had to struggle through a real London 'pea-souper' of a fog as they made their way to Buckingham Palace to receive their seals of office from Edward VII on 11 December 1905. Sir Henry was a sick man of 69, worn down with nursing his dying wife. Still, he accepted office and sought support for his new administration in the election of January 1906. The result was astounding. The Liberals gained 377 seats, while the Conservatives and Liberal-Unionists secured only 157. The Liberal manifesto had made little mention of social or land reform, yet despite everything the English weather, fate, and the political opposition could throw at the Liberals, theirs turned out to be the administration which in its desire for justice found the power to tear at the very heart of the British constitution. A century of reform was reaching its climax. In the wings was the Labour movement, to which 47 members of parliament were connected in 1906. Thirty of these were in the Labour Representation Committee, which almost immediately called itself the Labour Party.

FOURTEEN

The battle for Rent and Welfare
Part II: 1906 onwards

Health is the first good lent to men; A gentle disposition then; Next, to be rich by no by-ways; Lastly, with friends t' enjoy our days. (Robert Herrick, *Hesperides,* 1648)

The Britain of today looks, feels and *is* very different from that of 1900, but not in one most fundamental respect. While all sorts of emblazons of class have been taken down or left to fade where they stand, the ancient edifice still rests on its original foundations. Running through the whole is that vein of injustice which gives British society its peculiar characteristics. This vein has entered the bedrock of all other nations that have replicated the fundamentals of the British political economy.

The nation has devoted much of the past century attempting to remove social inequities, what Sidney and Beatrice Webb described in 1913 as "not so much the inequality of income ... as the resultant inequality of power over human lives" (Webb and Webb, 1913, p 14). As the first issue of the *New Statesman* summarised the challenges in that year:

> We are fully conscious of the difficulties which lie before those who seek to find a solvent for the almost infinitely complex problems of our 20th century social organisation. But for the fruits of the patient study of a generation of economists and sociologists, the attempt could not be made. Even today there are enormous gaps in our knowledge – gaps which no amount of goodwill on the one hand or social discontent on the other can of themselves help to fill. The remedying of the social defects of which we are all so painfully aware depends no doubt primarily upon the existence of a determination to remedy them; but it depends also, and no less emphatically, upon our knowing exactly how to set about it. (*New Statesman*, 12 April, 1913, p 5)

The *New Statesman* long ago ceased to be 'new', but this old editorial comment is as apposite today for 'New Labour' as it was for the newborn

Labour Party in 1913. Precisely because Old Labour went about tackling the problems the wrong way, New Labour seeks another as yet indistinctive approach today.

In his speech to the New Labour Party at the Brighton Conference on 30 September 1997, Prime Minister Tony Blair said: "I'll tell you: my heroes aren't just (Old Labour heroes) Ernie Bevin, Nye Bevan and (Clement) Attlee. They are also (John Maynard) Keynes, (William) Beveridge and (David) Lloyd George. Division among radicals almost 100 years ago resulted in a 20th century dominated by Conservatives. I want the 21st century to be the century of the radicals" (*The Times*, 1 October, 1997, p 9). But the 20th century *was* in many ways dominated by the radicals who reduced the power of the House of Lords, nationalised coal, rail and steel, and shaped the modern Welfare State. The division among the radicals to which Tony Blair referred did have profoundly negative consequences for Britain's fortunes, but not least because the popular radicalism in 20th century politics accomplished little more than a trade-in of old embellishments for new.

The old embellishments are easily reconjured by perusal of the columns of *The Times* newspaper of those days; here, for example, is a piece written during the famous general election of 1906:

> It is befitting that Mr Walter Long ... should, on his rejection by the electors of South Bristol (a seat he had held since 1900), find refuge in (South Dublin) a Leinster constituency: for his maternal grandfather, the Right Hon Wentworth Fitzwilliam Hume-Dick, of Hume-wood, county Wicklow, represented in the House of Commons from 1852 until 1880 that part of the same province which lies to the immediate south of South Dublin. Unlike the late Lord Fitzwilliam, who before his succession to the peerage was returned as a Liberal ... Mr Long's Irish ancestor was an old-fashioned Conservative. He was on terms of intimate friendship with Lord Beaconsfield, from whose uncle, Benjamin Disraeli, his father, Mr Hume, of Hume-wood, inherited the house in Fitzwilliam-street, Dublin, occupied for some time by an uncle of Lord Halsbury's, Mr (afterwards Sir Ambrose Hardinge) Gifford, who, until his appointment as Chief Justice of Ceylon, was a practising barrister at the Four Courts. (*The Times*, 29 January, 1906, p 10)

Why this pedigree, and any connection with Fitzwilliam Street in Dublin should have qualified Mr Long for a seat in the House of Commons, despite rejection by South Bristol, is difficult to understand these days, but it counted for much in 1906. Walter Long was, all importantly, the inheritor of the family estate of 14,000 acres at Road Ashton in Wiltshire, not far from Trowbridge, though by 1906 he had sold more than 5,000 acres as he moved into other forms of property at home and abroad and assumed directorships of English firms.

The Times openly regretted the loss of the landed governing class from parliament, writing during the same general election: "One of the most regrettable incidents so far ... is the defeat of Sir William Hart Dyke ... If re-elected, this survivor of the steadily diminishing band of county magnates sent to Westminster would have enjoyed the distinction, which fell to Sir Michael Hicks Beach (now Lord St Aldwyn) on the death of his kinsman, Mr W Brainston Beach, in 1901, of being the 'Father of the House of Commons" (*The Times*, 22 January, 1906, p 10). The Right Hon Sir W Hart Dyke had been defeated in Dartford, Kent, by the Labour candidate J Rowlands. Times were indeed changing.

The embellishments erected to display the wealth, power and status of the landed constituency and re-enforce that deference expected from the governed classes have been largely peeled away and replaced by the insignia of the Welfare State. The change of appearance should not be mistaken for anything other than a genuine national desire to right old wrongs. But the vein of injustice engrained within the edifice itself, the real cause of much that needs to be put right in order to narrow the gaps in health between rich and poor, remains untouched. As the *New Statesman* remarked long ago, "remedying of social defects ... depends ... upon our knowing exactly how to set about it" (*New Statesman*, 12 April, 1913, p 5). Face-lifts and aspirations are not enough.

Rent has for centuries been the secretive and obscure way, or as Herrick preferred, the 'by-way', to riches. Walter Long, the Right Hon Wentworth Fitzwilliam Hume-Dick of Hume-wood, Sir William Hart Dyke and others of the Edwardian governing class knew exactly what it was, and were certainly aware that it was not synonymous with the commercial rent due to them as property owners. So also did Karl Marx, John Stuart Mill, Arnold Toynbee, Henry Mayers Hyndman, Sidney and Beatrice Webb, Bernard and Helen Bosanquet, Henry George and Winston Churchill. Even more impressively perhaps, so did many a great-grandfather of the ordinary working man of today. Rent was the stuff of political philosophy in those days, a 'hot potato' that persuaded economists to revamp their discipline so as to play down its significance, diminish the fervour of the working classes and accommodate the new corporate businessman (Gaffney, 1994).

Rent formed a battleground over which the party that desired to 'conserve' the old ways and the radicals for change fought tooth and nail; the battleground on which, to Tony Blair's regret, the radicals were divided, allowing the Conservatives to force the breach and win through. Has New Labour learned from the fortunes of Victorian and Edwardian 'New Unionism', 'New Liberalism' and 'Nascent Labour'? It was not so much that the radicals were divided by the strength of Conservatism; they were never united behind reform of Rent. Radicalism was a cauldron of ideas for social and political reform, a hotchpotch of ingredients which often did not blend at all well, but out of which were spooned British Social Democracy and Welfare Capitalism. Both have in large measure preserved over-privilege and failed the under-privileged, which is why New Labour seeks the constructive reform of both systems. As we move on from the 20th century we have yet to confront the significance of Rent. Nothing less offers any prospect of genuine relief for dependent and under-privileged families in modern Britain or stands any chance of bringing their life expectancy closer to the standard set by independent and wealthier families. Yet another round of 'crisis funding' for deprived areas and struggling services simply will not do. We shall pick up the history in 1906.

The Edwardian era and its reformers

Faced with the opposition of the Conservative Party and the landed interest in parliament, the scepticism of Socialists, the popularity of eugenic and Malthusian views in influential quarters, and the revisionism of the 'new economics', those Edwardians advocating land reform for justice were forced to operate on several fronts, stretching their limited financial resources. The first blow of fate, however, fell not against them but the new parliamentary opposition. Joseph Chamberlain suffered a paralytic stroke on 11 July 1906. Men like Winston Churchill (then a Liberal) and Lloyd George were left to get on with the business of social reform, which Chamberlain had neglected for some years. Lord Crewe had warned in 1905: "the Liberal Party is on trial as an engine for securing social reform – taxation, land, housing ... It has to resist the Independent Labour Party claim to be the only friend of the workers" (Wood, 1982, p 398). In 1907, Churchill wrote to the *Westminster Review*: "minimum standard of wages and comfort, insurance in some effective form or other against sickness, unemployment, old age – these are the questions and the only questions by which parties are going to live in future" (Wood, 1982, p 398).

Initially the Liberal Cabinet was slow to take a leadership role, partly because of the condition of their leader. Campbell-Bannerman attended the House of Commons only for questions; otherwise he was at his wife's bedside. By October 1906 he was suffering from bouts of hypertensive heart failure, forcing him to take his medicines into the House. Nevertheless, he accepted two Bills from the Labour group, one allowing local authorities to provide free school meals and the other granting unions immunity in the event of strikes. Both measures became law in December 1906 (free meals for needy pupils was first advocated by the Board of Trade in 1697!). Asquith managed to introduce the distinction between unearned and earned income into his Budget of 1907. That November, however, Campbell-Bannerman had a hectic round of engagements during a visit of the German Emperor Wilhelm to Windsor. On the 13th he was found collapsed in his host's home. He never recovered, being confined to Downing Street from mid-February 1908. The Cabinet was without their leader, rendering many decisions impossible until Campbell-Bannerman's death on 22 April. Herbert Asquith then took charge.

Despite the administration's difficulties, Britain's first non-contributory old age pension scheme was introduced on 1 January 1909. Single people aged 70 years or more received 5 shillings (5s) a week and couples 7 shillings and 6 pence (7s 6d) a week in order to reduce the threat of the workhouse. Those who had been imprisoned in the previous 10 years, or failed to work according to ability, or received an annual income of more than £31 a year, did not qualify.

With Asquith as premier, Lloyd George moved to Chancellor of the Exchequer and Churchill to President of the Board of Trade. They were under strong influences. The radical wing of the party, numbering about 50 members, did not accept that Capital was the primary generator of wealth in the industrial economy. Quite obviously its own generation was dependent upon the application of Labour to Land, no matter how this link was obscured by the many intermediate steps in the productive process. The radicals also emphasised the distinction between the private and social origins of wealth, and the responsibility of government to secure Rent for public purposes even though current law condoned its retention in private hands. Outside government, William Beveridge was pressing for reforms in the labour market.

Beveridge not attracted to possibilities for Rent reform

In October 1905, Beveridge had been recruited to the Conservative daily newspaper, the *Morning Post*, the editor Fabian Ware wishing to influence Conservative opinion on social reform, a 'big issue' of the day. Ware was allied to Joseph Chamberlain and Alfred Milner in his views. He believed that in the light of the experience of the Boer War further imperialist expansion depended upon the nurturing of a 'true imperial race'. Imperial greatness needed social reconstruction in Britain, possibly along eugenic lines, to create a dominant race. Beveridge was certainly no Conservative, but saw in the columns of this paper a way to influence the influential. At 26 he had moved into journalism and was organising classes for the Workers' Educational Association, founded by Albert Mansbridge a few years before. In addition, he was preparing an academic study of unemployment and working five hours daily for the Central (Unemployed) Body. His acquaintances were very catholic, including Sydney and Beatrice Webb, Karl Pearson, Francis Galton and Sydney Buxton.

Beveridge's ideas for social reform began to gel in these early years of Campbell-Bannerman's and Asquith's Liberal administrations, but apparently he was never seriously attracted by the ideas of Henry George or other land reformers. In a letter to his mother dated 8 June 1902, while at Balliol College, he had begun, "My dearest Mother, Tawney read a paper on the 'Taxation of site values' at his or my society which provoked very keen discussion" (Beveridge Papers, IIa). Any interest shown by these men in those years must have been fleeting as they moved on in pursuit of their preferred causes in education and employment for the labouring classes.

Beveridge has been called a 'New Liberal' of the Edwardian age, but he neither belonged to the Liberal party nor upheld the radical theories of its land reformers. In 1906 he wrote in the *Morning Post*, "The Liberal Party ... is sick to death ... it is a party of negations" (Harris, 1977, p 86), quite an extraordinary comment (even if written for Conservative consumption) on the party of Lloyd George and Campbell-Bannerman. He must have been aware of Campbell-Bannerman's speech of 21 December 1905, given in London's Albert Hall: "We desire to develop our own undeveloped estate in this country – to colonise our own country – to give the farmer greater freedom and greater security; to secure a home and career for the labourers ... We wish to make the land less of a pleasure-ground for the rich, and more of a treasure-house for the nation ... There are fresh sources

to be taxed ... I include the imposition of a rate on ground (ie site) values"
(Douglas, 1976, p 135).

Beveridge was probably disappointed with senior Liberals such as the
jaded Lord Rosebery, given to depression and insomnia since the death
of his wife and loss of office in 1895 during a serious bout of influenza
(James, 1963, p 369). In 1902, in another letter to his mother, Beveridge
wrote of Lord Rosebery's "innate incapacity to lead the Liberal Party ...
he is far too critical and too little contriving ... criticising every other
proposal as unpractical ... the only justification for a statesman is that he
should be able to deal with practical difficulties" (Letter to Annette
Beveridge, 14 March, 1902, Beveridge Papers IIa). Beveridge preferred
to be a free thinker, finding something of appeal in the radicalism of
Liberalism, the imperialism of Milner, and the Socialism of the Webbs.
Under the influence of the Webbs he accepted their concept of Socialism,
with subordination of private interests to those of the State and society,
but he never became a practising convert. Industrial nationalisation did
not appeal to him apart from municipal 'gas and water' Socialism as a
way of helping poorer regions. Like the Webbs, however, he favoured a
paternalistic bureaucracy of enlightened men and women, detached and
unsentimental in their resolve to discipline society where previously it
had been left to the 'blind play' of conflicting interests (Harris, 1977,
p 87).

Beveridge pinned his hopes for progress not on political ideology but
on education of workers. In an organised labour market with its exchange
system, working men could perhaps acquire a little capital. He mistrusted
the intrusion of the Labour movement into labour affairs, though
welcoming its commitment to social reform. He believed that the politics
of Labour, arising out of the poverty of the working class, were, "materialist,
self-interested and incapable of reaching high political ideals" (Harris,
1977, p 94), a charge Labour of course levelled at the Conservative middle
and upper classes. This aloofness from organised labour, the impression
he gave of paternalistic and educated wisdom, did not endear him to
Labour or union leaders. They distrusted his ideas on social policy, based
on the notion that he and experts like him could organise the labour
market to the liking of the labourers themselves, without sentimentally
protecting the less competent from the disadvantages of their 'inferiority'.

To Beveridge's mind, poverty was not incurable in the classical
Malthusian sense, nor was there necessarily any need for unthinking
devotion to the dogma in private property. He accepted that modern
industrial society could generate sufficient wealth to abolish poverty –

the problem was to devise effective and just means of distribution. In the *Morning Post* of 15 May 1908 he sided with Alfred Marshall, pre-empting Professor Arthur Pigou (Pigou, 1920; Galbraith, 1987, p 212) by some 12 years when he argued that the 'marginal utility of money' did decline with increasing personal wealth, contrary to classical economic thought. Beveridge told his readers that the 'last pound' of a rich man's income brought him much less happiness than the 'last pound' of the income of the poor, and on this ground he supported progressive taxation (introduced by Lloyd George in 1914). He held out at that time (but not in later years) against a statutory minimum wage on the grounds that this would drive many 'marginal' workers on low income completely off the labour market and convert low pay to no pay. He rejected means-testing for relief, arguing that wherever the line was drawn the system would be unfair to those just above it and likely to create disincentives for the working class (Harris, 1977, p 97) – an argument still heard today outside government. For Beveridge, Capitalism was unrivalled at creating wealth but it also created poverty by distributing this wealth unfairly. He sought ways of redistributing wealth without discouraging savings and thrift, undermining incentives to accept work, or reducing the difference in rewards going to the efficient and inefficient. His solution was a state-organised system of insurance to protect against the worst consequences of poverty without interfering with the efficiency of wealth creation.

Beveridge's commitment to the labour exchange system and social insurance to protect the vulnerable in the labour market was more or less assured by his visit to Germany in September 1907 (which had over 4,000 exchanges by that time). Here a system financed by contributions from the worker, the employer and the State provided earnings-related maintenance of income at times of sickness, when there was permanent medical disability, and in old age. He greatly disliked Lloyd George's scheme of non-contributory old age pensions for 'deserving' citizens. The law of gratification of desires with least exertion seemed for him to be displayed by the Leicestershire miners in the immediate abandonment of their voluntary superannuation scheme, because otherwise they would have disentitled themselves to the new non-contributory pension. Why work to put aside for the future if to do so results in the loss of what the State would give for no labour? He argued strongly for a contributory scheme to encourage work and savings, for which the State should promptly establish the necessary machinery.

In June 1906, Beveridge wrote an article in the *Morning Post* showing clearly his acceptance that impoverishment of working class life was a major cause of sickness and early death. Infant mortality differed between rich and poor parts of the country and between rich and poor families in a way which was manifestly related to external physical conditions. He dismissed the eugenic argument: "Infant mortality is neither a symptom nor a result of racial degeneration ... the vast bulk of all children are born physically sound – the national stock is *not* tainted, it is the environment before and after birth that counts" (Harris, 1977, p 103). This was not to deny that some diseases were inherited, and he was not entirely persuaded that there was not an element of genetic inheritance in anti-social behaviour, but even if based in fact this had nothing to do with the separate effect of impoverishment on health. What troubled Beveridge and many others was that so much of this impoverishment of the labouring classes was man-made. His colleague Richard Tawney wrote:

> In so far as poverty arises from the niggardliness of nature or the natural defects of human character, it is an evil, but it is not a grievance. What gives it its sting, what converts economic misery into a political issue or a moral problem, is the conviction that the poverty of the modern world, since it is co-existent with riches, is unlike the natural poverty of the colonist, the fisherman or the peasant, in being a social institution ... Social poverty is merely one outward expression, impressive because it appeals to the eye, of the power over the lives of mankind which modern industrialism confers upon those who direct industry and control the material equipment upon which industry and social life depend ... Hunger and cold cause misery, but men do not revolt against winter or agitate against the desert. The fundamental grievance is that the government of industry and the utilisation of both capital and land are autocratic. (Tawney, 1963, p 102)

The advent of national insurance in Britain

Germany served not only to illustrate the possibilities in a labour exchange system, but also to encourage more serious consideration of social insurance in Britain. W H Dawson of the Board of Trade had written supportively on the German system in 1896 (Harris, 1977, p 168). Lloyd George would have known of this interest while President of the Board, and in August 1908 as Chancellor of Exchequer he went to Germany to gain first-hand experience. Churchill was equally enthusiastic, and within weeks of Lloyd George's return the preparatory work for the necessary Bills was shared between the two ministers. Churchill took unemployment insurance while Lloyd George at the Treasury took sickness and disability insurance. Churchill put Beveridge and Hubert Llewellyn Smith on to the job, and by December 1908 a scheme was ready for Cabinet. 'Less eligibility' was still there, Churchill explaining that unemployment benefit would be kept low so as to "imply a sensible and even severe difference between being in work and out of work". Lloyd George was not ready with health and disability insurance, however, having to deal with the vast entrenched interests of the Friendly Societies, the industrial insurance companies and other agencies which together held private policies for 12 million people.

While waiting for the Treasury, the Board of Trade looked further into its own scheme. Employers, employees and the taxpayer were all to dip into their pockets to cover the unemployment insurance fund: employers because they would profit from the preserved working capacity of the workforce; the State because the community had always assumed some responsibility for the able-bodied pauper; and the employee because he was the principal beneficiary. Payments were to be standardised (flat rate rather than earnings-related), to remove the need for means-testing with all its connotations of the Poor Law (Harris, 1977, p 172). Higher paid but out of work adults were likely to have savings to fall back on, in any case. Among the criticisms was the fear that the employers' contributions would simply be recouped by higher prices and lower wages, thereby reducing consumption and depressing trade, throwing men out of work. Nevertheless, a draft Bill was presented to Cabinet in April 1909. The cost to the taxpayer was put at £1 million annually, allowing for periodic unemployment of up to 16% at times.

There was great concern, as there still is today (Department of Social Security, 1998), to avoid the social insurance cheat, and Beveridge spent much time devising ways to close loopholes. No benefits would be payable to men who resigned from their employment, to men on strike (here the unions stepped in with strike pay), or to men sacked for misconduct. To catch the habitually unemployed, benefits were not to be paid until regular work had been performed in an insurable trade for at least six months, after which benefit would cover one week's unemployment for every five contributions. On the other hand, no man would be expected to accept a job for less than the going rate. A major difficulty had arisen in another quarter, however. Lloyd George was proposing to include in his Budget of 1909 (the People's Budget) a small measure of Rent collection (land taxation) to help raise revenue to cover old age pensions, unemployment insurance and anticipated sickness benefit. A major constitutional crisis loomed because the Conservative opposition was delaying its passage.

The constitutional crisis precipitated by land taxation

Lloyd George had two major Budgetary concerns in early 1909. He had to lay the foundations of tax reform to finance his long term plans for state-operated social security, and he needed to find the money to build battleships to match the shipbuilding programme of Admiral von Tirpitz, Secretary of State for the German navy. His long-standing interest in land reform and opposition to some British institutions left him in no doubt about what lay ahead. Indeed, events during the first three years of the Liberal administration had made the position only too clear. In 1906 the government had adopted a private member's Land Tenure Bill, by which tenants received additional rights of compensation for improvements they made to their properties and for damage to crops inflicted by the landlord's game. Many Conservatives were in strong opposition, but because farmers were pleased the Bill passed both houses virtually unscathed. With land taxation, however, it was a different story.

Large scale landownership is particularly obvious in Scotland, where as recently as 1980 as much as a quarter of land, over two million hectares (nearly 5 million acres), was in the possession of 100 landlords. Altogether, 340 families, a mere one thousandth of the population, owned between them 64% of Scotland. The Duke of Buccleuch owned 110,000 hectares, Lord Seafield 75,000 hectares, and the Duke of Roxburgh nearly 40,000 hectares (McEwen, 1981). Henry George was well known to the Duke of Buccleuch's ancestors. On 15 February 1884 the *New York Tribune* had written: "The late Duke of Buccleuch died with a hearty contempt for Mr Henry George's wild schemes of disorder and confiscation, and in his will arranged for the management of his estates for 1,300 years to come". In April of the same year, the Duke of Argyll (family estate in 1980 totalling 30,000 hectares) published an article entitled 'The Prophet of San Francisco' in the *Nineteenth Century*, denouncing George as a 'preacher of unrighteousness'. The editor gave George the honour of a reply, published as 'The Reduction to Iniquity' in July 1885. This debate between George and the titular chief of the Clan Campbell was circulated around Scotland as a pamphlet, *The peer and the prophet*. Against the background of crofter uprisings in the Western Isles at that time, the argument had only succeeded in raising George's popularity with the people (Geiger, 1939, p 49).

The Liberals tested the water in 1907 by introducing a Bill for the valuation of Scottish land. The Scottish people were generally enthusiastic about site value taxation, and some Conservatives had shown sympathy towards the idea with respect to local taxation in Glasgow. But with recent events in Scotland still fresh in their minds the Lords threw out the Scottish Land Valuation Bill. Another Scottish Land Valuation Bill, proposed in 1908, was wrecked on amendments. Not even two Bills to promote smallholdings in Scotland, designed to discourage emigration to North America, could get passed their Lordships. So the Liberals withdrew to re-think strategy, and their answer was Lloyd George's Budget of 1909. There was no going back. Keen though he was on Beveridge's plans for labour exchanges and unemployment insurance, Winston Churchill had declared in 1907 that land reform was the most important and certainly the most fundamental part of constructive Liberal social policy. Campbell-Bannerman had billed Scottish land valuation as an indispensable preliminary step for his government's programme of reform (*Liberal Magazine*, 1907, pp 255-8). In the country, the United Committee for the Taxation of Land Values (founded in 1889) was co-ordinating its land campaign, distributing over 50 million leaflets between 1907 and 1911.

Lloyd George stressed that, although valuation of the nation's land was an essential prerequisite for site value taxation, "It would be impossible to secure the passage of a separate Valuation Bill during the existence of the present parliament owing to the opposition of the Lords, and therefore the only possible chance which the government have of redeeming their pledges in this respect is by incorporating proposals involving land valuation in a Finance Bill. On the other hand, it must be borne in mind that proposals for valuing land which do not form part of the provision for raising revenue in the financial year for which the Budget is introduced would probably be regarded as being outside the proper limits of a Finance Bill by the Speaker of the House of Commons" (Douglas, 1976, p 143). With little option, Lloyd George decided to wrap up the first step in his land programme in his Budget, hoping thereby to out-manoeuvre the Upper House by sending up to the Lords measures they would wish to throw out, but presenting these in a form which by convention they ought to pass, however begrudgingly.

Lloyd George proposed to the Cabinet a tax of 1d in the pound (0.4%) on the capital value of land, which for the first two years would be collected only on vacant land, ground rents and mining royalties. Householders and practically all agricultural land were to be excluded at this stage. In addition, when land was sold at an increased price or leased for more than 14 years the increment in value would be taxed at 20%. Similarly, when valued land was inherited, the legatee would pay 20% on any increment in value at the date of transfer. In the case of land held by corporate bodies, the Increment Value Duty was to be assessed every 15 years. These land taxes were expected to raise about £500,000 of a total revenue of almost £13 million (less than 4%). Lloyd George had a fight on his hands with some members of his own Cabinet, and when the Budget was introduced on 29 April 1909 the land tax had been reduced to ½d in the pound. However, a Reversion Duty was added, so that landowners would pay 10% of any increment in land value when a lease fell in to their advantage.

Some 'land taxers' were disappointed that the Chancellor appeared to have veered from Georgist principles, but it is doubtful whether George himself would have proceeded differently if in Lloyd George's shoes on that Budget day. Nobody could have got a Valuation Bill through the Upper Chamber. Even in the Lower Chamber the Conservatives gave the Finance Bill a very rough passage. During his speech of four and a half hours, the Chancellor infuriated the opposition not only with his proposed taxes on landowners, but by his demonstration that enough revenue could be gathered in for purposes of social reform and naval defence without resorting to import duties of the kind favoured by Joseph Chamberlain. At the end of his speech he said: "This is a War Budget. It is for raising money to wage implacable warfare against poverty and squalidness. I cannot help hoping and believing that before this generation has passed away we shall have advanced a great step towards that good time when poverty and wretchedness and human degradation which always follows in its camp will be as remote to the people of this country as the wolves which once infested its forests" (*Hansard*, 29 April, 1909; Lee, 1996, p 39). As if to provide a reprise for Lloyd-George's refrain to close almost a century of welfare politics, Prime Minister Tony Blair declared in 1999: "Our historic aim will be for ours to be the first generation to end child poverty. It will take a generation. It is a 20 year mission, but I believe it can be done" (White, 1999).

Under great strain, and inflicted once more with bouts of neuritis, Lloyd George struggled throughout the summer and autumn to get his Finance Bill through the House of Commons. By the time the Bill passed the Commons on 4 November 1909 by 379 votes to 149, there had been 554 divisions, Lloyd George voting in 462, Asquith in 202 and Churchill in 198. It reached the Upper House some five months behind schedule, and on 30 November the Lords took the unprecedented step of vetoing the Bill by 350 to 75. Lloyd George's strategy had in one sense failed, yet in another succeeded. The Liberals had been provided with the opportunity to take their cause to the country. Eight Unionist lords, Boston, de Saumerez, Emly, James of Hereford, Monteagle, Peel, Torphichen and Rolls, had probably foreseen what was ahead should the Lords take this course of action, but their vote for the Bill was of no avail. The House of Commons regarded the Lords' action as unconstitutional, and so parliament was dissolved. Polling started on 15 January 1910 and lasted for one week.

The election was fought on the Budget's taxes against reinstatement of import duties, and on the powers of the House of Lords. The south of the country was not so supportive as the north and the Liberals were returned to power with only three seats more than the Conservatives. Thus the Liberals now needed the support of the Labour Party's 40 members and the Irish Nationalist Party's 82. The Finance Bill was reintroduced, and approved by the Lower House with the support of the small parties. It then went through the Lords without resistance and received Royal Assent on 29 April 1910. Arthur Balfour's plan to thwart the Liberals in collusion with Lord Lansdowne, leader of the Conservatives in the Lords, had backfired. Foreseeing such intrigue, Campbell-Bannerman had as early as 1907 carried a resolution in the Commons: "in order to give effect to the will of the people as expressed by their elected representatives, the power of the other House to alter or reject Bills passed by this House must be so restricted by law as to secure that within the limits of a single parliament the final decision of the Commons should prevail" (Wood, 1982, p 405). The treatment metered out to the People's Budget was the last straw.

The Parliament Act of 1911

The question now faced by Asquith was precisely what shape reformation of the Lords should take. Testing the water with a series of resolutions, he finally sought the end of the power of the Upper House to use an absolute veto to thwart the wishes of the democratically elected Lower House. However, on 6 May 1910 Edward VII unexpectedly collapsed and died, and a stunned nation went into mourning. King George V called a constitutional conference of both leading parties, but by October it was floundering. The king was reluctant to flood the Upper House with newly created Liberal peers in order to get Bills through the Lords, but on 16 November agreed to do so on condition that the Parliament Bill was put to a second general election. The Lords proposed that a change in their political composition was an answer, but this would have left untouched the absolute veto. The conference finally broke down and Asquith dissolved parliament on 28 November. Polling commenced on 2 December and was completed by the 20 December. The outcome was another narrow majority for the Liberals, who promptly introduced their Parliament Bill in February 1911. Once more the opposition picked at every word, tabling more than 900 amendments. Eventually, however, the Bill was carried on its third reading on 15 May. The Lords then tabled amendments unacceptable to the government, returning the Bill to the Commons on 6 July. Lloyd George met Arthur Balfour and Lord Lansdowne on 18 July to tell them in no uncertain terms of the king's promise to create peers of the government's choosing if the Bill was in danger. Asquith had his list of prospective Liberal peers at the ready, including Thomas Hardy, Baden-Powell, Bertrand Russell and James Barrie (Lee, 1996, pp 68-71).

Some days later the Duke of Westminster hosted a group of rebellious peers nicknamed the 'diehards' at Grosvenor House. There they swore to fight to the bitter end. As Lord Selbourne put it, "The question is, shall we perish in the dark, slain by our own hand, or in the light, killed by our enemies?" (Dangerfield, 1966, p 63). However, Lord Landsdowne met with 200 Conservative and Unionist peers on the same day to advise that the Bill should be let through. On 24 July, Asquith stood in the Commons for fully 30 minutes while the Conservative opposition yelled at him with taunts such as 'Who killed the king?'. Balfour sat motionless. The government's backbenchers then gave as good as their Prime Minister had received, and for the first time since 1893 the Speaker invoked standing order 21, suspending the House because of grave disorder. Debate was not resumed until 8 August when the Lords' amendments were finally rejected by a substantial majority. On return to the Lords, after two days debate, the Bill was finally passed by 131 to 114.

From then on, any Money Bill, so defined by the Speaker of the Commons, should become law one month after receipt by the House of Lords. Other Bills, except those extending beyond the maximum duration of a parliament, should become law despite rejection by the Upper House if they passed through the Lower House in three successive sessions in not under two years. A parliament's life was also reduced from seven to five years. This new arrangement still left the Lords with powers to kill a Bill introduced in the last two years of a parliament. Nevertheless, if returned for a second term of five years, a government could then be sure of securing legislation which met with approval in the Commons.

The Liberals now saw their opportunity to secure the land reforms and social reforms they wanted, the Irish Nationalists were more than ever confident of securing Home Rule, and the Labour Party had had its prospects improved by the Lords' defeat. There was further relief for Labour members when for the first time all members of parliament were salaried at £400 a month. For the Liberals, however, with five full years ahead of them, this was the time to move forward with their reforms. As Austen Chamberlain had said to Arthur Balfour after the election of January 1910, "the Budget was popular and the Lords were not. The electors ... voted against the Lords, and, above all, against landlords" (Douglas, 1976, p 149). But for the opposition this was the time for counter-strategies. The Conservatives chose to give ground on the question of reform to local taxation, in the hope of deflecting charges of complete intransigence, thereby enabling their party to throw its weight against any new national taxation based on land values. As Austen Chamberlain put it in March 1910: "... if we do nothing the Radical party will sooner or later establish their national tax, and once established in that form any Radical Chancellor in need of money or any Socialist Chancellor in pursuit of the policy of the nationalisation of the sources of production will find it an easy task to give a turn of the screw ... On the other hand if this source of revenue, such as it is, is once given to the municipalities, the Treasury will never be able to put its finger in the pie again, and the Chancellor of the Exchequer will have no temptation to screw up taxes from which he derives no advantage" (Douglas, 1976, p 150).

The resistance of the legal profession to a land register

The Liberal government had to demonstrate before the next election that the Land reforms which had created such a constitutional battle over two years were in fact worth the candle. However, on 18 May 1911, Lloyd George concluded that the land valuation needed to prepare the way for the tax would not be completed until 1915 at the earliest. If the government delayed the introduction of a Bill beyond 1913, and lost the next election, everything might be scuppered. The opposition created mayhem over Home Rule, deflecting the focus of the government and the electorate, and the land reform movement was hard pressed to keep valuation in the forefront of public debate. By-elections in 1912 in Norfolk, Yorkshire and Staffordshire all went to 'land taxers', leaving little doubt about the continued popularity of these proposed measures in the country. In other by-elections, Liberal candidates lacking commitment to land reform were defeated. To maintain the momentum the government set up a Land Enquiry Committee, which in 1913 recommended the establishment of a Ministry of Lands, a minimum wage for agricultural labourers and acquisition of land for housing and allotments. The release of this report coincided with the start of the Liberals' Land Campaign, meant to sustain interest up to the next election. This massive effort was backed by about 300,000 posters, 10 million pamphlets and 100 meetings daily around the country. Speeches on the land proposals by Lloyd George at Swindon, Winston Churchill in Manchester and Asquith in Leeds were received with great public enthusiasm (Douglas, 1976, p 160).

The bulk of the nation's Rent was in urban areas and here the Land Enquiry Committee had much more difficulty, being subjected to intense lobbying. The land nationalisers of the Wallace tradition wanted acquisition with compensation, but their policy had no satisfactory answer to the question, "If the owner's title is a just one, then on what grounds can his land (as against the Rent) be confiscated; if unjust, then why compensate?". The reformers of Georgist persuasion were afraid that the government would be over-cautious. In the event, the Urban Report of April 1914 did not recommend immediate introduction of a national land tax, instead limiting its proposals to pilot schemes of land reform by local authorities in favour, testing both 'nationalisation' and land value taxation (Douglas, 1976, pp 162-3). This report met with less public reaction, partly because of headlines whipped up by those opposed to Home Rule in Ireland. Lloyd George had feared just such a Conservative strategy. In 1913, at the start of the Land Campaign, he told the government chief whip: "The Tory press have evidently received instructions from headquarters to talk Ulster to the exclusion of land. If they succeed we are 'beat' ..." (Douglas, 1976, p 164).

The Tory press was of less concern to Lloyd George than his professional brethren in the Law Society and their loathing of land registration. Enthusiasm for a register came from two sources. There were bedfellows of *The Economist*, not concerned with the morality of bundling up Rent with other rights and privileges in land – only that a register would facilitate the land market. Then there were those land reformers who needed a register as a preliminary to removal of Rent from the bundle.

In their resistance to a land register the conveyancers set themselves in opposition to both movements.

On 15 June 1909, Mr Brickdale of the land Registry sent a proposal to the Lord Chancellor for a unified department to handle land registration, land value taxation and the necessary ordnance survey as a prelude to development of a unified system across the nation. Lloyd George was involved in discussions which eventually led to a "Scheme for the formation of a Domesday Office for England and Wales amalgamating the Land Registry and Land Values Departments, and ultimately (perhaps) the Cadastral Survey also" (Offer, 1977, p 508), proposals for which were circulated to Cabinet in 1910. However, the resultant Report of the Royal Commission on Land Transfer, published in February 1911, was heavily weighted by the opinions of solicitors who approved compulsory registration in principle but set out an assortment of reasons to go slowly. Nevertheless, the German Kataster was approved of and the County Veto came in for criticism, so work continued on two Bills for the extension of Land registration (Offer, 1977).

In July 1911 the Land Transfer Bills came before the House of Lords, the month that the Parliament Bill came back to their lordships for reconsideration. Passions were running extremely high, and Land Transfer was debated in the middle of the fervour, the 'diehard' Conservative and Unionist peers fearing the end of life as they knew it. Lord Loreburn, the Liberal Lord Chancellor, stated that it was a scandal that solicitors charged £4 million annually as the price for conveyancing. This high cost obstructed the 'diffusion of property' among an enlarging circle of landholders, frustrating those in the market. The atmosphere compelled the Law Society to recommend 'rationalisation and simplification' to its members. However, matters took a turn for the worse for reformers when Lord Loreburn's ill health forced his retirement as Lord Chancellor in 1912. Into his shoes stepped the professional conveyancer, Lord Haldane.

Richard Burden Haldane, later Viscount Haldane, British Liberal statesman, had been Minister for War between 1905 and 1912. In his new role he commenced to thwart the land reform movement within his own party, probably out of misplaced professional loyalty. By 1913, Haldane had introduced two new Bills in the House of Lords – the Real Property Bill (concerned with the reform of customary tenures – copyholds) and the Conveyancing Bill. The latter was to limit legal title to fee simple and leasehold, with all other interests such as trusts to be protected by cautions on the title. This simplified the solicitor's work, but left their scales of remuneration unchanged; in other words less work for the same money

(Offer, 1977, p 511). The Law Society was pleased and recommended the measure to its membership.

Then came the First World War, and afterwards the growth of small property ownership as an objective of government. Before 1914 fewer than 10% of households owned their houses, but by 1938 this figure had been trebled. House building enjoyed an unprecedented boom and more than one million houses previously rented were offered for owner-occupation. Home-ownership acquired a status that had not existed prior to 1914; before this time even many of the wealthy rented from private landlords. The market was assisted by the expansion of mortgage schemes to accommodate the limited financial status of this new proprietorship, and by the change in conveyancing practices. Only when legal practice permitted rapid transfer of a small plot of land with a State guarantee of title were banks and building societies willing to arrange a mortgage on the security of a property. The Land Registry served this purpose well, leaving the ancient landed estates undisturbed until their owners released parcels by sale into this new 'middle-class' debt-financed market.

Conveyancing practices came before the Land Transfer Sub-Committee set up by the Ministry of National Reconstruction in 1919. The lawyers resisted the abolition of the 'County Veto', but a Law of Property Bill was finally forged for nation-wide registry of title, simplified but *still* private conveyancing, and Haldane's reduction of legal estates to freehold and leasehold. The Bill also recommended abolition of the ancient principle of primogeniture on intestacy.

Lord Birkenhead stated, "this Bill will do more for the land-owning and land-acquiring class than any Bill which has been before your Lordships' house for many years ... the whole (existing) process (of land transfer) is irrational to a degree that I cannot describe. Nothing can remedy this except registration of title ..." (Offer, 1977, p 517). But suddenly, just when the lawyers seemed to be approaching some form of compromise agreement, the landowners' pressure group, the Land Union, set up in 1910 to oppose land valuation, became alarmed that land registration might soon become a reality. Opposition rapidly intensifying, the compromise demanded before acceptance of the Bill was an initial public enquiry into land registration and subsequent entry into the statute books only on approval of both Houses of Parliament, by vote to be taken in 10 years time.

The Law of Property Bill was sweetened for the new Labour Party by an amendment which repealed the clause in the Trades Union Act of

1871 that had forbidden the purchase or lease of more than one acre of land by a trade union. The Bill was finally passed in 1922, but enactment was delayed for three years. Land registration was swept aside by the demand for preliminary public enquiry and in 1925 solicitors received a 33% rise in conveyancing scale charges. Thus the land transfer monopoly was secure, the costs of conveyancing to the solicitor were reduced by simplifying procedures, the costs to the client were considerably increased, and the practice remained one of private treaty. With the boom in mass debt-financed proprietorship, the solicitors' profession had renewed appeal after 1925, but the administrative foundation for collection of Rent as public revenue had been blown sky-high by the profession that practised the law. The implications of the Act for mortgagors and mortgagees (who would pay a 'land tax'?) have been discussed in Chapter 6. The whole episode was strangely reminiscent of Henry VIII and his clash with the common law lawyers almost 400 years previously.

To witness between 1909 and 1925 the painful pregnancy, threatened abortions, and finally the birth of the sickly and post-mature Law of Property Act must have been distressing for Lloyd George. The defeat of land registration was nonsensical. For much of his time in the Liberal Party Lloyd George had struggled to establish a land register rather like the German Kataster as a prerequisite to the collection of Rent, albeit on a small scale, at least initially. Landholders, however, were determined to hold tenaciously to Rent, and conveyancers clung to an archaic system to protect their income. For these reasons both lawyer and client colluded to resist the land register. As Lord Campbell had told the House of Lords a generation earlier, "There is an estate in the realm more powerful than either your Lordships or the other House of Parliament, and that (is) the country solicitors" (Spring, 1977).

Given his professional background, David Lloyd George would have had no misapprehension about Lord Campbell's meaning. Added to this, he wore no rose-tinted spectacles when he looked at the urban landlord. Addressing the House of Commons on 29 April 1909, Lloyd George described what had happened in Woolwich. In the parish of Plumstead, land had been let for agriculture at £3 per acre in 1845, when the estate of 250 acres was worth £750 per annum. At 20 years purchase of the rent, its selling price was £15,000. Then the Arsenal was developed in Woolwich, creating a demand for 5,000 houses. The result was that in 1909 the same acreage brought the landlord £14,250 per annum. Following the government initiative to develop the Royal Arsenal, the ground landlord had collected an income of £1 million in ground rents owing to associated housing development. Furthermore, in accordance with the usual terms of leasehold, in 20 years all the houses were to revert to the landowner's family, bringing in another £1 million without spending a penny. Lloyd George's proposal to take 20% of this 'unearned increment' for the exchequer (a figure he was subsequently forced to reduce substantially) brought gasps of disbelief from the Conservative and Unionist benches (*Hansard*, 29 April, 1909).

The launch of national site valuation, 1910

Lloyd George had desires to base reform both of local taxation and imperial (central or national) taxation on land reform. In December 1910, campaigning in Deganwy, near Llandudno, he said, "I know something about valuation. I had a good deal of experience of valuation in the days when I was practising down at Portmadoc ... One thing especially struck me ... I have never seen a tradesman let off without paying on the full valuation, but I have seen many a mansion let off at a tenth of its value ... I am more concerned for the poor man at the bottom than the man at the top ... When we get the complete valuation we shall have a basis then for readjusting the burden of local taxation" (Short, 1989, p 6).

In his Finance (1909–1910) Act, Lloyd George pushed the boat out by empowering the commissioners of the Inland Revenue to, "cause a valuation to be made to all land in the United Kingdom, showing separately the total value and the site value respectively of the land, and in the case of agricultural land the value of the land for agricultural purposes where that value is different from the site value. Each piece of land which is under separate occupation, shall be separately valued, and the value shall be estimated as on the thirtieth day of April nineteen hundred and nine" (Finance Act, 1910, section 26.1).

There had been only one precedent to this valuation exercise, that of the Domesday Book itself, also assembled for purposes of taxation on the order of William the Conqueror in 1086. Once the land was valued it would be liable to duty on the 'increment value', defined as the amount (if any) by which the site value at the occasion of transfer exceeded the original site value as of 30 April 1909 (section two). Owner-occupiers of less than 50 acres (20 hectares) were exempt from the tax, though not from the valuation exercise, provided their land's annual total value did not exceed £75 per acre. The valuation would also provide the basis of the Reversion Duty, Undeveloped Land Duty, and the Mineral Rights Duty (sections 13 to 15, 16 to 19, and 20 to 24 of the Act respectively).

On 29 April 1910, the day that the Finance Act became law, a circular was sent to every solicitor in the country, the Inland Revenue having anticipated the Bill's eventual success. The regulations relating to collection and recovery of duty in cases of land transfers and leases were distributed at the same time. Up to that date, the Valuations Office had been staffed by 61 employees who attended to valuations for death duties. New professionals were therefore recruited, the first Chief Valuer being Sir Robert Thompson, succeeded in 1911 by Sir Edgar Harper. England and Wales were organised into 14 divisions, each under a superintendent valuer. Divisions were then partitioned into districts with their district valuers, each with his own staff. Mineral valuers were appointed, and the Board of the Inland Revenue met regularly to discuss cases which raised issues of principle.

The basic unit within each of the 118 districts was the pre-existing income tax parish (sometimes a single Poor Law parish, sometimes part of such a parish) established by the Inland Revenue under the Taxes Management Act of 1880. Each income tax parish had its land valuation officer, almost always an assessor of the income tax with the necessary local knowledge. In all, some 7,000 land valuation officers were recruited for the work. The next step was the compilation of the Valuation Book, which got off to a start by copying the necessary details from the Schedule A registers of the income tax. Other properties had to be individually identified. Each property was given a number, and it was in August, in the middle of the constitutional conference of 1910, that Lloyd George faced another uproar when the Inland Revenue issued its famous 'Form Four' to all owners listed in the Valuation Book. The bulk of the questions on this form had in fact been asked of occupiers of property for the previous 60 years. Now, however, for the first time, it was not the occupier's duty to respond, but the owner of the land, who was asked to identify himself or herself. There was a separate Form Three for 'statutory companies' such as the railways and docks, a Form Five for whenever mineral rights duty was likely to be levied, and a Form Six for owners of unworked minerals. There was also a Form Eight to trace owners through agents and rent payers. By April 1911 over 90% of the 10.5 million forms sent out had been returned, at a cost in wages to the land valuation officers of £174,000 pounds (about £6 million at 1993 prices) (Short, 1989, p 12).

Among the details entered onto Form Four was whether the land was freehold, copyhold or leasehold, and if copyhold the name of the manor. If the land of an owner-occupier, that person was asked to state the annual rent obtainable if let to a yearly tenant keeping it in repair. Details of the last sale (if any) within 20 years of 13 April 1909 were to be disclosed, together with capital expenditure on the land since that time. This information was transcribed into the valuers' field books, each hereditament covering four pages. The provisional valuations were then sent to the owners. Back in the district office the largest available Ordnance Survey sheets were spread out and marked to show the boundaries of each property. Provided no appeal was made within 60 days, the property was numbered on the map to indicate finalisation of the valuation. The giant Ordnance Survey sheets, to a scale of one in 500 for urban areas, are now in the Public Record Office or with local archivists, released under the Public Records Act of 1958. The Valuation Books are also in local archives, saved because they were consulted for many years after the repeal of the land clauses in 1920.

The Finance Act and the valuations provoked landholders to combine as the Land Union to thwart the statute law. Their main course of action was to resort to the courts. The Inland Revenue suffered several important setbacks, culminating in the Norton Malreward case of 28 February 1914. Norton Malreward lies off the main road between Bristol and Shepton Mallet in Avon. Here arose a dispute in which Mr Justice Scrutton found the whole basis upon which the Inland Revenue was valuing agricultural land to be invalid. The court ordered alternative methods of valuation which were impractical, bringing the Inland Revenue to a temporary halt. The government's Revenue Bill of 1914 attempted to overcome these difficulties, but, with war looming, never became law. In August, E.G. Pretyman, Conservative member of parliament and one of the Land Union, argued that men with the necessary knowledge for local valuation were being mobilised and that the exercise should therefore be suspended indefinitely. Nevertheless, the Inland Revenue pressed ahead, valuing 20 million acres (8 million hectares) of agricultural land after 1914 (Short, 1989, p 7).

World war destroys the land reform movement

With the First World War all questions of land reform were shelved. This expression of national solidarity, for the common purpose of defeating the enemy, led to popularisation of Socialist policies along the lines of Labour Party proposals. What did the war do for Rent reform? To say that the movement was set aside would be an understatement! The movement fell apart, the reason being that the Liberal Party fell apart.

The Liberal Party fell apart because Asquith proved less than equal to the task of leadership in war, and Lloyd George left his party behind. Being no respecter of party boundaries, Lloyd George pursued coalition and the establishment of specialist ministries to cope with the demands of mobilisation. His ruthless drive brought Britain through to victory; he was 'the man who won the war', but at the cost of the demise of the Liberal Party and his own career. Rent reform as a concept survived intact, for no party had shown the identification of Rent with public income to be in any way flawed. Rent reform as a movement, however, was badly wounded.

This episode said much about practical politics in Britain and its conflicts with political morality. When Lloyd George became Prime Minister in 1916 he forged a coalition of men he trusted from among his own party, the Conservatives, and Labour. This act by its very nature left some Liberals more favoured than others, weakening bonds in the party. Politicians were quick to criticise when the going was not to their liking. Many of Lloyd George's actions threatened the standing of some of his pre-war supporters. He was Prime Minister, but Asquith was still leader of the Liberal Party. Asquith had not forgotten that Lloyd George's resignation in early December 1916 (after Asquith had decided not to form a small Cabinet Committee to improve direction of the war effort) culminated in Asquith himself being obliged to resign, Lloyd George then taking over the helm. Lloyd George's subsequent War Cabinet did not contain Asquith. Some Liberals considered Asquith to have been treated badly and sided with him. Some pro-Rent reform Liberals now sat with Lloyd George in the coalition government, while others sat with Asquith. Others who were not only Rent reformers but also pacifists found more comfort cooperating with pacifists in the Labour Party (Douglas, 1976, pp 169-70). They resented Lloyd George's part in the decision to declare war in 1914. There were also Liberals who cherished the notion of civil liberty, bruised by conscription and the regulation of labour during the war. Some disliked the way Lloyd George had appeared to embrace the 'national efficiency' doctrine of the far right, even going so far as to have Lord Milner in his coalition government.

When the German army collapsed, Lloyd George decided his best chance politically was to stay with the coalition. Much needed to be done to restore the country now that peace was secured and he naturally favoured tackling the work ahead in the way that had proved so successful in wartime. The Conservatives also favoured coalition. They had not won an election since 1900 and even then only on the 'khaki vote' of

Boer War patriotism. The Representation of the People Act of February 1918 had given full adult enfranchisement to men from age 21 years and to women from 30 years (women were enfranchised on the same basis as men in 1928). All parties were unsure of the voting intentions of this new mass electorate, more than double its previous size. Staying in coalition would give some power at least, provide time to get the measure of the new electorate, and keep their Liberal opponents split. Thus the post-war coalition was a marriage of convenience from which, crucially, the Labour Party withdrew, fired by its increasing strength and anxious to stand foursquare behind its Socialist manifesto. The Labour Party had been split on entry into the war but, unlike the Liberals, had united by the Armistice.

Lloyd George set about trying to ensure parliamentary seats for Liberals loyal to himself and his coalition programme. The Conservatives agreed not to oppose about 150 Liberals in the forthcoming election. They and approved Conservative candidates were given what the remaining Liberals called 'the coupon', an official letter of support signed by Lloyd George and Bonar Law (Cuthbert, 1994, p 176). This was an unholy alliance. Lloyd George was a staunch advocate of some form of Home Rule for Ireland, while Bonar Law so opposed the Liberal's Home Rule Bill before the war that he had declared menacingly, 'there were things stronger than parliamentary majorities'. A man like Bonar Law would have no sympathy with Rent reform. In the event, the election result sowed the seeds of disaster for Lloyd George.

The Independent Liberals (ie non-coalition) secured only 28 seats, Asquith and other senior Liberals losing theirs. Lloyd George's coalition could depend on at least 526 members of parliament, but the ratio of Conservatives and Irish Unionists to Coalition Liberals was about three to one. Thus *de facto*, the Liberal Lloyd George found himself leading a hybrid party of predominantly Conservative persuasion. Politically, he was ensnared! The Labour Party, with 57 seats and nearly 2.5 million votes, were now the real opposition.

Then in February 1920 Asquith was returned to the Commons in a by-election victory, and several Coalition Liberals went over to their old leader. Lloyd George recognised that a successful administration pursuing popular issues was his only hope of survival, and loyal ministers worked on issues of immediate appeal. Addison, as Minister at the new Ministry of Health, introduced a Housing Act in 1919, launching a programme of house building by local authorities which served as a model for decades to come. At the Board of Education, Herbert (HAL) Fisher, formerly vice-chancellor of Sheffield University, handled the complex Education Act of 1918. The Ministry of Labour, with Dr T J Macnamara as Minister, extended unemployment insurance to virtually all manual workers, and added dependants' allowances in 1921.

Under post-war stresses, cracks soon appeared in the coalition. Even worse, by 1921 the nation was in yet another disruptive economic slump, necessitating unemployment relief works. The Treasury, City of London financiers, the Federation of British Industries and sections of the press cried out for cutbacks in public spending. The nature of privatised Rent (see Chapter 3) ensured that Christopher Addison's housing programme sent prices through the roof and, given the state of the economy, the scheme was halted within the year. Expansion of education was also curtailed, while unemployment insurance soared. Addison resigned and Labour shouted about 'broken promises'. Everybody had talked about a new beginning, discarding pre-war practices, but by 1921 the old domestic battle lines were being redrawn. The Conservatives demanded the restoration of laissez-faire in private enterprise and the trade unions demanded the restoration of pre-war wage bargaining. Industrial strikes flared up as employers cut wages to lower costs. In 1921 nearly 86 million days of work were lost in this way. On top of all this Lloyd George had the Irish problem and continuing problems with external affairs in Europe. He got into serious trouble when, beached without party funds, he attempted to re-launch by selling honours in return for donations (knighthoods cost around £10,000, or about £110,000 at 1993 prices). Honours in return for financial support had been (and remains) a longstanding practice in party politics, but many were upset to see them exposed as yet another commodity. What goes up must eventually come down, and Lloyd George was being seen less and less as an asset to the Conservatives. At a meeting in the Carlton Club on 19 October 1922 the Conservatives voted to contest the next general election as an independent party. Lloyd George, now without the Liberals and Conservatives, promptly resigned.

The Conservative repeal of Lloyd George's land reforms

With the Liberal party scuppered and its old captain shipwrecked, Rent reform drifted into the backwater of politics where it has remained almost forgotten. In 1914, barely eight years previously, there were 4,760 men valuing land for the Inland Revenue. By the end of 1915, 1,000 of them had enlisted and another 2,600 had been dismissed (Douglas, 1976, p 169). As they were dispersed, so was the party that had created the need for them. Lloyd George had some notable land reformers in his coalition but they were outweighed by the Conservatives. In 1918 the party conferences both of Labour and the National (ie Coalition) Liberals declared in favour of land value 'taxation', but in view of the political and economic turmoil ahead this was whistling in the wind. No longer was there political unity behind an enthusiastic and capable leadership. The Rent reform movement and the Liberals had lost their financial backing while the coffers of the Labour Party had swollen rapidly. Labour was at least talking of land taxation, and as a result former land reforming Liberals drifted over to the Independent Labour Party during 1919. Labour stood for nationalisation, however, not site value taxation and Rent reform, so the drifters were doomed. Furthermore, the lack of commitment of these former Liberals to Labour's 'clause IV' made them unwelcome candidates for the Parliamentary Labour Party. Those of Georgist persuasion were now well and truly in disarray.

In April 1919 the Coalition Cabinet appointed a Select Committee to examine the whole system of land valuation and the attached taxes introduced before the war. With the Unionist Pretyman on one side of the committee, an ardent enemy of land taxation, and Liberal land taxers such as P W Raffan on the other, the committee could not even agree on its terms of reference and disbanded even before getting started (Douglas, 1976, p 178). Lloyd George must have known that Conservative opposition within his own coalition and the self-interest of the conveyancing lawyers predicted this outcome. Those set on abandonment of the system were never going to see eye to eye with those wishing to bring it up to date.

By 1920 the way was unimpeded for the Conservative Austen Chamberlain, second only to Bonar Law in his party hierarchy and Chancellor of the Exchequer, to propose abolition of the existing land duties and the valuation system. David Lloyd George was placed in the extraordinary position of witnessing *his own* Chancellor propose demolition of Liberal legislation and of being impotent to do anything about it, because the new electorate created in 1918 had returned, in effect, a Conservative majority with a Liberal Prime Minister. Chamberlain argued that the system was complicated and yielded little tax, and therefore should go. Lloyd George could have argued that what had taken root should be nurtured, not abandoned before it had time to bear fruit. One does not uproot a sapling simply because it has failed to yield the crop of a mature tree.

Land reformers scattered about the House of Commons stood up to criticise the Conservatives' land proposals. Asquith said, "I still believe, as my Chancellor of the Exchequer said in February 1914, in the necessity, first of all, of the valuation, and next, as a consequence of that valuation, as a proper purpose to which it should be applied, the taxing for public purposes, both imperial (national) and local, of the site value of land. Further, it has always been to me one of the great recommendations of the valuation and taxation of land that land may be acquired by the community at the same rate and upon the same terms upon which it was taxed". To which the land reformer Colonel Wedgewood remarked, "I only regret that you did not do it while you were in power". Asquith rose to reply, "We were doing it; we were on the point of doing it, in the spring of 1914 ... by legislation. Then came the war in August of that year which made such legislation impossible". Austen Chamberlain accused Asquith of hypocrisy; of not having been "an early or an enthusiastic convert to the principle of these taxes". Asquith cut him down with the reply that he should "apply to the Prime Minister (Lloyd George) and ask his views on that" (Douglas, 1976, p 180).

The government won the vote and the land clauses were repealed, but few Coalition Liberals could bring themselves to enter the same division lobby as their Conservative colleagues. Thirteen crossed the floor to join Asquith and 100 abstained. Coalition though there was, this was a Conservative dismemberment of Rent reform. Lloyd George presided over this dismemberment, powerless to prevent the slaughter of his own child.

When Lloyd George resigned in 1922, Bonar Law created a new administration composed mainly of former junior ministers, the 'second XI' as this Cabinet was called. The subsequent election of 1922 was another disaster for Lloyd George when 38% of the electorate voted Conservative, giving the party 345 out of 615 seats, with Labour taking 30% and 142, respectively. In the following election of December 1923 Labour took 31% of votes and 191 seats to form its first government, albeit a minority one.

Picking up the pieces: land reformers after 1920

Party politics during 1924 was particularly shabby, bringing the Labour government down by October. In the ensuing election the Conservatives gained considerable ground, Labour lost many seats, and the Liberals were down to about 40 members of parliament. Truly out in the wilderness, Lloyd George attempted to reunite his party. The strain of the previous five years had exhausted him, bringing on his frequent nervous reactions, but he was willing to try again. On 7 June 1921, in the middle of the recession, he had written to Bonar Law, "I have had a temporary breakdown ... much to my disappointment it is only temporary ...". In August of that year he was ill with a dental abscess, a potentially dangerous condition in the pre-antibiotic era. In March 1922, aged 59, lacking success in his efforts to sponsor reconciliation in Europe, and charged by some Liberals and Conservatives with intensifying class conflict, he wrote, "It is difficult to rest with all these 'crises' hurtling about your head. I have had today a return of those neuralgic pains that worried me" (L'Etang, 1969, p 65). His resignation brought little improvement in health.

Still, site value taxation as an idea was by no means dead. Lloyd George was elected Chairman of the Parliamentary Liberals, and used his personal political fund to set up the Liberal Land Committee. One of its reports, *Towns and the land* (known as the Brown Book), laid considerable emphasis on site value rating. Asquith (now Lord Oxford) called a special conference of the Liberals in February 1926 at which site value rating was top of the agenda. The Labour Party continued to talk of land nationalisation with freeholds being turned over to the state in return for compensation to the landlords in the form of Land Bonds. Then in April 1929 Ramsay MacDonald made a speech at the Albert Hall promising that a Labour government would tax land values (Douglas, 1976, p 195). Labour's manifesto for the election of that year included a programme of 'national development' very close to that set out in Lloyd George's report, *Britain's industrial future* (the Yellow Book) published the year before. Labour declared, "The Party will deal drastically with the scandal of the appropriation of land values by private landowners. It will take steps to secure for the community the increased value of land which is created by industry and the expenditure of public money" (Douglas, 1976, p 195).

Rentholding since 1880

Secrecy on the one side and disinterestedness on the other with respect to the monopolisation of Rent means that there remain huge uncertainties as to exactly who constitutes this monopoly and what is the true value of the national Rent. Certainly the landed aristocracy is not as it was, and many thousands of families who once would have rented are now owner-occupiers of their homes, but neither change has been as extensive as might seem.

In 1880, the estates of 331 great landholders covered almost one quarter (more than seven million acres) of England. In this group there were 43 magnates who between them held 8% of the country. The 1,032 greater gentry owned another 19% of the Land. Thus 1,363 individuals claimed for themselves 43% of the country. Large landholding was most marked in the north of England, where these families held more than half of the 3.8 million acres. But many rural properties became weighed down with debt following the great agricultural depression of the 1880s. So what did landholders do with their estates over the next 40 years? Some of the landed gentry, dependent upon rural Rent alone, were ruined and lost their properties. Landholders with urban income from town property, banking, brewing, harbours and mines, especially those of the peerage, came through rather better, but many divested themselves of parts of their estates to accommodate demands for industrial sites and housing development on the urban fringe.

With threats of land taxation or nationalisation, land sales increased between 1910 and 1922. One estimate put the sales at over 800,000 acres (324,000 hectares) up to 1914 (Thompson, 1963, p 322). Then, between 1918 and 1922, over 25% of land in England and Wales changed ownership (Clemenson, 1982, p 111). Some of this upheaval was due to deaths of owners within the commissioned ranks during the war. The Public Schools Club recorded that 800 of its members, mostly landed, died in action (Lejeune, 1972, p xvi). In some families double bereavements meant death duties in quick succession. However, land sale means land transfer; there were many willing buyers ready to take over the title to Rent. The bundle was as secure as ever. Sometimes the estate was sold in one lot; sometimes it was broken up. Sometimes only peripheral farms or secondary parts of the estate were sold off to leave the core in healthier financial shape. After debt clearance the balance was invested in stocks and shares, thereby returning in part to land.

The Wyvill family kept their ancestral estate at Constable Burton in the North Riding but sold off the 4,000 acre Denton Park Estate in 1902. The Antrobus family let go of almost all their 6,400 acre Abbey estate (Wiltshire) in 1915. Lord Derby sold just over 4,000 acres of outlying land in Burscough (Lancashire) in 1916. The Earl of Pembroke sold over 8,000 acres on the outskirts of his Wilton estate (Wiltshire) in 1918. Urban land was also transferred after 1918, often to property speculators. In London the area of land owned by the aristocracy diminished, though an informed commentator remarked, "The idea that these ancient estates have been broken up and scattered by taxation is largely a myth" (Marriot, 1967, p 80).

The trend over the 20th century has been for individual landholding of large tracts to be replaced with landholding by public, institutional or corporate organisations. Standing alongside the monarchy, the landed aristocracy, the public schools, Oxford and Cambridge universities and the established Church of England there are now the banks, insurance companies, pension trusts and property companies. These hugely wealthy organisations invest as Rentholders for security and the certainty of profit in the long term.

Nevertheless, one late 20th century survey of 500 estates that had extended to 3,000 acres or more in 1880 showed that survival had been remarkably strong, considering the turnover in the land market. Of 124 estates originally of 10,000 acres or more, 25% were still in this category in 1980. Of 500 estates originally of 3,000 acres or more, 34% were still of 1,000 acres or more. Half of the original 500 families in the survey still possessed some of their original estate, although in many cases it had been diminished (Clemenson, 1982, pp 118-19). Where increases in agricultural productivity materialised these sometimes offset the effects of lost acreage, especially when what was sold off had been land of poorer quality. Such studies as these are rare, however, and hampered by secrecy. A report of 1979 declared, "It is disturbing that so little is known about ... ownership ... of agricultural land and that governments should have to take decisions, which may have far-reaching effects ... on the basis of incomplete or non-existent data" (Committee of Enquiry into the Acquisition and Occupancy of Agricultural Land, 1979, p 109).

Turning to the urban centres, there is nowhere better to examine than London. Moth-eaten though the fabric of the old landed estates is these days in central London, the extent to which it survives is striking. Walk on the north side of Oxford Street from Marble Arch and you are in the Portman Estate, about 100 acres of the land originally given to Lord Chief Justice Portman in 1533 by Henry VIII. Walk on the other side and you are in the 100 acre Mayfair Estate of Gerald Grosvenor, Duke of Westminster, whose inheritance goes back to 1677. Walk further down Oxford Street and to the north is the Howard De Walden Estate of another 100 acres, surrounding Harley Street (an heiress of the Duke of Newcastle married a Harley). Regent's Park has belonged to the Crown since the time of Henry VIII. The length of Regent Street, through Piccadilly and into the Haymarket and St James, is mostly Crown Estate, as also is the Millbank Estate surrounding the Tate Gallery. Belgravia, 200 acres of

Regency London, also belongs to the Grosvenor family. Cross over Sloane Street from Belgravia and you are in Viscount Chelsea's 100 acre Cadogan Estate.

The inheritance that has taken a hammering is the Bedford Estate of the Russell family to the east of Tottenham Court Road. Once offering up sufficient rents to support the establishment of the stately home at Woburn Abbey, the main remnant now runs between Tottenham Court Road and Gower Street. What had the Gowers to do with the Bedfords? The expansion of the great estates of the Duke of Sutherland (Leveson-Gowers) was achieved partly by alliances through marriage. Disraeli is said to have remarked that the Leveson-Gowers "had made it good by its talent for absorbing heiresses" (Richards, 1973, pp 5-13). Thomas Gower of Stittenham, Yorkshire, married a co-heiress of Sir John Leveson of Trentham, Staffordshire in 1689. The heir, Sir John Leveson-Gower, married the daughter of the Duke of Rutland. Granville Leveson-Gower, first Marquis of Stafford, was connected by marriage to the Dukes of Bedford and Bridgewater. This process went on until by 1880 the Leveson-Gowers, by then Dukes of Sutherland, owned more than 1.3 million acres in England and Scotland.

Walk west from Marble Arch on the north side of Bayswater Road, opposite Hyde Park, and you are on lands owned by the established Church of England. Not long ago this vast estate stretched north to Maida Vale, but much north of Paddington Station has now been sold and the proceeds re-invested. The Church Commissioners achieved notoriety in the 1980s when their reinvestments in commercial property collapsed following the burst of a 'property bubble', leaving the Church in considerable financial difficulty for a while. Church Commission land is scattered all over central London.

Once, the City of London, the City of Westminster and Southwark across the River Thames were discrete areas of occupation. The City of London has always been owned by its merchants, and one acre of land in this area is worth a king's ransom. Each trade within the ancient walls had its own livery company. How much wealth in land is held by these companies is anybody's guess, but the Merchant Taylors, the Drapers, the Carpenters, the Vintners, the Leathersellers, the Grocers, the Goldsmiths, the Mercers and the Cutlers must hold vast fortunes. The governing body is the City Corporation, which owns about 200 of the City's 677 acres. The Corporation holds the freeholds of its land through three estates. The Cash Estate and the Bridge House Estate are privately owned, and the revenue of the latter is spent on the City's bridges. The Planning

Estate is owned by the Corporation in its role as local authority. Revenue from this Estate goes to the Inner London Education Authority, and a substantial sum is used to subsidise poorer neighbouring local authorities. The Cash Estate owns the City's markets as well as land on either side of Bond Street between the Grosvenor Estate and the Crown Estate. There is also land much further out purchased for the enjoyment of Londoners by an Act of 1875, including Epping Forest, Highgate Wood, Burnham Beeches near Beaconsfield, and other parks.

Britain's public schools also own considerable areas of land as part of the ancient establishment. Eton College, Dulwich College, Tonbridge School, Rugby School, Bedford School and Christ's Hospital are to varying extent London landholders. So, in summary, London's landed establishment has loosened but far from lost its grip on the highest Rent in the nation (Green, 1986, pp 9-59). There has always been an inevitable fluidity in the landed establishment as families failed, fell upon hard luck, or suffered a profligate heir, while others were always prepared to step into the ranks. For example, the Earl of Iveagh (the Guinness family) owns about 24,000 acres in Norfolk, Viscount Leverhulme (the soap magnate) owned about 100,000 acres of Cheshire, and the Vesty family (who supplied the beef to the troops of the First World War) owns about the same in Scotland. According to the Royal Commission on the Distribution of Income and Wealth, in 1976 the richest 1% of the population owned 52% of British land, and the top 3% an astonishing 74% (Royal Commission on the Distribution of Income and Wealth, 1979), though much of this was rural and of low economic productivity.

From an analysis of estate duties on almost 3,000 thousand estates in the 1950s, the conclusion was reached that to consider the large country estate as a phenomenon that had passed into English history would be premature (Denman, 1957, p 122). Burke's *Landed gentry* commented in 1965, "the Landed Gentry has not just survived, it has recovered ...Those who had faith in the future and kept their Land, perhaps at considerable sacrifice, have been extremely well-rewarded. Today, with Land worth £200 an acre, the owner of a 5,000 acre estate is a millionaire" (Bence-Jones, 1965). To which the response must be that provided the million is earned equitably, and no one is impoverished by the holding of Rent, there can be no complaint. The article, entitled 'The Trust of Landowning', devoted much space, however, to advice on tax avoidance:

> There are various reliefs from taxation offered to the landowner, such as the Statutory Repairs Allowance, the Maintenance Claim, and the

Capital Expenditure Claim. A farm loss can be charged to surtax ... Opening the house to the public is a help ... there is a great advantage of being able to set the cost of running one's house – over and above what is allowed under the Maintenance Claim – against taxation, as a business loss ... There are certain ... reliefs from death duties which benefit the Landed Gentry. The duty on timber trees is not payable until they are cut and sold ... More and more people are making over estates to their heirs to avoid death duties ... And there is complete exemption on property made over in consideration of marriage. A few years ago the nephew and heir of a Gloucestershire landowner married in a hurry and sooner than had been planned to enable his uncle, who was dying, to make over the estate to him and save all duty. (Bence-Jones, 1965)

Of course it had always been possible to lower the incidence of taxes by dividing ownership between man and wife and by gradually transferring land during the owner's lifetime.

One more attempt at site value taxation, 1931-1934

The Great Depression was well advanced by 1931, when unemployment was to pass the 2.5 million mark or about 21% of the workforce. Overseeing the crisis was a Labour minority government led by Ramsey MacDonald, dependent on the Liberals for power. Chancellor of the Exchequer Philip Snowdon faced a severe Budgetary deficit, unemployment benefit having more than tripled to over 3% of national income in four years. He took two measures. First, in February, he appointed a committee under Sir George May to advise the government. Second, in his April Budget he re-introduced land valuation and a small land tax to help raise much needed revenue: "There shall be charged ... a rate of 1d for each pound of the land value of every unit of the land in Great Britain" (Lawrence, 1957, p 177). Despite the economic calamity facing the nation, the defenders of private Rentholding were at daggers drawn the moment 'site valuation' was uttered. On 4 July, with debate on the Finance Bill raging, *The Times* declared, "when the Socialist party possesses an independent majority they will be able without delay to convert an irksome tax into an instrument of confiscation" (*The Times*, 4 July, 1931). Still, with the Lords' claws now drawn, the Bill became law in early July, land valuation included. On 15th of that month *The Times* printed the words of Stanley Baldwin, the Conservative leader who had played a major role in the disruption of Lloyd George's earlier coalition: "I can say one thing about it … that if we get back into power that tax will never see daylight" (*The Times*, 15 July, 1931). On the very same day, the May Committee issued the report which brought down the Labour administration within weeks. Insisting that the Budget should be balanced not by extra taxation but mainly by cuts in public expenditure, there could be only one interpretation. The families of unemployed working men were to be called upon for sacrifice rather than those of Rentholders. Unemployment benefit needed to be cut by 10% from 17s 0d to 15s 3d week. Convulsed by this proposal, Labour's Cabinet was split. MacDonald resigned on 24 August, and the king asked him to lead a National government to handle the crisis. MacDonald quickly found himself corralled in a Conservative dominated coalition, he and Snowdon being neutered as had been Lloyd George. Within weeks unemployment benefit was cut. The Conservative Chancellor of the Exchequer Neville Chamberlain, half brother of Austen and son of Joseph, suspended all work on site valuation on 8th December. By 1934 the land tax had disappeared completely.

Apart from very misguided Labour legislation in the financial provisions of the Town and Country Planning Act of 1947, quickly repealed and only a distraction to recall, virtually nothing has been heard of Rent for public revenue over the past 50 years. A Departmental Committee on Site Value Rating was appointed in 1947, its members deliberating for more than four years. The outcome was a favourable minority report and a negative majority report, objections in which were largely overturned by repeal of the poorly thought through provisions of the Town and Country Planning Act. Members of Parliament spoke up for Rent collection from time to time; George Brown (created a life peer in 1970), speaking in Bristol in 1954, said that it was far better to have 'taxation of site values' rather than land nationalisation. Land nationalisation would imply the payment of many millions of pounds in compensation. What was important was not technical ownership but the benefit derived from land for the community (*Cooperative News*, 27 February, 1954).

Let us give the final say not to Stanley Baldwin, Neville Chamberlain, or George Brown but to that Nobel laureate for physics, Albert Einstein. In the climactic year of 1931, Einstein was preparing to write his work *My Philosophy*. On 8 October he wrote, "I read the largest part of the book by Henry George (*Progress and poverty*) with extraordinary interest, and I believe that in the main points the book takes a stand which cannot be fought, especially as far as the cause of poverty is concerned" (*Land and liberty*, March–April, 1932, p 35).

'Let Curzon Holde what Curzon Helde', read the motto of the family of George Nathaniel Curzon of Kedleston, eldest son of 4th Baron Scarsdale, the man passed over for premiership of the Conservative Party in 1923. How aptly and honestly this dynastic aphorism, almost a war cry, declared what landed aristocracy was all about. There was no grand design in what generations of the Rentholding constituency pursued, only a primitive urge to claim for themselves what in a much earlier age the State had entrusted to the stewardship of the progenitors of their type. Over a millennium the guardians of the nation's Rent elected themselves through their courts and parliament to be the owners of this wealth. The estates of the Victorians and Edwardians are no longer what they were, but Rent remains as securely bound as ever in that bundle entitled land, a fact of far more significance than the descent of the hereditary peerage from the House of Lords on 11 November 1999.

The hereditary peers voted themselves out of power, the Bill passing by 221 to 81. Lord Wedgewood was all for rejection of any Bill to deny him a seat and a vote in the House. Lord Strathclyde urged his fellow Tory peers to avoid constitutional crisis by abstaining in the final vote, just as had George Nathaniel Curzon during those critical days in August 1911. Strathclyde prevailed. As Carlyle or Cobbett might have written, the Rent eaters of the old sort may now be defunct as legislators, but the legislation of their forefathers survives. More worryingly, the ancient Minotaur may have decayed in tooth and claw, but was it easy prey for a more terrible mutant of the species? Has Capitalism grown into a monster more voracious and cannibalistic of its own and lesser kind than anything seen before, skulking in its labyrinth talking up bull markets? Has ermine been doffed and a less conspicuous pinstripe donned?

Carlyle wrote, "in this world of ours which has both indestructible hope in the Future, and an indestructible tendency to persevere in the Past, must Innovation and Conservation wage their perpetual conflict" (Carlyle, undated, p 34). There are many who hope for a better life, better health and better life expectancy for their own, their communities, the poor, the unemployed, and those who fail to qualify as a 'human resource' in today's labour market. Their drawback is society's perseverance with privatisation of Rent, the lethal legacy it has yet to throw off. Is our Social Democracy up to the challenges within our brand of Welfare Capitalism? Future generations would wish it so, for as Carlyle also wrote, "what generous heart can pretend to itself, or be hoodwinked into believing, that Loyalty to the Moneybag is a noble Loyalty? Mammon, cries the generous heart out of all ages and countries, is the basest of known Gods, even of known Devils" (Carlyle, undated, p 604).

Bibliography

Acheson, D. (1998) *Independent Inquiry into Inequalities in Health*, London: The Stationery Office.

Ackerknecht, E.H. (1981) *Rudolf Virchow*, NY: Arno Press.

Aquinas, T. (1959) 'Summa Theologica', in A.P. d'Entrèves (ed) *Aquinas: Selected political writings*, Oxford: Basil Blackwell.

Argyll, J.G.E.H.D.S. Campbell, 9th Duke of (1892) *Viscount Palmerston, K.G. by the Marquis of Lorne*, London: Sampson Low, Marston.

Ashton, T.S. (1946) 'The relation of economic history to economic theory', *Economica*, vol NS13, p 86.

Bank of England (1998) *Minutes of the monetary policy committee meeting*, 15 July.

Banks, M.H. and Jackson, P.R. (1982) 'Unemployment and risk of minor psychiatric disorder in young people: cross-sectional and longitudinal evidence', *Psychological Medicine*, vol 12, pp 789-98.

Banks, R. (ed) (1989) *Costing the earth*, London: Shepheard-Walwyn.

Barber, W.J. (1991) *A history of economic thought*, London: Penguin.

Barnett, J. (1982) *Inside the Treasury*, London: Andre Deutsch.

Bassett, S. (1989) 'In search of the origins of Anglo-Saxon kingdoms', in S. Bassett, *The origins of Anglo-Saxon kingdoms*, London: Leicester University Press.

Bateman, J. (1971) *The Acre-ocracy of England. Retitled English aristocracy in the nineteenth century*, London: Leicester University Press.

Bean, J.M.W. (1968) *The decline of English feudalism 1215-1540*, NY: Manchester University Press, Barnes and Noble Inc.

Bence-Jones, M. (1965) 'The trust of landowning', in *Burke's Landed Gentry*, *vol 1*, London: Burke's Peerage Ltd.

Best, G. (1971) *Mid-Victorian Britain*, London: Fontana Press.

Bethune, A. (1997) 'Unemployment and mortality', in F. Drever and M. Whitehead (eds) *Health inequalities*, London: The Stationery Office, Series DS no 15, pp 156-67.

Beveridge Papers (IIa), Letter to Annette Beveridge, 14 March 1902. Deposited in the London School of Economics Library.

Beveridge Papers (IIa). Deposited in the London School of Economics Library.

Blane, D. and Drever, F. (1988) 'Inequality among men in standardised years of potential life lost, 1970–93' *British Medical Journal*, vol 317, p 255.

Blaug, M. (1964) 'The poor law report re-examined', *Journal of Economic History*, vol 24, pp 229-45.

Blaug, M. (1997) *Economic theory in retrospect*, Cambridge: Cambridge University Press.

Board of Trade (1917-1939) *Statistical abstract for the United Kingdom*, London: HMSO.

Board of Trade (1932) *Statistical abstract for the United Kingdom for each of the fifteen years 1913 and 1917 to 1930, Seventy-fifth number*, London: HMSO.

Board of Trade (1939) *Statistical abstract for the United Kingdom for each of the fifteen years 1913 and 1924 to 1937, Eighty-second number*, London: HMSO.

Body, R. (1982) *Agriculture: The triumph and the shame*, London: Semple Smith.

Booth, C. (1887) 'The inhabitants of Tower Hamlets (school board division), their condition and occupations', *Journal of the Royal Statistical Society*, vol 50, pp 326-401.

Botting, B. (1997) 'Mortality in childhood', in F. Drever and M. Whitehead (eds) *Health inequalities*, London: The Stationery Office, Series DS no 15, pp 83-94.

Boulton, J. (1997) 'Going on the parish: the parish pension and its meaning in the London suburbs, 1640-1724', in T. Hitchcock, P. King, and P. Sharpe (eds) *Chronicling poverty. The voices and strategies of the English poor, 1640-1840*, London: Macmillan.

Brown, A.L. (1981) 'Parliament, c1377-1422', in R.G. Davies and J.H. Denton (eds) *The English parliament in the middle ages*, Manchester: Manchester University Press.

Burnett, J. (1986) *A social history of housing 1815-1985*, London: Methuen.

Cairncross, A.K. and Weber, B. (1956-7) 'Fluctuations in building in Great Britain, 1785–1849', *Economic History Review*, 2nd series, vol 9, pp 283-97.

Cairnes, J. (1874) *Some leading principles of political economy*, London: Macmillan.

Campbell, D.A., Radford, J.M.C. and Burton, P. (1991) 'Unemployment rates: an alternative to the Jarman index?', *British Medical Journal*, vol 303, pp 750-55.

Carlyle, T. (undated) *History of the French Revolution*, London: Ward, Lock and Co.

Carnegie, A. (1962) 'The gospel of wealth and other timely essays', in E.C. Kirkland (ed) MA: Belknap Press of Harvard University Press.

Carvel, J. (1999) 'University drop-out rates reflect class roots', *The Guardian*, 3 December.

Cavanaugh, F. (1996) *The truth about the national debt*, MA: Harvard Business School Press.

Central Statistical Office (1949-96) *Annual abstract of statistics*, nos 86-132, London: HMSO.

Central Statistical Office (1995) *Social Trends 25*, London: HMSO.

Chadwick, E. (1842) *Report on the sanitary condition of the labouring population of Great Britain*, London: W. Clowes for HMSO.

Chamberlain, J. (1883) 'Labourers' and artisans' dwellings', *Fortnightly Review*, February.

Chandaman, C.D. (1975) *The English public revenue 1660-1688*, Oxford: Clarendon Press.

Chandola, T. (1998) 'Social inequality in coronary heart disease: a comparison of occupational classifications', *Social Science Medicine*, vol 47, pp 525-33.

Charles, E. (1935) 'The effect of present trends in fertility and mortality upon the future population of England and Wales', London and Cambridge Economic Service Special Memorandum, no 40, August, cited in P. Hall, H. Land, R. Parker, and A. Webb (eds) (1975) *Change, choice and conflict in social policy*, London: Heinemann.

Clark, J.B. (1925) *The distribution of wealth*, London: Macmillan.

Clark, P. and Langford, K. (1996) 'Hodge's politics: the agricultural labourers and the third reform act in Suffolk', in N. Harte and R. Quinault (eds) *Land and Society in Britain, 1700-1914*, Manchester: Manchester University Press.

Clemenson, H.A. (1982) *English country houses and estates*, London: Croom Helm.

Coats, A.W. (1990) 'Marshall and ethics', in R. McWilliams Tullberg (ed) *Alfred Marshall in retrospect*, Aldershot: Edward Elgar Publishing, pp 153-77.

Cole, O. and Farries, J.S. (1986) 'Rehousing on medical grounds, an assessment of its effectiveness', *Public Health*, vol 100, pp 229-35.

Commission for Racial Equality (1984) *Race and housing in Liverpool: A research report*, London: CRE.

Committee of Enquiry into the Acquisition and Occupancy of Agricultural Land (1979) Report, Cmnd 7599, London: HMSO.

Commission of Enquiry into the State of Large Towns and Populous Districts (1844) First Report, Appendix, London: HMSO.

Constantine, S. (1992) *Lloyd George*, London: Routledge.

Coomber, V. (1996) *The Admission of the elderly into the Tonbridge Union workhouse 1880-1930*, University of London MSc thesis.

Coppin, N. (1993) *Landscaping and revegetation of china clay wastes*, London: HMSO.

Cornfield, P.J. (1996) 'The rivals: landed and other gentlemen', in N. Harte and R. Quinault (eds) *Land and Society in Britain, 1700-1914*, Manchester: Manchester University Press.

Coupland, R. (1923) *Wilberforce: A narrative*, Oxford: Clarendon Press.

Cox, B.D., Huppert, F.A. and Whichelow, M.J. (1993) *The Health and Lifestyle Survey: seven years on*, Aldershot: Darmouth.

Crook, A.D.H. (1986) 'Privatisation of housing', *Environment and Planning*, vol 18.

Curwen, M. and Devis, T. (1988) 'Winter mortality, temperature and influenza: has the relationship changed in recent years?' *Population Trends*, vol 54, pp 17-20.

Cuthbert, D.D. (1994) 'Lloyd George and the Conservative Central Office 1918-22', in A.J.P. Taylor (ed) *Lloyd George. Twelve essays*, Aldershot: Gregg Revivals.

Dangerfield, G. (1966) *The strange death of Liberal England*, London: MacGibbon and Kee.

Daunton, M.J. (1996) 'The political economy of death duties: Harcourt's Budget of 1894', in N. Harte and R. Quinault (eds) *Land and Society in Britain, 1700-1914*, Manchester: Manchester University Press.

Davenport, H.J. (1910) 'The single tax in the English Budget', *Quarterly Journal of Economics*, vol 24, pp 279-92.

Daveri, F. and Tabellini, G. (1997) 'Unemployment, growth and taxation in industrial countries', *Discussion paper series, no 1681*, London: Centre for Economic Policy Research.

Davey Smith, G. and Dorling, D. (1996) '"I'm all right, John": voting patterns and mortality in England and Wales 1981-92', *British Medical Journal*, vol 313, pp 1573-77.

Davey Smith, G., Shipley, M.J. and Rose, G. (1990) 'Magnitude and causes of socioeconomic differentials in mortality: further evidence from the Whitehall Study', *Journal of Epidemiology and Community Health*, vol 44, pp 265-70.

Denman, D.R. (1957) *Estate capital*, London: Allen and Unwin.

Department of Employment (1983) *Family expenditure survey*, London: HMSO.

Department of Health (1991) *The health of the nation: a consultative document for England and Wales*, London: DHSS.

Department of Health (1992) *The health of the nation – a strategy for health in England*, London: HMSO.

Department of Health (1998) *Our healthier nation – A contract for health*, Cm 3852, London: The Stationery Office.

Department of Social Security (1998) *New ambitions for our country: A new contract for welfare*, Cm 3805, London: The Stationery Office.

Department of the Environment (1961) *Homes for today and tomorrow*, London: HMSO.

Dickens, C. (1950) *The dealings with the firm of Dombey and son: Wholesale, retail and for exportation*, London: Oxford University Press.

Digby, K.E. (1897) *An introduction to the history of the law of real property, with original authorities*, Oxford: Clarendon Press.

Donnison, D. (1982) *The politics of poverty*, Oxford: Martin Robertson.

Douglas, F.C.R. (undated) *Karl Marx's theories of surplus value and land rent*, Hastings: Battle Instant Press.

Douglas, R. (1976) *Land, people and politics. A history of the land question in the United Kingdom, 1878-1952*, London: Allison and Busby.

Dove, P.E. (1854) *The elements of political science, book 2*, Edinburgh: Johnstone and Hunter.

Dowell, S. (1965) *A history of taxation and taxes in England*, London: Frank Cass and Co.

Drever, F., Bunting, J. and Harding, D. (1997) 'Male mortality from major causes of death' in F. Drever and M. Whitehead (eds) *Health inequalities*, London: The Stationery Office, Series DS no 15, pp 122-42.

Drever, F. and Whitehead, M. (eds) (1998) *Health inequalities*, London: The Stationery Office, Series DS no 15.

Drever, F., Whitehead, M. and Roden, M. (1996) 'Current patterns and trends in male mortality by social class (based on occupation)', *Population Trends*, vol 86, pp 15-20.

Duncan, B., Rumel, D., Zelmanowicz, A., Mengue, S.S., Dos Santos, S. and Dalmaz, A. (1995) 'Social inequality in mortality in Sao Paulo State, Brazil', *International Journal of Epidemiology*, vol 24, pp 359-65.

Economic Trends (1986) November, London: The Stationary Office.

Economic Trends (1994) December, London: The Stationary Office.

Elliot, S. (1969) 'The Cecil family and the development of 19th century Stamford', *Lincolnshire History and Archaeology*, vol 4, pp 27-31.

Elton, G.R. (1973) *Reform and renewal: Thomas Cromwell and the common weal*, London: Cambridge University Press.

Ely, R.T. (1938) *Ground under our feet. An autobiography*, NY: Macmillan.

Engels, F. (1993) *The condition of the working class in England*, Oxford: Oxford University Press.

Esam, P. (1987) 'The bottom line: Has Conservative social security protected the poor?', in A. Walker and C. Walker (eds) *The growing divide: a social audit, 1979-1987*, London: Child Poverty Action Group.

Feder, K. (1994) 'Public finance and the cooperative society', in F. Harrison (ed) *A philosophy for a fair society*, London: Shepheard-Walwyn.

Feldstein, M. (1977) 'The surprising incidence of a tax on pure rent: a new answer to an old question', *Journal of Political Economy*, vol 85, pp 349-60.

Ferrie, J.E., Shipley, M.J, Marmot, M.G, Stansfield, S. and Davey Smith, G. (1995) 'Health effects of anticipation of job change and non-employment: longitudinal data from the Whitehall II Study', *British Medical Journal*, vol 311, pp 1264-69.

Fetter, F.A. (1935) 'Capital', in E.R.A. Seligman (ed) *Encyclopaedia of the social sciences*, NY: Macmillan.

Fitch, R. (1995) 'The new poor laws', *The Village Voice*, 10 January, pp 29-32.

Fletcher, R. (1971) *John Stuart Mill: A logical critique of sociology*, London: Michael Joseph.

Floud, R., Wachter, K. and Gregory, A. (1990) *Height, health and history. Nutritional status in the United Kingdom, 1750-1980*, Cambridge: Cambridge University Press.

Forbes, T. (1979) 'By what disease or casualty: the changing face of death in London', in C. Webster (ed) *Health, medicine and mortality in the 16th century*, Cambridge: Cambridge University Press.

Fowler, H.W. and Fowler, F. (eds) (1990) *The concise Oxford dictionary of current English*, Oxford: Oxford University Press.

Fox, A.J. and Goldblatt, P. (1982) 'Socioeconomic differentials in mortality 1971-75', *Office of Population Censuses and Surveys Series LS*, London: HMSO.

Fraser, D. (1984) *The evolution of the British welfare state*, London: Macmillan.

Frey, J.J. (1982) 'Unemployment and health in the United States', *British Medical Journal*, vol 284, pp 1112-13.

Friedman M. (1968) 'The role of monetary policy', *American Economic Review*, vol 58, pp 1-17.

Gaffney, M. (1994) 'Neo-classical economics as a stratagem against Henry George', in M. Gaffney and F. Harrison (eds) *The corruption of economics*, London: Shepheard-Walwyn.

Gaffney, M. (1997) 'Alfred Russel Wallace's campaign to nationalise land: How Darwin's peer learned from John Stuart Mill and became Henry George's ally', *American Journal of Economic Sociology*, vol 56, pp 609-15.

Galbraith, J.K. (1987) *Economics in perspective: a critical history*, MA: Houghton Mifflin.

Galbraith, J.K. (1996) *The good society – The humane agenda*, London: Sinclair-Stevenson.

Gates, P. (1943) *The Wisconsin pinelands of Cornell University,* NY: Cornell University Press.

Gayer, A.D., Rostow, W.W. and Schwartz, A.J. (eds) (1953) *The growth and fluctuation of the British economy 1790-1850*, Oxford: Clarendon Press.

Geiger, G.R. (1933) *The philosophy of Henry George*, NY: Macmillan.

Geiger, G.R. (1939) *Henry George. A biography*, London: Henry George Foundation of Great Britain.

General Register Office (1913) *Seventy-fourth annual report of the registrar general of births, deaths and marriages in England and Wales (1911)*, London: HMSO.

George, H. (1941) *The Irish land question*, NY: Robert Schalkenbach Foundation.

George, H. (1947) *The condition of labour. An open letter to Pope Leo XIII*, London: Land and Liberty Press.

George, H. (1979) *Progress and poverty*, NY: Robert Schalkenbach Foundation.

George, H. (1981) *The science of political economy*, NY: Robert Schalkenbach Foundation.

George, H. (undated) *Why the landowner cannot shift the tax on land values*, NY: Robert Schalkenbach Foundation.

Giles, C. and Johnson, P. (1994) 'Tax reform in the UK and changes in the progressivity of the tax system, 1985-95', *Fiscal Studies*, vol 15, pp 64-86.

Goldblatt, P. (1989) 'Mortality by social class, 1971-1985', *Population Trends*, vol 56, pp 6-15.

Goldthorpe, J.H. (1987) *Social mobility and class structure in modern Britain*, Oxford: Clarendon Press.

Gorgas, W.C. (1915) 'Economic causes of disease', in W.C. Gorgas and L.J. Johnson, *Two papers on public sanitation and the single tax*, OH: Joseph Fels Fund of America.

Grayson, J.P. (1985) 'The closure of a factory and its impact on health', *International Journal of Health Services*, vol 15, pp 69-93.

Green, S. (1986) *Who own's London?*, London: Weidenfeld and Nicolson.

Griffith, W. (1949) *A hundred years. The board of inland revenue*, London: HMSO.

Groundwork Foundation, The (1996) *The post-industrial landscape: a resource for the community, a resource for the nation?*, Birmingham: The Groundwork Foundation.

Habakkuk, H.J. (1950) 'Marriage settlements in the eighteenth century', *Transactions of the Royal Historical Society*, 4th series, vol 32, p 18.

Hahn, R.A., Eaher, E., Barker, N.D., Teutsch, S. M., Sosniak, W. and Kriejer, N. (1995) 'Poverty and death in the United States – 1973 and 1991', *Epidemiology*, vol 6-7, pp 490-97, 453-54.

Halevy, E. (1951) *A history of the English people in the nineteenth century*, London: Benn Bros.

Hall, C. (1805) *The effects of civilisation on the people in European states*, London: Printed for the Author.

Hall, P., Land, H., Parker, R. and Webb, A. (eds) (1975) *Change, choice and conflict in social policy*, London: Heinemann.

Halsbury's Statutes of England and Wales (1987), vol 37, London: Butterworths.

Hamlin, C. (1995) 'Could you starve to death in England in 1839? The Chadwick-Farr controversy and the loss of "social" in public health', *American Journal of Public Health*, vol 85, pp 856-66.

Hammond, J.L. and Hammond, B. (1932) *The town labourer 1760-1832. The new civilisation*, London: Longman Greens.

Hansard (1909) vol IV, 536, 29 April.

Haralambos, M. and Holborn, M. (1990) *Sociology. Themes and perspectives*, London: Unwin Hyman.

Harding, S. (1995) 'Social class differences in mortality of men: recent evidence from the OPCS Longitudinal Study', *Population Trends*, vol 80, pp 31-37.

Harding, S., Bethune, A., Maxwell, R. and Brown, J. (1997) 'Mortality trends using the Longitudinal Study', in F. Drever and M. Whitehead (eds) *Health inequalities*, London: The Stationery Office, Series DS no 15, pp 143-55.

Harris, J. (1972) *Unemployment and politics. A study of English social policy 1886-1914*, Oxford: Clarendon Press.

Harris, J. (1977) *William Beveridge: A biography*, Oxford: Clarendon Press.

Harrison, F. (1983) *The power in the land. An inquiry into unemployment, the profits crisis and land speculation*, London: Shepheard-Walwyn.

Harrison, F. (1998) *The losses of nations*, London: Othila.

Harrison, J.F.C. (1971) *The early Victorians, 1832-1851*, London: Weidenfeld and Nicholson.

Hattersley, L. (1997) 'Expectation of life by social class', in F. Drever and M. Whitehead (eds) *Health inequalities*, London: The Stationery Office, Series DS no 15, pp 73-82.

Hazlitt, W. (1906) *The spirit of the age, or contemporary portraits*, London: George Bell.

Hill, C. (1954) 'The Norman yoke', in J. Saville (ed) *Democracy and the labour movement*, London: Lawrence and Wishart.

Hobson, J.A. (1895) 'The meaning and measure of unemployment', *Contemporary Review*, vol 67, pp 415-32.

Hoeker-Drysdale, S. (1992) *Harriet Martineau. First woman Sociologist*, Oxford: Berg.

Holdsworth, W.S. (1924) *A history of English law*, vol 4, London: Methuen and Co.

Hollingworth, T. (1965) 'A demographic study of the British ducal families', in D. Glass and D. Eversley (eds) *Population and history*, London: Edward Arnold.

Holt, J.C. (1972) 'Politics and property in early medieval England', *Past and Present*, vol 57, p 12.

Holt, J.C. (1981) 'The prehistory of parliament' in R.G. Davies and J.H. Denton (eds) *The English parliament in the middle ages*, Manchester: Manchester University Press.

Holt, J.C. (1992) *Magna Carta*, Cambridge: Cambridge University Press.

Hopton, J.L. and Hunt, S.M. (1996) 'Housing conditions and mental health in a disadvantaged area in Scotland', *Journal of Epidemiology and Community Health*, vol 50, pp 56-61.

Hoskins, W.G. (1985) *The making of the English landscape*, London: Penguin.

House, J.S., Lapkowski, J.M., Kinney, A.M., Mero, R.P., Kessler, R.C. and Herzog A.R. (1994) 'The Social stratification of ageing and health', *Journal of Health and Social Behaviour*, vol 35, pp 213-34.

Howell, R. (1976) *Why work? A challenge to the chancellor*, London: Conservative Political Centre.

Hoyle, R.W. (1998) 'Taxation and the mid-Tudor crisis', *Economic History Review*, vol 51, pp 649-75.

Hudson, J. (1996) *The formation of the English common law*, London: Longmans.

Hudson, M. (1997) *Where did all the land go? The Fed's new balance sheet calculations*, NY: Robert Schalkenbach Foundation.

Hudson, M. and Feder, K. (1997) 'Real estate and the capital gains debate', Working paper 187, Annandale-on-Hudson, NY: Jerome Levy Economic Institute, Bard College.

Huggett, F.E. (1978) *Victorian England as seen by Punch*, London: Sidgwick and Jackson.

Humphreys, N.A. (1887) 'Class mortality statistics', *Journal of the Royal Statistical Society*, vol 50, pp 255-92.

Hurstfield, J. (1955-56) 'The profits of fiscal feudalism, 1541-1602', *Economic History Review*, 2nd Series, vol 8, pp 53-61.

Hyndman, H.M. (1911) *The record of an adventurous life*, London: Macmillan.

Ilersic, A.R. (1960) *Parliament and commerce. The story of the association of British chambers of commerce. 1860-1960*, London: Association of British Chambers of Commerce and Newman Neame.

Inter-Departmental Committee on Physical Deterioration (1904), *House of Commons parliamentary papers*, vol 32, pp 1-93.

James, R.R. (1963) *Rosebery. A biography of Archibald Philip, fifth earl of Rosebery*, London: Weidenfeld and Nicolson.

Jevons, W.S. (1905) *The principles of economics and other papers*, London: Macmillan.

Jin, R.L., Shah, C.P. and Svoboda, T.J. (1995) 'The impact of unemployment on health: a review of the evidence', *Canadian Medical Association Journal*, vol 153, pp 529-40.

Johnson, E. (1986) *Charles Dickens. His tragedy and triumph*, London: Penguin.

Jozan, P.E. and Prokorskas, R. (1997) *Atlas of leading and 'avoidable' causes of death in countries of central and eastern Europe*, Budapest: Hungarian Central Statistical Office.

Justice (1884) 'Land Restoration League', 5 April.

Kaplan, G.A., Pamuk, E.R., Lynch, J.W., Cohen, R.D. and Balfour, J.L. (1996) 'Inequality in income and mortality in the United States: analysis of mortality and potential pathways', *British Medical Journal*, vol 312, pp 999-1003.

Kay, J.A. and King, M.A. (1990) *The British Tax System*, Oxford: Oxford University Press.

Kee, R. (1982) *Ireland. A history*, London: Abacus.

Kennedy, B.P., Kawachi, I. and Prothrow-Stith, D. (1996) 'Income distribution and mortality: cross-sectional ecological study of the Robin Hood Index in the United States', *British Medical Journal*, vol 312, pp 1004-7, 1194.

Kennedy, W. (1913) *English taxation, 1640-1799. An essay on policy and opinion*, London: G. Bell.

Kennedy, W. (1964) *English taxation, 1640-1799*, London: Frank Cass and Co.

Keynes, J.M. (1924) 'Alfred Marshall, 1842-1924', *The Economic Journal*, vol 34, pp 311-17.

Keynes, J.M. (1940) *How to pay for the war*, London: Macmillan.

Knight, F. (1953) 'The fallacies of the single tax', *The Freeman*, pp 809-11.

Kunst, A.E., Groenhof, F., Mackenbach, J.P. and the EU Working Group on Socioeconomic Inequalities in Health (1998) 'Occupational class and cause specific mortality in middle aged men in 11 European countries: comparison of population based studies', *British Medical Journal*, vol 316, pp 1636-41.

Kynaston, D. (1995) *The City of London*, London: Chatto and Windus.

L'Etang, H. (1969) *The pathology of leadership*, London: William Heinemann.

Lancet, The (1843), 'Editorial', ii, pp 657-61.

Lancet, The (1942) 'Editorial', ii: pp 623-4.

Lawrence, E.P. (1957) *Henry George in the British Isles*, MI: Michigan State University Press.

Leather, P. (1994) *Papering over the cracks*, London: National Housing Forum.

Lee, G. (1996) *The people's Budget. An Edwardian tragedy*, London: Henry George Foundation.

Lejeune, A. (1972) 'Gentleman's estate' in *Burke's Landed Gentry*, London: Burke's Peerage Ltd.

Locke, J. (1948) *The second treatise of civil government*, and *A letter concerning toleration*, J.W. Gough (ed), Oxford: Basil Blackwell.

Longmate, N. (1974) *The workhouse*, London: Temple Smith.

Lynch, J.W., Kaplan, G.A. and Shema, S.J. (1997) 'Cumulative impact of sustained economic hardship on physical, cognitive, psychological and social functioning', *New England Journal of Medicine*, vol 337, pp 1889-95.

M'Gonigle, G.C.M. and Kirby, J. (1936) Poverty and Public Health, London: Victor Gollancz.

Mc Briar, A.M. (1987) *An Edwardian mixed doubles. The Bosanquets versus the Webbs. A study in British social policy 1890-1929*, Oxford: Clarendon.

McCleary, G.F. (1953) *The Malthusian population theory*, London: Faber and Faber.

McCord, C. and Freeman, H.P. (1990) 'Excess mortality in Harlem', *New England Journal of Medicine*, vol 322, pp 173-77.

McDonough, P., Duncan, G.J., Williams, D. and House, J. (1997) 'Income dynamics and adult mortality in the United States, 1972 through 1989', *American Journal of Public Health*, vol 87, pp 1476-83.

McEwen, J. (1981) *Who owns Scotland?*, Edinburgh: Edinburgh University Student Publication/Polygon Books.

McKeganey, N. (1994) 'AIDS and HIV infection within Scotland; current state of the epidemic and future areas of need', *Health Bulletin*, vol 52, pp 260-77.

Mackenbach, J.P. (1995) 'Social inequality and death according to late-medieval death dances', *American Journal of Public Health*, vol 85, pp 1285-95.

Malthus, T.R. (1821) *Principles of political economy considered with a view to their practical application*, MA: Wells and Lilly.

Malthus, T.R. (1909) *An essay on the principle of population*, London: Macmillan.

Mann, J.M., Tarantola, S.J.M. and Netter, T.W. (1993) *Aids in the world 1992*, MA: Harvard University Press.

Mann, T. (1895) *The programme of the I.L.P and the unemployed*, Clarion Tract no 6, London: Clarion Newspaper Co.

Marriott, O. (1967) *The property boom*, London: Hamish Hamilton.

Marshall, A. (1891) *Principles of economics*, London: Macmillan.

Marshall, A. (1909) 'Rates and taxes on land values', *The Times*, 16 November.

Marshall, J.D. (1961) 'The Nottinghamshire reformers and their contribution to the new poor law', *Economic History Review*, 2nd series, vol 13, pp 382-96.

Martikainen, P.T. and Valkonen, T. (1996) 'Excess mortality of unemployed men and women during a period of rapidly increasing employment', *Lancet*, vol 348, pp 909-12.

Martineau, H. (1877) *Autobiography, with memorials by Maria Weston Chapman*, vol 1, London: Elder.

Maxwell, R.J. (1981) *Health and wealth*, Lexington: Lexington Books.

Mihill, C. (1995) 'Poor suffer more illness than rich', *The Guardian*, 24 October.

Mill, J.S (1876) *Principles of political economy*, Peoples Edition, London: Longman, Green and Co.

Milsom, S.F.C. (1976) *The legal framework of English feudalism*, Cambridge: Cambridge University Press.

Ministry of Construction (1945) *Housing*, Cmd 6609, London: HMSO.

Ministry of Health (1920) *Consultative council on medical and allied services. Interim report on the future provision of medical and allied services*, London: HMSO.

Ministry of Health (1920-21 to 1929-32) *Annual local taxation returns, England and Wales*, London: HMSO.

Ministry of Health (1921) *Second annual report, 1920–1921*, London, HMSO.

Ministry of Health (1933-39) *Local Government Financial Statistics, England and Wales. Part I: Poor relief*, London: HMSO.

Ministry of Health and Department of Health for Scotland (1944), *A national health service*, Cmd 6502, London: HMSO.

Mitchell, B.R. (1962) *Abstract of British historical statistics*, Cambridge: Cambridge University Press.

Morley, J. (1905) *The Life of William Gladstone*, London: Macmillan.

Morris, J. (1979) *Heaven's command. An imperial progress*, London: Penguin.

Morris, J.K., Cook, D.G., Shaper, A.G. (1994) 'Loss of employment and mortality', *British Medical Journal*, vol 308, pp 1135-39.

Moser, K., Goldblatt, P., Fox, J. and Jones, D. (1990) 'Unemployment and mortality', in P. Goldblatt (ed) *Longitudinal study 1971-1981: mortality and social organisation*, London: HMSO.

Moser, K.A., Goldblatt, P.O., Fox, A.J. and Jones, D.R. (1987) 'Unemployment and mortality: comparison of the 1971 and 1981 longitudinal study census samples', *British Medical Journal*, vol 294, pp 86-90.

Myers, A.R. (1981) 'Parliament, 1422-1509', in R.G. Davies and J.H. Denton (eds) *The English parliament in the middle ages*, Manchester: Manchester Univeristy Press.

National Federation of Housing Associations (1985) *Inquiry into British housing*, The evidence, January 1985, Report July 1985.

Nearing, S. (1915) 'Land values increase in American cities', *The Public*, p 1151.

Newman, O. and Foster, A. (1995) *Prices and income in Britain 1900-1993*, NY: Gale Research International.

Newsholme, A. and Stevenson, T.H.C. (1906) 'The decline of human fertility in the United Kingdom and other countries as shown by corrected birth-rates', *Journal of the Royal Statistical Society*, vol 69, pp 34-87.

Nissel, M. (1987) *People count. A history of the General Register Office*, London: HMSO.

Norton-Taylor, R. (1982) *Whose land is it anyway? Agirculture, planning and land use in the Bristish Countryside*, Wellingborough: Turnstone Press.

Offer, A. (1977) 'The origins of the Law of Property Acts 1910-25', *The Modern Law Review*, vol 40, pp 505-22.

Office of Population Censuses and Surveys (1984), *Census 1981: Economic activity, Great Britain*, London: HMSO.

Office of Population Censuses and Surveys (1988) *General Household Survey 1988*; London, HMSO.

Office of Population Censuses and Surveys (1992), *Census 1991: Report for Great Britain, part 2*, London: HMSO.

Office of Population Censuses and Surveys (1996) *Population Trends 83*, London: HMSO, p 59.

Olivier, S. (1896) *Capital and land*, Fabian Tract no 7, London: The Fabian Society.

Ormerod, P. (1994) *The death of economics*, London: Faber and Faber.

Ormrod, W.M. (1995) *Political life in medieval England, 1300-1450*, NY: Martin's Press.

Paine, T, (1948) *The age of reason*, NJ: Citadel Press.

Paine, T. (1969) *Rights of Man*, London: Penguin.

Paine, T. (1976) *Common sense*, London: Penguin.

Paine, T. (1987) 'Agrarian Justice', (1795), *The Thomas Paine Reader*, Harmondsworth: Penguin.

Palmer, R.C. (1985) 'The origins of property in England', *Law and History Review*, vol 3, pp 1-50.

Pamuk, E. R. (1985) 'Social class inequality in mortality in 1921 to 1972 in England and Wales', *Population Studies*, vol 39 pp. 17-31.

Parker, H. (1995) *Taxes, benefits and family life. The seven deadly traps*, London: Institute of Economic Affairs.

Parker, J. and Layard, R. (1996) *The coming Russian boom. A guide to new markets and politics*, NY: Free Press.

Pater, J.E. (1981) *The making of the national health service*, London: King Edward's Hospital Fund for London.

Patten, S.N. (1908) 'The conflict theory of distribution', *Yale Review*, vol 17, pp 156-84.

Pease, E.R. (1916) *The history of the Fabian Society*, London: A C Fifield.

Pelling, H. (1967) *Social geography of British elections 1855-1910*, London: Macmillan.

Pelling, H. (1976) *A history of British trade unionism*, London: Macmillan.

Perrenoud, A. (1975) 'L'inegalité sociale devant la mort à Gènève au XVII ème siècle', *Population*, vol 30, pp 211-43.

Perrins, B. (1995) *Introduction to land law*, London: Cavendish.

Phelps Brown, H. (1991) *Egalitarianism and the generation of inequality*, Oxford: Clarendon Press.

Phillips, A.W. (1958) 'The relation between unemployment and the rate of change of money wage rates in the United Kingdom, 1861-1957', *Economica*, vol NS25, 283-99.

Pierson, P. (1994) *The dismantling of the welfare state? Reagan, Thatcher and the politics of retrenchment*, NY: Cambridge University Press.

Pigou, A.C. (1920) *The economics of welfare*, London: Macmillan.

Pigou, A.C. (ed) (1925) *Memorials of Alfred Marshall*, London: Macmillan.

Platt, S.D., Martin, C.J., Hunt, S.M. and Lewis, C.W. (1989) 'Damp housing, mould growth, and symptomatic health state', *British Medical Journal*, vol 298, pp 1673-78.

Plucknett, T.F.T. (1956) *A concise history of the common law*, London: Butterworth.

Plumb, J.H. (1957) 'The organisation of the Cabinet in the reign of Queen Anne', *Transactions of the Royal Historical Society*, 5th series, vol 7, pp 137-157.

Plumb, J.H. (1967) *The growth of political stability in England, 1675-1725*, London: Macmillan.

Poor Law Commission (1834) *Report of the Poor Law Commissioners*, London: HMSO.

Prandy, K. (1990) 'The revised Cambridge scale of occupations', *Sociology*, vol 24 pp 629-55.

Pugh, M. (1988) *Lloyd George*, London: Longmans.

Pumphrey, R.E. (1959) 'The introduction of industrialists into the British peerage: a study in adaptation of a social institution', *American Historical Review*, vol 65, pp 1-16.

Redfearn, D. (1992) *Tolstoy. Principles for a new world order*, London: Shepheard Walwyn.

Registrar General (1925) *Census of England and Wales 1921*, London: HMSO, Table 2.

Reid, S.L. (1895) *Lord John Russell*, London: Sampson Low.

Ricci, D.M. (1969–70) 'Fabian Socialism: a theory of rent as exploitation', *Journal of British Studies*, vol 9, pp 105-121.

Richards, D. (1989) *The Land Value of Britain 1985–1990*, London: Economic and Social Science Research Association.

Richards, E. (1973) *The leviathan of wealth*, London: Routledge and Kegan Paul.

Richards, P.G. (1975) *The reformed local government system*, London: George Allen and Unwin.

Roseveare, H. (1969) *The Treasury: The evolution of a British Institution*, London: Allen Lane The Penguin Press.

Routh, G. (1980) *Occupation and pay in Great Britain 1906-1979*, London: Macmillan.

Routh, G. (1987) *Occupations of the People of Great Britain, 1801-1981*, London: Macmillan.

Rowbotham, M. (1998) *The grip of death. A study of modern money, debt slavery and destructive economics*, Charlbury: Jon Carpenter.

Rowntree, B.S. (1906) *Poverty. A study of town life*, London: Longmans, Green and Co.

Rowntree, B.S. (1941) *Poverty and progress. A second social survey of York*, London: Longmans, Green and Co.

Royal Commission on Land Transfer (1909) *First report*, C 4510, Appendix, London: HMSO.

Royal Commission on Local Taxation (1899), C 958, London: HMSO.

Royal Commission on the Distribution of Income and Wealth (1979), report no 7, London: HMSO.

Royal Commission on the Housing of the Working Classes (1885) *First Report*, Parliamentary Paper.

Royal Commission on the Poor Laws and Relief of Distress (1909) *Majority report*, London: HMSO.

Sawyer, P.H. (1968) 'Anglo-Saxon charters: an annotated list and bibliography', cited in O. Hooke (1990) *The Anglo-Saxon landscape of North Gloucestershire*, Friends of Deerhurst Church.

Schomburg, W. (1992) *Lexikon der Deutschen Steur-und*, Munchen: Zollgeschichte.

Scottish Office (1992) *Scotland's health: a challenge for all*, Edinburgh: HMSO.

Secretary of State for Social Services (1985) *Reform of social security*, Cmnd. 9517, London: HMSO.

Seligman, E.R.A. (1895) *Essays on taxation*, NY: Macmillan.

Shaw, G.B. (1930) *Socialism: Principles and outlook; and Fabianism*, Fabian Tract no 233, London: The Fabian Society.

Shepherd, J. and Abakaks, A. (1992), *The national survey of vacant land in urban areas of England, 1990*, London: HMSO.

Short, B. (1989) 'The geography of England and Wales in 1910: an evaluation of Lloyd George's "Domesday" of landownership', *Historical Geography Research Series no 22, Institute of British Geographers*.

Sidgwick, H. (1883) *Principles of political economy*, London: Macmillan.

Simpson, A.W.B. (1986) *A History of the land law*, Oxford: Clarendon.

Slack, P. (1977) 'The local incidence of epidemic disease: the case of Bristol 1540-1650', *The Plague Reconsidered, Local Population Studies*, Suppl, pp 49-62.

Slack, P. (1988) *Poverty and policy in Tudor and early England*, London: Longman.

Slack, P. (1992) 'Dearth and social policy in early modern England', *Social History of Medicine*, vol 5, pp 1-17.

Slater, G. (1913) 'A historical outline of land ownership in England', in Land Enquiry Committee, *The Land: the report of the Land Enquiry Committee*, London: Hodder and Stoughton.

Smith, A. (1986) *The wealth of nations*, books 1-3, London: Penguin.

Smith, J. and Harding, S. (1997) 'Mortality in women and men using alternative social classifications', in F. Drever and M. Whitehead (eds) *Health inequalities*, London: The Stationery Office, Series DS no 15, pp 168-83.

Smith, R. (1985) 'Occupationless Health', *British Medical Journal*, vol 291, pp 1024-27, 1338-41, 1563-66.

Smith, S. and Wied-Nebbeling, S. (1986) *The shadow economy in Britain and Germany*, Anglo-German Foundation for the Study of Industrial Society.

Social Exclusion Unit, The (2000) *National strategy for neighbourhood renewal: a framework for consultation*, London: Cabinet Office.

Solow, R.M. (1997) 'How to treat intellectual ancestors', in H. James Brown (ed) *Land use and taxation*, MA: Lincoln Institute of Land Policy.

Spring, D. (1996) 'Willoughby de Broke and Walter Long, English landed society and political extremism, 1912-1914', in N. Harte and R. Quinault (eds) *Land and Society in Britain, 1700-1914*, Manchester: Manchester University Press.

Spring, E. (1977) 'Landowners, lawyers, and land reform in nineteenth-century England', *American Journal of Legal History*, vol 21, pp 40-59.

Spring, E. (1993) *Law, land and family. Aristocratic inheritances in England, 1300 to 1800*, NC: University of North Carolina Press.

Sraffa, P. and Dobb, M.H. (eds) (1951) *The works and correspondence of David Ricardo*, vol 1, Cambridge: Cambridge University Press.

Statutes of the Realm (by command of George III, 1810), held by the Library of the Corporation of London, Guildhall, vol 1, 1826.

Stedman Jones, G. (1971) *Outcast London. A study in the relationship between classes in Victorian society*, Oxford: Clarendon Press.

Stevens, L. and Lee, S. (eds) (1973) *Dictionary of national biography,* vol 8, Oxford: Oxford University Press.

Stevenson, T.H.C. (1923) 'The social distribution of mortality from different causes in England and Wales 1910-1912', *Biometrika*, vol 15, pp 382-400.

Stigler, G.J. (1969) 'Alfred Marshall's lectures on Progress and poverty', *Journal of Law and Economics*, vol 12, pp 181–226.

Stiglitz, J.E. (1977) 'The theory of local public goods', in M.S. Feldstein and R.P. Inman (eds) *The economics of public services*, London: Macmillan.

Stone, L. and Stone, J.C.F. (1984) *An open elite? England 1540–1880*, Oxford: Clarendon Press.

Survey of Personal Incomes, 1984–85, London: HMSO, 1987.

Tawney, R.H. (1963) *The radical tradition. Twelve essays on politics, education and literature*, London: George Allen and Unwin.

Temple, W. (1976) *Christianity and Social Order*, London: Shepheard-Walwyn.

Thompson, F.L. (1977) 'Britain', in D. Spring (ed) *European landed elites in the nineteenth century*, Baltimore.

Thompson, F.M.L. (1958–9) 'English landownership: the Ailesbury Trust 1832-56', *Economic History Review*, 2nd series, vol 11, pp 121-132.

Thompson, F.M.L. (1963) *English landed society in the nineteenth century*, London: Routledge and Kegan Paul, pp 218-20.

Thorne, S.E. (1959) 'English feudalism and estates in land', *Cambridge Law Journal*, November, p 201.

Tideman, N. and Plassmann, F. (1998) 'Taxed out of work and wealth: the costs of taxing labor and capital', in F. Harrison (ed) *The losses of nations*, London: Othila.

Timmins, N. (1996) *The five giants. A biography of the welfare state*, London: Fontana.

Toller, T.N. (1898) *An Anglo-Saxon dictionary*, Oxford: Clarendon Press.

Townroe, B.S. (1928) *The slum problem*, London: Longmans, Green and Co.

Townsend, P., Davidson, N. and Whitehead, M. (1992) *Inequalities in health*, London: Penguin Books.

Toye, J. (1997) 'Keynes on population and economic growth', *Cambridge Journal of Economics*, vol 21, pp 1–26.

Toynbee, A. (1884) *'Progress and poverty' A criticism of Mr Henry George*, London: Kegan Paul, Trench and Co.

United Nations (1948) General Assembly resolution 217 A (III), UN Document A/810 at 71.

van Rossum, C.T.M., Shipley, M.J., van de Mheen, H., Grobbee, D.E. and Marmot, M.G. (2000) 'Employment grade differences in cause specific mortality. A 25 year follow up of civil servants from the first Whitehall study', *Journal of Epidemiology and Community Health*, vol 54, pp 178-84.

Virchow, R.L.C. (1879) *Gessamelte Abhandlungen aus dem Gebiete der offenlichen Medicin und der Seuchenlehre*, vol 1, Berlin: A. Hirschwald.

Wadsworth, M.E.J. (1991) *The imprint of time: Childhood, history and adult life*, Oxford: Oxford University Press.

Walberg, P., McKee, M., Shkolnikov, V., Chenet, L. and Leon, D.A. (1998) 'Economic change, crime, and mortality crisis in Russia: regional analysis', *British Medical Journal*, vol 317, pp 312-18.

Walker, F. (1887) 'The source of business profits', *Quarterly Journal of Economics*, vol 1, pp 281-2.

Wallace, A.R. (1908) *My life. A record of events and opinions*, London: Chapman and Hall.

Wannamethee, S.G. and Shaper, A.G. (1997) 'Socioeconomic status within social class and mortality: a prospective study in middle-aged British men', *International Journal of Epidemiology*, vol 26, pp 532-41.

Ward, W.R. (1953) *The English land tax in the eighteenth century*, London: Oxford University Press.

Weatherall, D. (1976) *David Ricardo. A biography*, The Hague: Martinus Nighoff.

Webb, B. and Webb, S. (1920) *The history of trade unionism*, London: Longmans.

Webb, S. (1907) *The Decline in the birth rate*, Fabian Tract no 131, London: The Fabian Society.

Webb, S. and Webb, B. (1913) 'What is Socialism?', *The New Statesman*, 12 April.

Webb, S. and Webb, B. (eds) (1974) *The poor law commission (1909) minority report, part II. The public organisation of the labour market*, Clifton: Augustus M Kelley.

Webster, C. (1988) *The health services since the war. Vol I. Problems of health care. The national health service before 1957*, London: HMSO.

Weich, S. and Lewis, G. (1998) ' Poverty, unemployment, and common mental disorders: population based cohort study', *British Medical Journal*, vol 317, pp 115-19.

Wennemo, I. (1993) 'Infant mortality, public policy and inequality – a comparison of 18 industrialised countries 1950–1985', *Sociology of Health and Illness*, vol 15, pp 429-46.

Wharton, J. (1875) *National self-protection*, PA: The Iron and Steel Association.

White, M. (1999) 'PM's deadline to end child poverty', *The Guardian*, 15 March, p 10.

Whitney, R. (1987) *House of Commons Hansard*, 6 April.

Wickens, D., Rumfitt, A. and Willis, R. (1995) *Survey of derelict land in England 1993. Vol 1 – Report*, London: HMSO.

Wilkinson, R.G. (1992) 'Income distribution and life expectancy', *British Medical Journal*, vol 304, pp 165-168.

Wilkinson, R.G. (1994) *Unfair Shares. The effects of widening income differences on the welfare of the young*, Ilford: Barnardo's.

Wilkinson, R.G. (1996) *Unhealthy societies: the afflictions of inequality*, London: Routledge.

Williamson, A. (1973) *Thomas Paine. His life, work and times*, London: George Allen and Unwin.

Wilson, A. and Mackay, G.S. (1941) *Old age pensions. An historical and critical study*, London: Oxford University Press.

Wilson, W. (1994) *Rothschild. A story of wealth and power*, London: Mandarin.

Wood, A. (1982) *Nineteenth century Britain, 1815-1914*, London: Longman.

Wood, M. (1990) *Domesday. A search for the roots of England*, London: BBC Books.

Woodham-Smith, C. (1982) *Florence Nightingale 1820-1910*, London: Constable.

Woodward, M., Shewry, M., Smith, W.C. and Tunstall-Pedoe, H. (1990) 'Coronary heart disease and socio-economic factors in Edinburgh and North Glasgow', *The Statistician*, vol 39, pp 319–29.

World Health Organization (1996) *World health statistics annual 1995*, Geneva: WHO A3-A9.

Wrigley, E. and Schofield, R. (1989) *The population of England, 1541-1871: a reconstruction*, Cambridge: Cambridge University Press.

Youings, J. (1991) *Sixteenth century England*, London: Penguin.

Youings, J. (1967) 'Landlords in England: The church', in J. Thirsk (ed) *The agrarian history of England and Wales, vol IV, 1500-1600*, Cambridge: Cambridge University Press.

Yuen, P. and Balarajan, R. (1989) 'Unemployment and patterns of consultation with the general practitioner', *British Medical Journal*, vol 298, pp 1212-14.

Index

subsidies 97
see also health education, state education
education acts 95, 97, 103
Einstein, Albert 431-2
election expenses 357-8
Ely, Richard 381-2
employment recruitment and class 15-16, 19, 100
see also full employment; unemployment enclosure 144-5, 350-3
Board of 352-3
Encumbered Estates Act (1848) 350
enfranchisement *see* parliamentary reform
Enrolments (1536), Statute of 233
entail, barring the 223
enterprise zoning 70, 71
eugenics, theories of 16-19, 136-7, 15
excise duties 260-2, 263, 269-70
see also licence duty
excise, taxation in lieu of rent 237-40

F

Fabian Society 389-90
family allowances 138
Family Endowment Society 137
family income supplement 292
Farr, Dr William 14, 301-2
Farre, J.R. 30
Feder, Kris 177, 178
Fee Grant Act (1891) 97
feoffee to use 225-7, 231-2
feudal obligations 216-18, 225-6, 235-6
feudalism *see* Norman feudalism
Franchise Act (1884) 356
free market economy, flaws in 95-7
free trade
in land 349-50
and the landholder 341-4
freehold 219
Friedman, Milton 89, 90, 134, 177
friendly societies and pensions 394
full employment, fears of 124

G

Galbraith, John Kenneth 39, 89
Galton, Francis 16-19, 22, 28
garden city movement 150, 157
George, Henry 31, *363-9*, 375-6, 377, 379, 392, 407
Georgists, the 370
Gladstone, William 262, 276-8, 355
Gorgas, William Crawford 31-2
government financing 266-8
Green, Thomas Hill 23
Greenwood Act (1930) 159
guardians of the poor 291-2

H

Haldane, Viscount 414
Hall, Dr C. 12
Harcourt, William 281, 282
health
education 105
iniquities or inequalities 8
local boards of 305-7
socio-economic factors 4, 10, 11, 45-7, 171-4
see also death rates; diseases; life expectancy
Health and Moral of Apprentices Act (1802) 339
health services
development of 106-10
voluntary 109
see also National Health Service; poor law
heir
at law 218-19, 221
surrogate 241-2
heiress
at law 240
threat of 221-2
see also land, inheritance of
Henry VIII, King 227
Holdsworth, William 233
home ownership *see* owner-occupation
honours, sale of 422
house
jobbers 146

Y